Pediatric Emergency Medicine

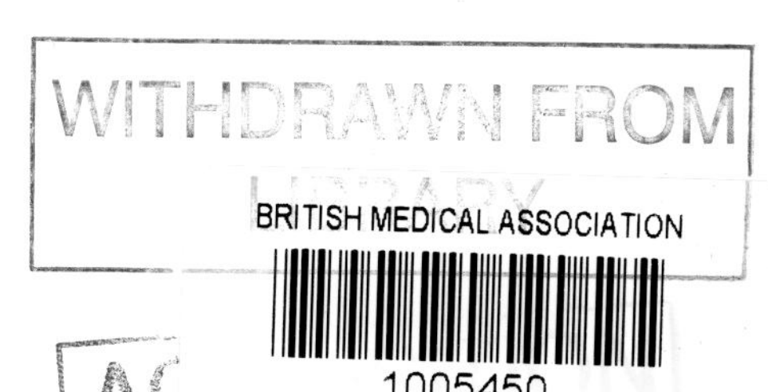

ILLUSTRATED CLINICAL CASES

Pediatric Emergency Medicine

Second edition

EDITED BY

ALISA McQUEEN
The University of Chicago Medicine
Comer Children's Hospital
Chicago, Illinois, USA

S. MARGARET PAIK
The University of Chicago Medicine
Comer Children's Hospital
Chicago, Illinois, USA

CRC Press
Taylor & Francis Group
Boca Raton London New York

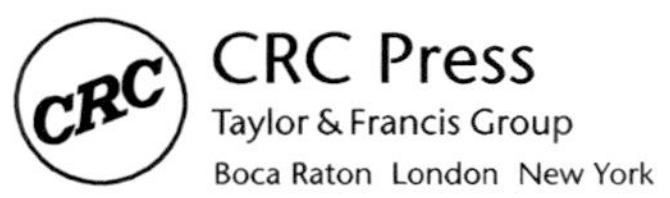

CRC Press is an imprint of the
Taylor & Francis Group, an **informa** business

CRC Press
Taylor & Francis Group
6000 Broken Sound Parkway NW, Suite 300
Boca Raton, FL 33487-2742

Printed on acid-free paper

International Standard Book Number-13: 978-1-4822-3029-1 (Paperback)
978-1-138-34649-9 (Hardback)

Visit the Taylor & Francis Web site at
http://www.taylorandfrancis.com

and the CRC Press Web site at
http://www.crcpress.com

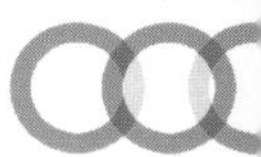

CONTENTS

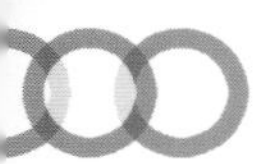

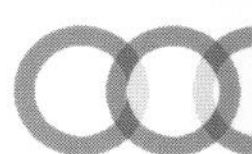

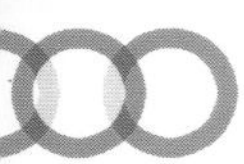

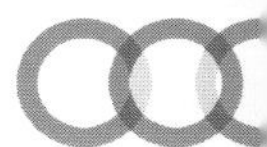

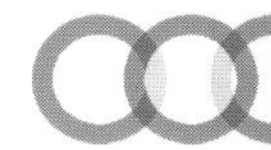

PREFACE

This book offers 200 clinical cases which present as emergencies. Congenital and acquired conditions affecting all body systems in infants and children are covered, including allergies, abuse, burns, fractures and other trauma, feeding problems, foreign bodies, genetic disorders, infections, poisoning, hematology, oncology, and much more. Cases appear in random order, reflecting actual practice in emergency medicine, and reinforcing skills in investigation, diagnosis, and treatment. It is superbly illustrated with high-quality radiographic images and photographs, and is indispensable for all health professionals dealing with emergencies involving children.

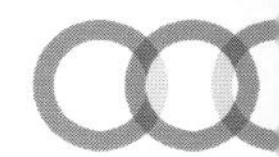

EDITORS

Alisa McQueen, MD, is Associate Professor of Pediatrics at the University of Chicago Comer Children's Hospital.

S. Margaret Paik, MD, is Associate Professor of Pediatrics at the University of Chicago Comer Children's Hospital.

Together, they oversee pediatric emergency medicine education for medical students, residents, and fellows in training.

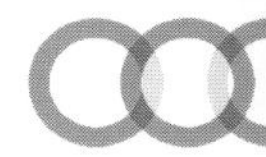

CONTRIBUTORS

Lauren Allister, MD
Hasbro Children's Hospital
Alpert Medical School of Brown University
Providence, Rhode Island

James Bistolarides, MD
Beaumont Health
Royal Oak, Michigan

Catherine H. Chung, MD, MPH
Inova Children's Hospital
Falls Church, Virginia

Michael Farnham, BA
Comer Children's Hospital
University of Chicago Medicine
Chicago, Illinois

Leah Finkel, MD
University of Illinois at Chicago
Chicago, Illinois

Michael Gottlieb, MD, RDMS
Rush University Medical Center
Chicago, Illinois

Jaimee Holbrook, MD
Comer Children's Hospital
University of Chicago Medicine
Chicago, Illinois

Timothy Ketterhagen, MD
Comer Children's Hospital
University of Chicago Medicine
Chicago, Illinois

Nina Mbadiwe, MD
Comer Children's Hospital
University of Chicago Medicine
Chicago, Illinois

Alisa McQueen, MD
Department of Pediatrics
Comer Children's Hospital
University of Chicago Medicine
Chicago, Illinois

Emily Obringer, MD
Advocate Children's Hospital
Oak Lawn, Illinois

S. Margaret Paik, MD
Department of Pediatrics
Comer Children's Hospital
University of Chicago Medicine
Chicago, Illinois

Barbara Pawel, MD
St. Christopher's Hospital for Children
Philadelphia, Pennsylvania

Veena Ramaiah, MD
Comer Children's Hospital
University of Chicago Medicine
Chicago, Illinois

Victoria Rodriguez, MD
Ann & Robert H. Lurie Children's Hospital of Chicago
Northwestern University Feinberg School of Medicine
Chicago, Illinois

Kevin R. Schwartz, MD
Massachusetts General Hospital
Harvard Medical School
Boston, Massachusetts

Justin Triemstra, MD
Central Maine Healthcare/Spectrum Health
Michigan State University
Grand Rapids, Michigan

Diana Yan, MD
Comer Children's Hospital
University of Chicago Medicine
Chicago, Illinois

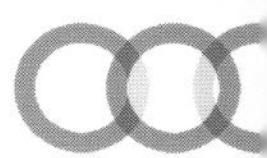

BROAD CLASSIFICATION OF CASES

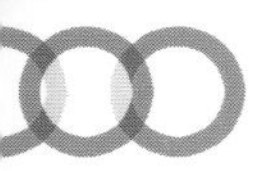

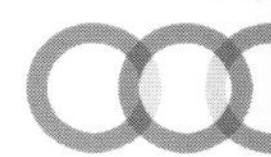

ABBREVIATIONS

ACE	angiotensin-converting enzyme
BSA	body surface area
CBC	complete blood count
CRP	C-reactive protein
CSF	cerebral spinal fluid
CT	computed tomography
CVA	costovertebral angle
CXR	chest x-ray
ECG	electrocardiogram
ED	emergency department
FFP	fresh frozen plasma
GC	gonorrhea
GCS	Glasgow Coma Score
GI	gastrointestinal
GSW	gunshot wound
GU	genitourinary
HSV	herpes simplex virus
IU	International Units
IV	intravenous
IVF	intravenous fluid
MRI	magnetic resonance imaging
NPO	nil per os
NSAIDs	nonsteroidal anti-inflammatory drugs
po	per os
PT	prothrombin time
PTT	partial thromboplastin time
RA	room air
RLQ	right lower quadrant
TBSA	total body surface area
UA	urine analysis
URI	upper respiratory infection
US	ultrasonography
UV	ultraviolet

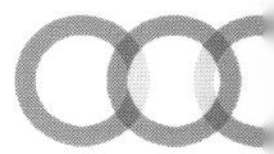

CASE 1

Timothy Ketterhagen

Questions

A 4-year-old boy presents to the emergency department because of "something in the back of his throat." Mother states that earlier today she was looking in the patient's mouth when he was yelling and she happened to notice "something in the back of his throat" that she had never seen before. The patient is otherwise doing well. Parents deny any ingestion of a foreign body. Mother denies any recent illnesses. The patient has been eating and drinking well without any difficulty. No fevers, vomiting, diarrhea, choking, difficulty breathing, drooling, or abdominal pain noted.

Physical exam reveals a well-appearing child. Vital signs are within normal limits for age. No stridor, wheezing, retractions, or drooling are noted. No foreign body is noted in the oral cavity. There are no oral lesions or masses noted. No neck masses or tenderness reported. When the patient opens his mouth fully, this view is seen. The physical exam is otherwise unremarkable.

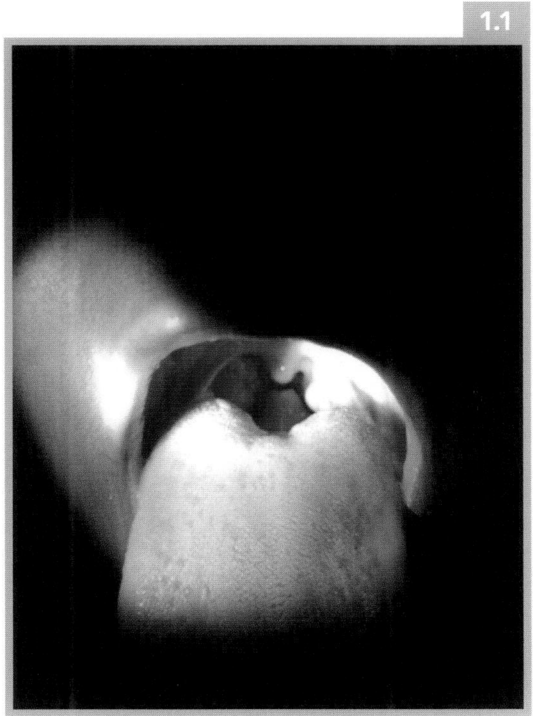

1.1

1. What is the explanation for this mother's concerns?
2. What is the Mallampati classification?

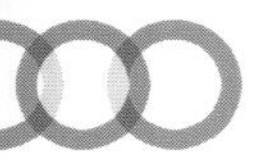

Answers

1. This mother is visualizing a normal epiglottis. The epiglottis can occasionally be visualized in children without any instrumentation. It is important to exclude foreign body ingestion, anatomical abnormalities, or infectious causes. This patient is healthy and in no distress.

2. The Mallampati classification is used to help predict the difficulty of an endotracheal intubation. There are four classes, with each class including specific oral cavity anatomy. Class I corresponds to an easier intubation, whereas class IV corresponds to a more difficult intubation.
    - Class I: Soft palate, uvula, fauces, pillars visible
    - Class II: Soft palate, uvula, fauces visible
    - Class III: Soft palate, base of the uvula visible
    - Class IV: Only hard palate visible

Keywords: head and neck/ENT, airway

Bibliography

Eberhart LHJ, Arndt C, Cierpka T, Schwanekamp J, Wulf H, Putzke C. The reliability and validity of the upper lip bite test compared with the Mallampati classification to predict difficult laryngoscopy: An external prospective evaluation. *Anesth Analg* July 2005;101(1):284–9.

Petkar N, Georgalas C, Bhattacharyya A. High-rising epiglottis in children: Should it cause concern? *J Am Board Fam Med* September–October 2007;20(5):495–6.

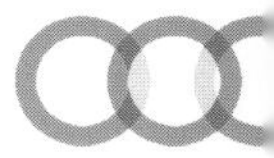

CASE 2

Timothy Ketterhagen

Question

The mother of a 10-day-old female brings her daughter to the emergency department because she has “swelling of her breasts.” The patient was born full-term, vaginal delivery, no complications. Mother was not taking any medications during the pregnancy and denies any current medication or drug use. Mother noticed the swelling over the past few days and it has been gradually increasing, but the patient otherwise seems to be doing well. The patient has been feeding well on breast milk, urinating well, and has returned to her birth weight. No fevers, breast discharge, or redness reported by mother.

Physical exam shows a well-appearing female infant and is unremarkable except for swelling under the bilateral nipples. Swelling is approximately 4 cm in diameter bilaterally, non-erythematous, not fluctuant, and is not warm to the touch. The swelling is mobile, presenting no nipple discharge, and non-tender. The genitalia are normal for age and there is no lymphadenopathy.

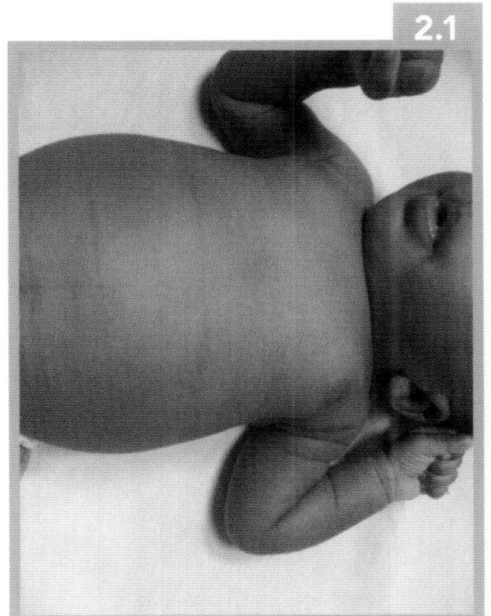

2.1

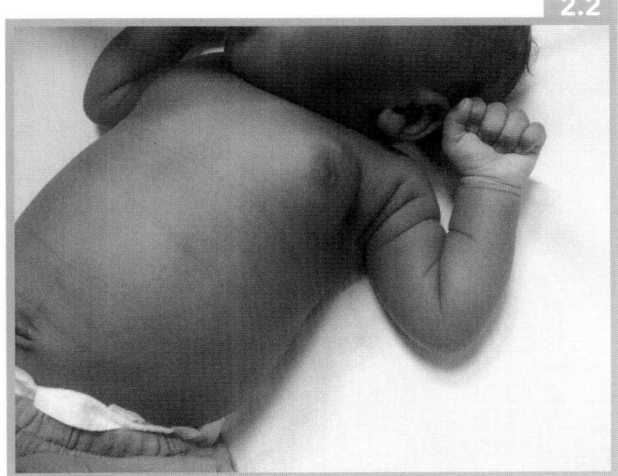

2.2

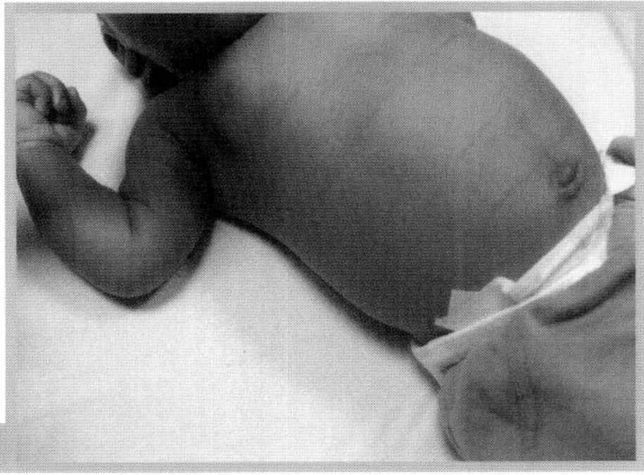

2.3

What workup should be performed in this patient?

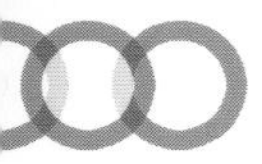

Answer

Neonatal gynecomastia is a common finding in both male and female infants in the first few weeks of life. The breast hypertrophy is related to stimulation from maternal hormones. Generally, no workup is necessary. Reassurance and education are often all that is required.

History and physical should focus on differentiating physiologic changes from infectious or structural abnormalities. The presence of fever, poor appetite, lethargy, warmth, erythema, or nipple discharge are concerning for mastitis or an abscess. The presence of secondary sexual characteristics could indicate the presence of an endocrinopathy. Benign lesions should be monitored every few months.

Keywords: neonate, dermatology, benign

Bibliography

Fleisher GR, Ludwig S, eds. *Textbook of Pediatric Emergency Medicine.* 6th ed. Philadelphia: Lippincott Williams & Wilkins, 2010.

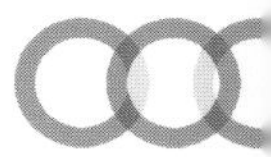

CASE 3

Timothy Ketterhagen

Questions

A 3-week-old female is brought to the emergency department by her father because her "breasts are swollen and red." The father states that he noticed the swelling about a week ago, but the patient looked well so he didn't think anything of it. However, for the past couple of days the swelling has increased, the skin turned red on the left nipple area, and the patient has been fussier than usual. Birth history is unremarkable. The patient has been growing well and feeding well. No fever or nipple discharge are reported.

Physical exam shows a crying, uncomfortable female infant. Vital signs are within normal limits. There is swelling beneath the bilateral nipples, approximately 4 cm in diameter. The left breast is erythematous, warm to the touch, and indurated. There is no purulent discharge from the nipple. Physical exam is otherwise unremarkable.

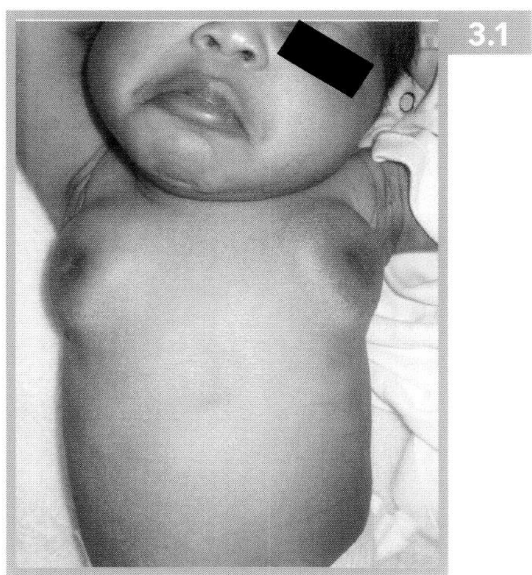

3.1

1. What is the diagnosis?
2. What is the management of this diagnosis?

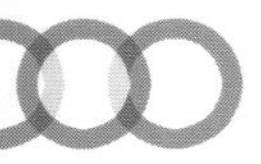

Answers

1. This patient has left-sided mastitis. Mastitis is an infection of the breast tissue. It is usually unilateral. The affected area may be swollen, tender, and warm to the touch. There may or may not be purulent drainage from the nipple and systemic symptoms (e.g. fever) are rare. Mastitis is most common in the first 2 to 5 weeks of life and *Staphylococcus aureus* is the usual causative organism. Girls are affected twice as often as boys. Mastitis must be distinguished from physiologic breast hypertrophy, which resolves spontaneously. The patient should also be evaluated for abscess formation.

2. Management of neonatal mastitis includes a thorough history and physical examination. CBC (complete blood cell), CRP (C-reactive protein), blood culture, and culture of any purulent drainage should be obtained. CSF (cerebrospinal fluid) culture should be obtained in a febrile, ill-appearing infant, or if younger than 28 days. The patient should be started on parenteral antibiotics with coverage against *Staphylococus aureus* and group A streptococcus. Consider surgical consultation if incision and drainage is indicated. The patient should be admitted for continued management.

Keywords: neonate, skin and soft tissue infection, do not miss

Bibliography

Fleisher GR, Ludwig S, eds. *Textbook of Pediatric Emergency Medicine.* 6th ed. Philadelphia: Lippincott Williams & Wilkins, 2010.

Hoffman RJ, Wang VJ, Scarfone R. *Fleisher & Ludwig's 5-Minute Pediatric Emergency Medicine Consult.* Philadelphia: Wolters Kluwer Health/Lippincott Williams & Wilkins, 2012.

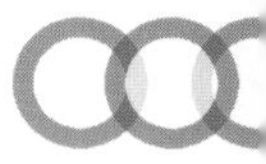

CASE 4

S. Margaret Paik

Question

An 11-year-old girl is brought to the emergency department from school after she complained of chest pain and shortness of breath. She was walking down the hallway when she suddenly felt her heart beating rapidly with a burning sensation in her chest. Her palms became sweaty. Her symptoms lasted about 5–10 minutes. The school nurse called emergency services. The girl denies any upper respiratory tract symptoms, fever, or previous history of a similar episode.

Her vital signs upon arrival to the emergency department are

BP 106/52
Pulse 86
Temperature 35.9°C (tympanic)
Respiratory rate 20
SpO_2 100% on room air

She is alert, answering questions appropriately, and well-appearing. Her lungs are clear to auscultation. There is a normal S1 and S2. No murmur is noticed. Her pulses are +2 bilaterally throughout. There is no hepatosplenomegaly, cyanosis, or edema.

Her ECG tracing shows the following:

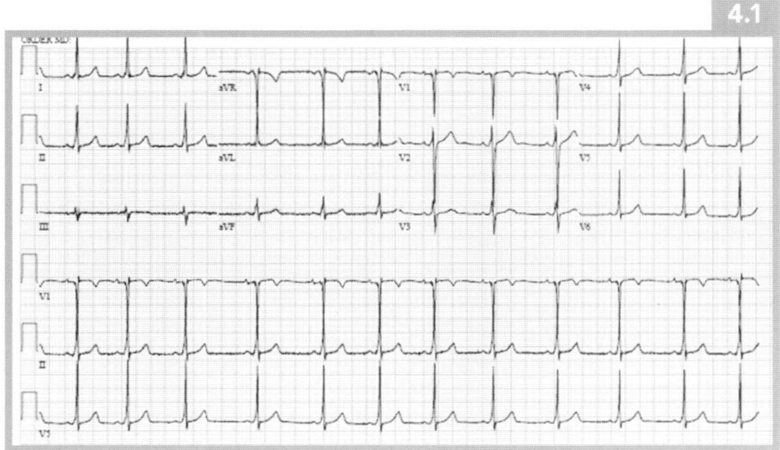

What is seen on her ECG?

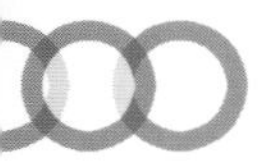

Answer

The PR interval is short at 116 ms and delta waves (initial slurring of the QRS complex) are seen in the leads. The short PR interval is due to rapid AV conduction. Causes of short PR interval include Lown-Ganong-Levine (LGL) syndrome and Wolff-Parkinson-White (WPW) syndrome. LGL is characterized by a short PR interval and normal QRS complex. WPW syndrome is the classic form of preexcitation with accelerated atrioventricular conduction through an accessory pathway, bypassing the AV node and episodes of tachydysrhythmias including supraventricular tachycardia (SVT), atrial flutter/fibrillation, or wide complex tachycardia. A wide QRS complex due to the delta wave is seen.

Symptoms can present at any age. Younger children can present with irritability, poor feeding, tachypnea, and pallor. An older child may complain of chest pain, palpitations, shortness of breath, and syncope. Patients can also present with severe cardiopulmonary compromise and cardiac arrest.

Initial treatment for SVT includes vagal maneuvers and IV adenosine. IV verapamil or diltiazem is used for some patients. IV procainamide or amiodarone is used if wide complex tachycardia is noted.

Keywords: cardiology, chest pain, ECG

Bibliography

Cain N, Irving C, Webber S, Beerman L et al. Natural history of Wolff-Parkinson-White syndrome diagnosed in childhood. *Am J Cardiol* 2013;112(7):961–5.

Park MK, Guntheroth WG. *How to Read Pediatric ECGs*. 4th ed. St. Louis: Mosby, 2006.

Zeng R. *Graphics-Sequenced Interpretation of ECG*. Singapore: Springer, 2016.

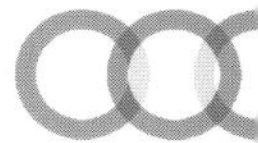

CASE 5

Leah Finkel

Question

A 7-month-old, full-term, healthy male presents with cough, congestion, and increased work of breathing. According to his mother, this is his third episode of "bronchiolitis." He takes albuterol at home as needed. On exam he is tachypneic. There are diminished breath sounds diffusely and he has some mild subcostal retractions. You decide to give him nebulized albuterol and order a chest x-ray. The albuterol does not improve his work of breathing.

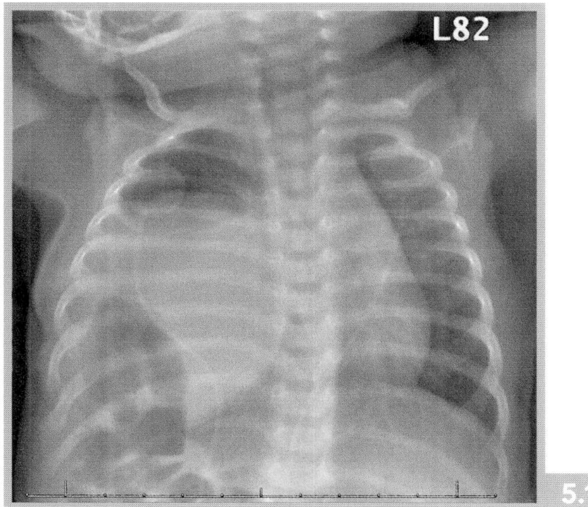

5.1

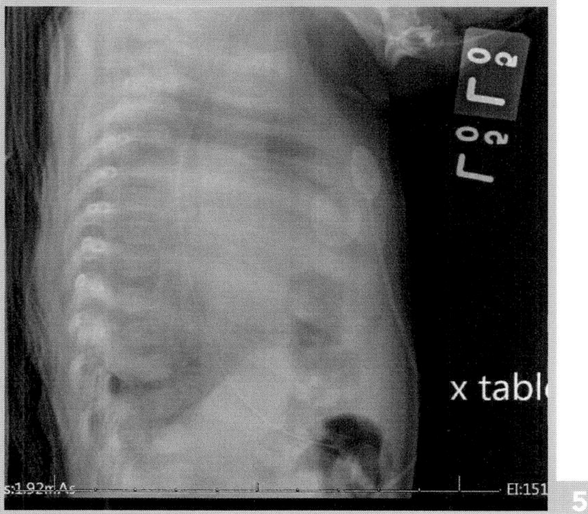

5.2

What do these radiographs display and how would you manage this?

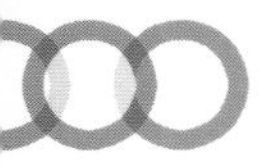

Answer

This radiograph shows a congenital diaphragmatic hernia (CDH). CDH occurs because of a diaphragmatic defect that occurs *in utero*, usually between weeks 8 and 10 of gestation. This defect then allows abdominal organs to herniate into the chest cavity, which causes the development of lung hypoplasia. Although lung hypoplasia is most significant on the side of the diaphragmatic defect, both lungs may be affected. CDH is more common on the left side compared to the right (about 85% versus 13%) and much less commonly may be bilateral. Right-sided defects are associated with higher mortality.

There is a high mortality associated with CDH within hours of life. It is typically diagnosed prenatally or in the immediate postnatal period. In the delivery room, bag mask ventilation should be avoided as this may worsen abdominal distension and compression of the lung. Management typically includes ventilation with low peak inspiratory pressures to minimize lung injury, nasogastric decompression with continuous suction to decompress abdominal contents, IV access, and blood pressure support.

Patients with delayed presentation of CDH may demonstrate respiratory or gastrointestinal complaints, including recurrent chest infections, respiratory distress, recurrent emesis, diarrhea, failure to thrive, and signs of acute hernia incarceration. CDH may be missed in this age because it is often thought of as a neonatal problem.

Keywords: pulmonary, gastrointestinal, cough, respiratory distress

Bibliography

Banac S, Ahel V, Rozmanić V, Gazdik M, Saina G, Mavrinac B. Congenital diaphragmatic hernia in older children. *Acta Med Croatica* 2004;58(3):225–8.

Haroon J, Chamberlain RS. An evidence-based review of the current treatment of congenital diaphragmatic hernia. *Clin Pediatr (Phila)* February 2013;52(2):115–24.

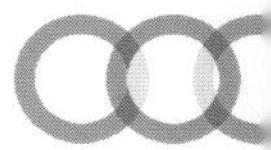

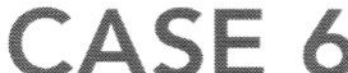

CASE 6

Alisa McQueen

Question

A mother brings her 9-month-old in for evaluation of blood in the diaper. She reports his stool this morning was completely red. He's otherwise been acting well with no fever, vomiting, or apparent abdominal pain. Physical examination is normal, including a benign abdomen and no anal fissures. The diaper is shown next.

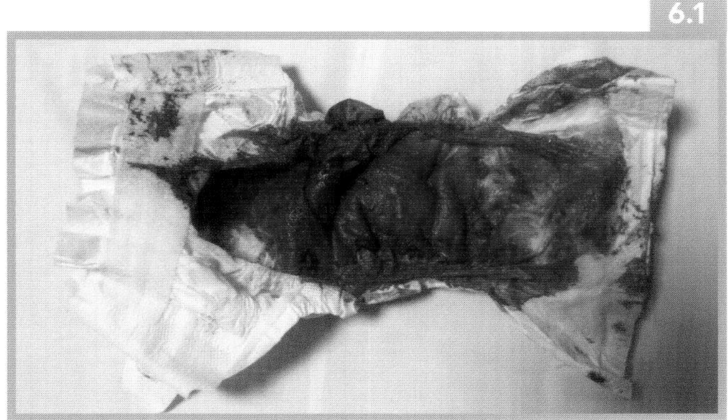

6.1

Hemoccult testing of the diaper contents is negative.

What entities can cause bloody appearance in stool?

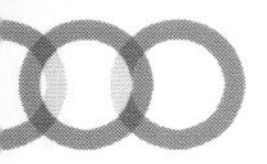

Answer

Several foods and medications can cause discoloration of the stool, and when red, often prompt emergency room visits for fear that the stool is bloody. These include foods which are artificially colored or naturally red, including beets, berries, and tomatoes.

This patient was taking cefdinir, an oral cephalosporin, which, in the presence of iron, causes oxidation of the iron and gives an apparently bloody appearance to the stool. This most commonly occurs in infants receiving iron supplements or iron-rich formula.

Keywords: medications, gastrointestinal, mimickers

Bibliography

Graves R, Weaver SP. Cefdinir-associated 'bloody stools' in an infant. *J Am Board Fam Med* 2008;21(3):246–8.
http://www.childrenscolorado.org/wellness/at_home/abdomen/stools-unusual-color.aspx.

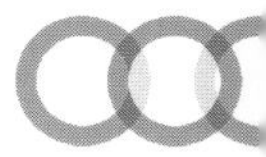

CASE 7

Timothy Ketterhagen

Question

A 4-day-old male infant is brought to the emergency department because of "bloody urine in the diaper." Parents noticed the discoloration after a diaper change earlier in the day, so they brought the patient in for evaluation. The patient is otherwise doing very well. The patient was born at 39 weeks via a normal, spontaneous, vaginal delivery. There were no complications and prenatal labs were normal. The patient went home with parents after a couple of days. The patient has been breastfeeding well, making approximately six to eight wet diapers and one to two non-bloody stools per day. Prior to this episode, the parents had not noticed any blood in the urine. There is no family history of any kidney problems. No fevers, vomiting, trauma, or lethargy are reported.

Physical exam shows a calm, well-appearing male infant. Vital signs are within normal limits for age. The patient is uncircumcised and genitalia are normal for age and sex. There are no rashes or lesions in the diaper region. There is no blood at the urethral meatus, no urethral discharge, and no anal fissures or bleeding. The physical exam is otherwise unremarkable.

7.1

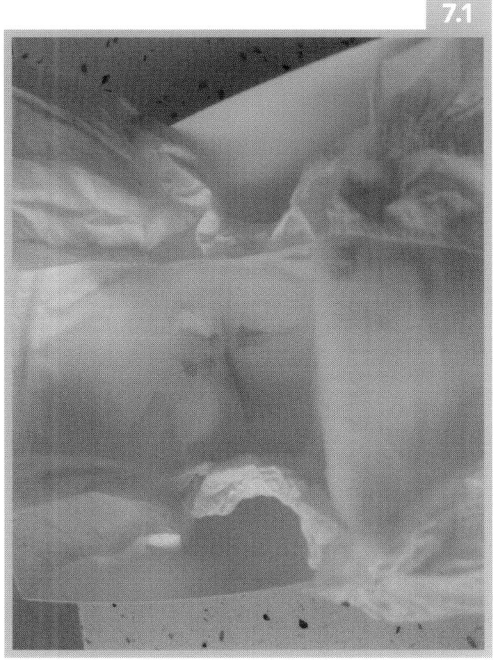

What should be considered in a newborn with apparent bloody urine?

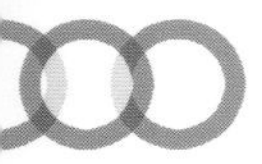

Answer

Bloody urine in an infant is never normal. However, red/orange urine may not be blood. This discoloration may be caused by the crystallization of uric acid in the urine. In the first few days of life, infants are at risk for dehydration caused by poor intake or maternal milk supply. This may lead to concentration of the urine and uric acid crystal formation, which gives the urine an orange or red hue. Parental education and correction of dehydration should be performed.

If the infant is otherwise well, vital signs are normal, and there are no systemic symptoms, then no further workup may be necessary. However, a urine dip may be performed to evaluate for blood in the urine or signs of infection. Gross hematuria may be caused by glomerular disease, urinary tract infection (UTI), trauma, or thrombosis. In older children, the ingestion of beets, blackberries, rifampin, ibuprofen, deferoxamine, or exposure to aniline dyes may cause urine to appear red or brown. Further workup may be warranted if there are any other concerning patient characteristics.

Keywords: neonate, mimickers, benign, hematuria

Bibliography

Hoffman RJ, Wang VJ, Scarfone R. *Fleisher & Ludwig's 5-Minute Pediatric Emergency Medicine Consult.* Philadelphia: Wolters Kluwer Health/Lippincott Williams & Wilkins, 2012.

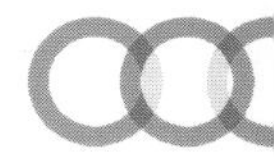

CASE 8

Timothy Ketterhagen

Questions

A father brings his 12-year-old daughter to the emergency department because she has had difficulty moving the left side of her face for the past 24 hours. The patient has had liquid dribbling out of the side of her mouth when she drinks and her left eye has felt dry. The patient denies any other neurologic changes or any trauma. Father reports that the patient had a cold a couple of weeks ago, but that she has improved. She also denies any drug use or recent travel. This is the first time the patient has displayed these symptoms.

On physical exam the patient is awake, alert, and in no distress. There is flattening of the nasolabial crease on the left side of the face. There is also decreased movement of the left corner of the mouth when she is instructed to smile. She is unable to wrinkle her left forehead and has diminished ability to fully close her left eyelid. The neurologic exam is otherwise unremarkable. The rest of the physical exam also reveals no abnormalities including no evidence of otitis media, parotid gland swelling, or mastoid tenderness.

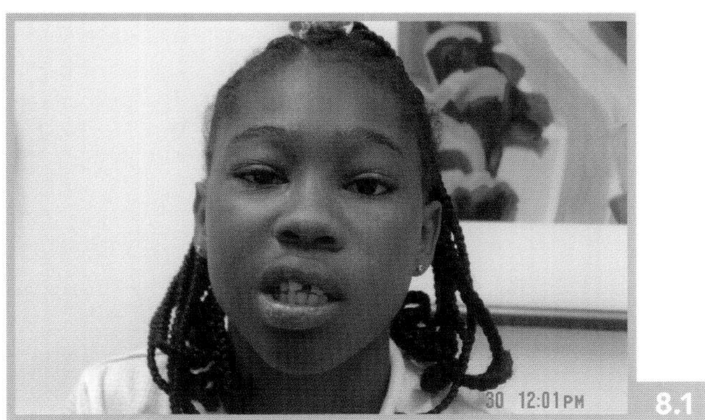

8.1

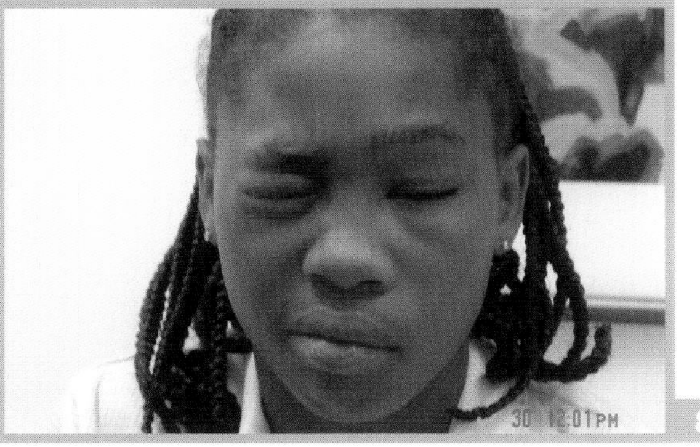

8.2

1. What workup is required for this diagnosis?
2. What is the treatment?

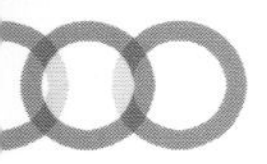

Answers

1. This patient is suffering from Bell's palsy, which is unilateral peripheral facial nerve palsy. The cause of Bell's palsy is unknown, although a history of a preceding upper respiratory infection or a reactivation of Epstein-Barr virus or HSV may be responsible. Bell's palsy is a clinical diagnosis. If paralysis is bilateral or ipsilateral forehead sparing is present, other diagnoses should be considered. The differential diagnosis includes stroke, multiple sclerosis, tumors, Lyme disease, Guillain-Barré syndrome, and Ramsay Hunt syndrome. A workup for these should be performed only if the diagnosis is uncertain. Brain imaging is indicated for gradual onset of symptoms (>48 hours), bilateral facial paralysis, or sparing of the ipsilateral forehead. Vesicles on the face, mouth, or ear are indicative of Ramsay Hunt syndrome, which is a reactivation of varicella zoster.

2. Treatment for Bell's palsy is controversial due to a lack of studies in children. However, supportive treatment including artificial tears, eye ointments, and patching at night should be performed in all patients to protect the cornea. Corticosteroids have shown some benefit in adults but have not been studied extensively in children. There is a lack of evidence to support the routine use of antivirals (e.g. acyclovir and valacyclovir) in children. Symptoms will resolve spontaneously in most children within 3 months.

Keywords: neurology, infectious diseases, signs and symptoms

Bibliography

Fleisher GR, Ludwig S, eds. *Textbook of Pediatric Emergency Medicine*. 6th ed. Philadelphia: Lippincott Williams & Wilkins, 2010.

Hoffman RJ, Wang VJ, Scarfone R. *Fleisher & Ludwig's 5-Minute Pediatric Emergency Medicine Consult*. Philadelphia: Wolters Kluwer Health/Lippincott Williams & Wilkins, 2012.

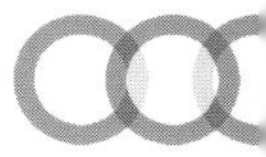

CASE 9

Timothy Ketterhagen

Question

The parents of a 12-month-old male bring him to the emergency department because of swelling in the right wrist. The parents noticed the swelling a couple of days ago, but it has not resolved, so they brought the patient in for evaluation. The parents deny any trauma and state that the patient has otherwise been acting normally. The patient was exclusively breastfed until 6 months but now also takes table foods. He does not take any daily vitamins. The patient has been urinating normally, no fevers reported, no vomiting or diarrhea, and the patient is in the 20th percentile for weight and 5th percentile for height. The patient is cruising, but not yet walking without support. Patient is otherwise meeting his developmental milestones. The patient was born at 34 weeks, but the birth history is otherwise unremarkable. The patient has missed several appointments with his pediatrician because of transportation problems.

Physical exam shows a non-toxic, alert male infant. Vital signs are within normal limits for age. Upon inspection of the extremities, there is swelling in the bilateral wrists and knees. The swollen areas are hard, non-fluctuant, non-tender, and non-erythematous. There also appears to be bowing of the lower extremities. The physical exam is otherwise unremarkable.

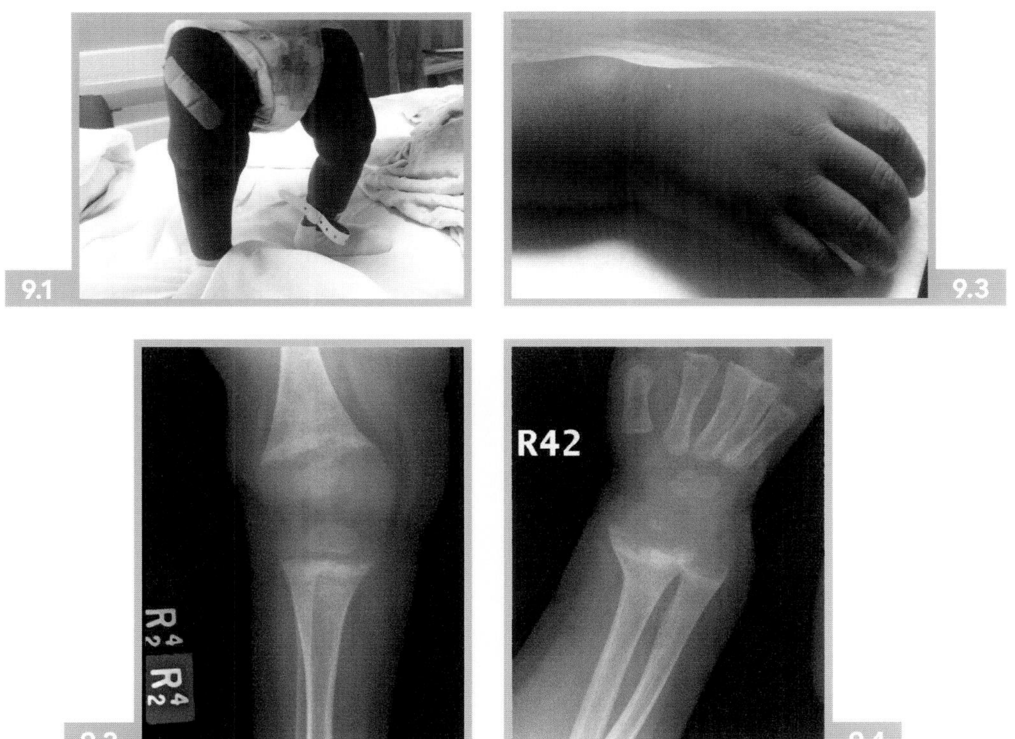

What is the diagnosis and etiology of the physical exam findings?

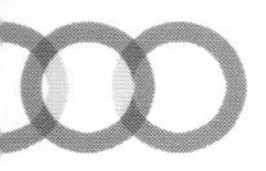

Answer

This patient is suffering from rickets, which is caused by vitamin D deficiency. Rickets is caused by the failure of mineralization of the bone matrix in growing bone due to a lack of vitamin D. Causes include inadequate dietary vitamin D, excess phosphate excretion, inability to form the active metabolite [1,25-$(OH)_2D_3$] of vitamin D, and excess accumulation of acid. The incidence of rickets has decreased since vitamin D supplementation in foods has increased. However, rickets may be seen in certain ethnic groups, premature infants, children with malabsorption problems, patients with decreased sunlight exposure, and patients with severe renal disease.

A thorough social and dietary history is helpful, as is a detailed family history. Children may present with skeletal deformities, skeletal pain, slippage of epiphyses, fractures, growth disturbances, seizures, hypotonia, or lethargy. Radiography is the test of choice to confirm the diagnosis. Characteristic findings include widening and irregularity of the epiphyseal plates, cupped metaphyses, fractures, and bowing of limbs. Calcium, phosphate, alkaline phosphatase, PTH (parathyroid hormone), and 25-hydroxyvitamin D levels may be obtained.

Treatment depends on the underlying disease. Dietary rickets may be treated with 1200–1600 IU of ergocalciferol daily until healing occurs. Radiographic improvement is generally seen by 2 weeks. The patient should then be continued on 400 IU of vitamin D to prevent recurrence.

Keywords: metabolic, orthopedics

Bibliography

Fleisher GR, Ludwig S, eds. *Textbook of Pediatric Emergency Medicine*. 6th ed. Philadelphia: Lippincott Williams & Wilkins, 2010.

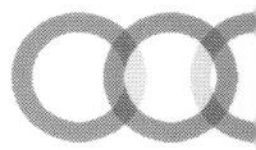

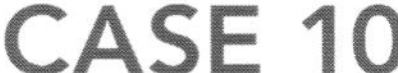

CASE 10

Michael Gottlieb

Questions

A 1-year-old uncircumcised boy presents with penile pain and swelling. His mother states that she gave him a bath before bed. After being put to bed, he began crying for an extended period of time. When she examined his diaper to change him, she noticed swelling as demonstrated in the following.

10.1

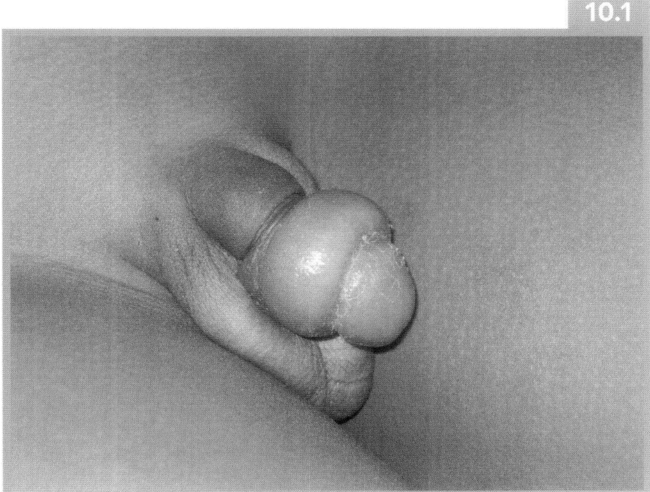

1. What is the diagnosis?
2. What are some strategies for treating this condition?

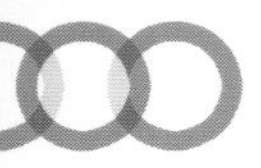

Answers

1. This patient has paraphimosis. Paraphimosis is a condition in which the foreskin is retracted behind the glans penis and becomes progressively edematous, leading to decreased blood flow to the glans. This is a medical emergency that requires reduction to preserve vascular supply to the glans. In contrast, phimosis is a medical condition where the foreskin is unable to be retracted over the glans. Although this latter condition often requires urologic follow-up, it is rarely associated with acute medical complications.
2. Paraphimosis may be treated with mechanical reduction or non-manipulative therapies. Mechanical reduction is performed by applying gentle and steady pressure to the retracted foreskin to decrease the edema while gently retracting the foreskin back over the glans. It is important to provide adequate analgesia with topical anesthetics or a dorsal penile block, as this can be very painful for the patient. Non-manipulative strategies include mannitol-soaked gauze, application of granulated sugar, cold compresses, and compression bandages.

Keywords: genitourinary, do not miss, procedures

Bibliography

Clifford ID, Craig SS, Nataraja RM, Panabokke G et al. Paediatric paraphimosis. *Emerg Med Australas* February 2016;28(1):96–9.

Dubin J, Davis JE. Penile emergencies. *Emerg Med Clin North Am* August 2011;29(3):485–99.

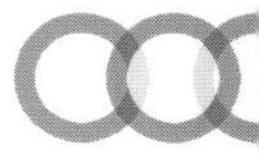

CASE 11

Timothy Ketterhagen

Question

The father of a 1-year-old boy brings him to the emergency department because his penis "doesn't look right." The patient started crying last night and did not sleep well. Today, the father reports that the patient has been crying uncontrollably. When the father went to change the patient's diaper, he noticed that the penis appeared swollen, so he brought him to the emergency department. The father denies any trauma. No fevers, foul-smelling urine, or rashes.

Physical exam shows a vigorous, crying child. Genitourinary exam shows swelling of a circumcised penis with an indentation circumferentially proximal to the glans. Upon closer inspection, what appears to be a hair is visualized on the shaft of the penis. The patient appears to have tenderness when the penis is manipulated. Testes are palpated bilaterally in the scrotum with no masses or lesions present. The physical exam is otherwise unremarkable. The penile exam is shown next.

11.1

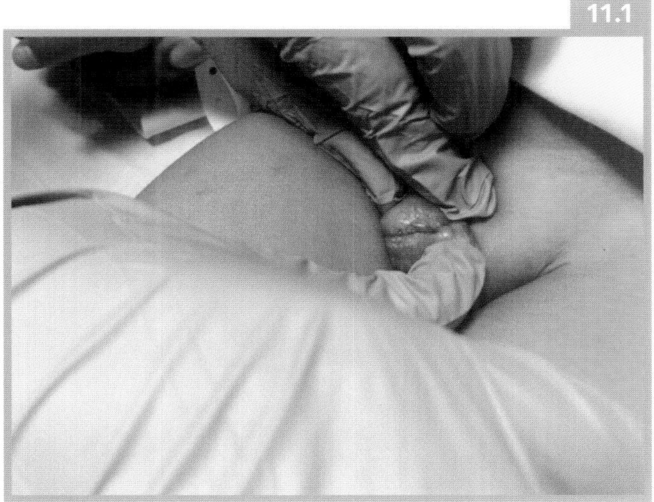

What are the steps that should be performed to treat a penile hair tourniquet?

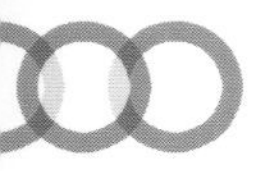

Answer

Tourniquet syndromes may lead to soft tissue injury, neurovascular bundle damage, urethral transection, or necrosis. Hair, threads, clothing, or a variety of other synthetic materials may cause tourniquet syndrome of the penis.

A thorough physical exam is required of any infant, but especially a patient who presents with uncontrollable crying. This includes the genitalia and all digits in order to detect tourniquet syndromes. The affected tissue may appear edematous, erythematous, and strangulated. The constricting material may be easily visualized or may be hidden by the surrounding swelling. Conditions such as trauma, insect bites, abscesses, paraphimosis, balanitis, or allergic reactions should be considered in a patient with similar examination findings.

Treatment of a penile hair tourniquet includes pain control through a penile block or parenteral medications. Procedural sedation may be required. Grasping the loose end of the string/hair and carefully unwrapping circumferentially or inserting a blunt probe under the fiber and cutting it with scissors or a scalpel may be performed to remove a superficial tourniquet. Incisions should be made at the 4- or 8-o'clock positions of the penis to avoid the dorsal neurovascular bundles. Hair removal creams may be applied, but will not work on synthetic fibers and may cause local irritation. Deeply embedded tourniquets may require consultation with a urologist if ischemia, urethral injury, or neurovascular injury is suspected, as operative management may be indicated. Suspected urethral injury may be assessed by retrograde urethrogram. A Doppler ultrasound may be used to evaluate for occlusions of the penile vasculature. Patients with uncomplicated removal and with no signs of ischemia may be discharged to follow up with a urologist in 24 hours and given family instructions to monitor for signs of ischemia.

Keywords: genitourinary, GU trauma, do not miss, procedures

Bibliography

McAninch SA, Letbetter SA. Hair tourniquet syndrome. In *Current Diagnosis & Treatment: Pediatric Emergency Medicine*, Stone CK, Humphries RL, Drigalla D, Stephan M, eds. New York: McGraw-Hill, 2015:477–8.

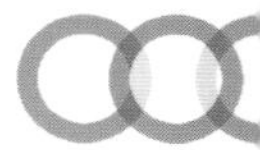

CASE 12

Timothy Ketterhagen

Questions

A 4-year-old female is brought to the emergency department because of a "lump in her groin." The parents noticed the swelling earlier in the day. The swelling increases in size when she cries. The patient is otherwise doing well. The parents deny any recent illnesses. The patient has been eating well and she is not complaining of any pain. The parents have never noticed this swelling before. No vomiting, diarrhea, rhinorrhea, fevers, abdominal pain, or dysuria are reported.

Physical exam shows a well-appearing child. Vital signs are normal. Her abdomen is soft, non-tender, non-distended, with no rebound or guarding and normal bowel sounds. No masses are palpated. On genitourinary (GU) exam, a painless inguinal swelling is noted on the right. The swelling is soft and mobile, but not reducible. There is no overlying erythema. The physical exam is otherwise unremarkable.

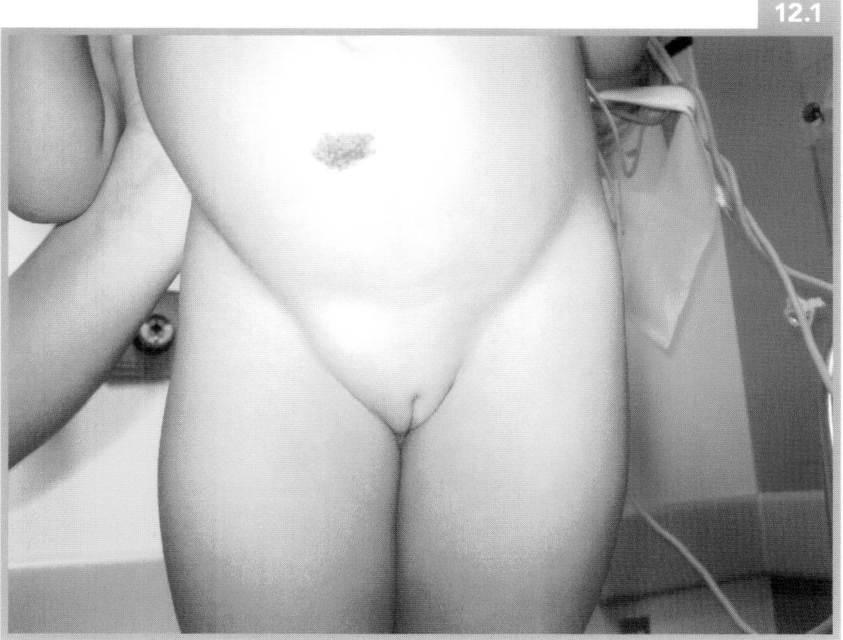

12.1

1. What is the diagnosis?
2. What diagnosis should not be missed in a female patient with an inguinal mass?

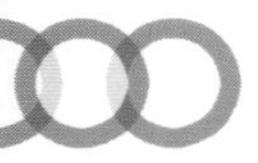

Answers

1. This patient has an inguinal hernia. Inguinal hernias are diagnosed based on physical exam and lab studies are not usually indicated. Many infants and children manifest with a bulge in the inguinal canal that occurs with crying or straining. This is usually caused by a loop of intestine extending into the hernia sac. Inguinal hernias are caused by a patent processus vaginalis in both males and females. If the patient is well-appearing, a manual reduction of the hernia may be attempted with adequate analgesia. Surgical consultation is recommended if manual reduction is unsuccessful.

2. In a female, it is important to consider that an ovary may have herniated and may be at risk for torsion. If a painful mass is present, incarceration or strangulation of a loop of bowel is also possible. The patient may also show signs of bowel obstruction, such as vomiting. In a toxic-appearing patient, emergent surgical consultation may be indicated following fluid resuscitation. When an inguinal mass is painless and irreducible, a recently incarcerated hernia (i.e. an ovary) or an enlarged lymph node is the most likely causes. Ultrasound may be helpful to evaluate blood flow to an ovary that cannot be reduced.

Keywords: gastrointestinal, mass, ultrasound

Bibliography

Fleisher GR, Stephen L, eds. *Textbook of Pediatric Emergency Medicine.* 6th ed. Philadelphia: Lippincott Williams & Wilkins, 2010.

Hoffman RJ, Wang VJ, Scarfone R. *Fleisher & Ludwig's 5-Minute Pediatric Emergency Medicine Consult.* Philadelphia, PA: Wolters Kluwer Health/Lippincott Williams & Wilkins, 2012.

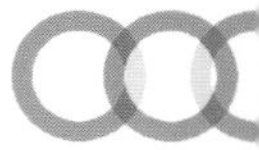

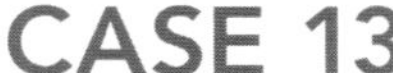

CASE 13

Barbara Pawel

Question

A 16-year-old male is brought to the emergency department with a gunshot wound (GSW) to his left chest. Tachycardia, hypoxia, and respiratory distress are noted. Lung exam reveals decreased breath sounds over his left chest.

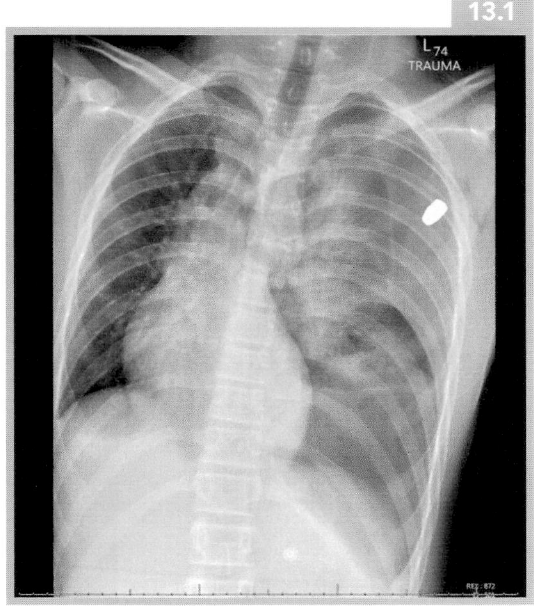

13.1

List the possible high-risk injuries with penetrating trauma to the thorax.

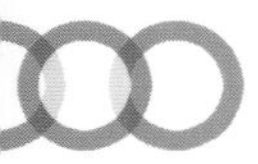

Answer

- Open, closed, or tension pneumothorax
- Hemothorax
- Cardiac tamponade
- Exsanguinating hemorrhage

Any penetrating trauma to the head, neck, chest, abdomen, or extremities proximal to the elbows or knees carries a high risk of significant injury and the need for surgical intervention. A full primary and secondary survey should be completed on all children with a mechanism of injury or a physical exam concerning for serious or multiple injuries. Life-threatening injuries should be identified and addressed during the primary survey.

Any type of pneumothorax can present with unilateral diminished breath sounds and subcutaneous air (crepitus) in the chest wall in addition to respiratory distress, tachypnea and tachycardia, pleuritic chest pain, and hypoxia.

A tension pneumothorax may also cause tracheal deviation, and if suspected and the patient is hemodynamically unstable, a needle thoracostomy should be performed with a 14–16 gauge angiocatheter followed by chest tube placement. Any pneumothorax involving >15% of lung volume is unlikely to resolve without chest tube insertion. An open pneumothorax will require a three-sided occlusive dressing and surgical intervention. A hemothorax will be dull to percussion and require early chest tube placement. Open thoracotomy may be needed and is based on initial/ongoing bloody drainage. Frequent re-assessments are necessary to rapidly identify decompensation pre- and post-interventions.

Keywords: penetrating trauma, procedures, do not miss, respiratory distress

Bibliography

American College of Surgeons Committee on Trauma. *Advanced Trauma Life Support (ATLS) Student Course Manual*. 9th ed. Chicago: American College of Surgeons, 2012.

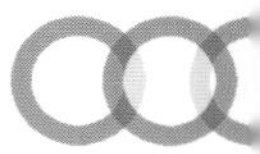

CASE 14

Michael Farnham and Timothy Ketterhagen

Questions

A mother brings her 14-year-old daughter into the emergency department. Her lips and cheeks are swollen and slightly itchy. Symptoms started to develop over the past few hours. The patient has a history of hypertension that is being managed by a nephrologist. She was recently started on a new medication for high blood pressure, but the mother cannot remember the name of it. The patient denies difficulty breathing or swallowing. No cough, rhinorrhea, vomiting, or diarrhea. No fever reported. No new soaps, detergents, or creams. No history of allergies. No recent illnesses.

Physical exam reveals a developmentally normal young girl in no apparent distress. Vital signs are normal. Head and neck exam reveals non-pitting edema to the face and lips. The patient's face also appears flushed. There is no tachypnea, stridor, or wheezing. The patient's hands appear minimally edematous, but no other edema is present. Abdominal exam is normal. No other rashes are noted. The physical exam is otherwise unremarkable.

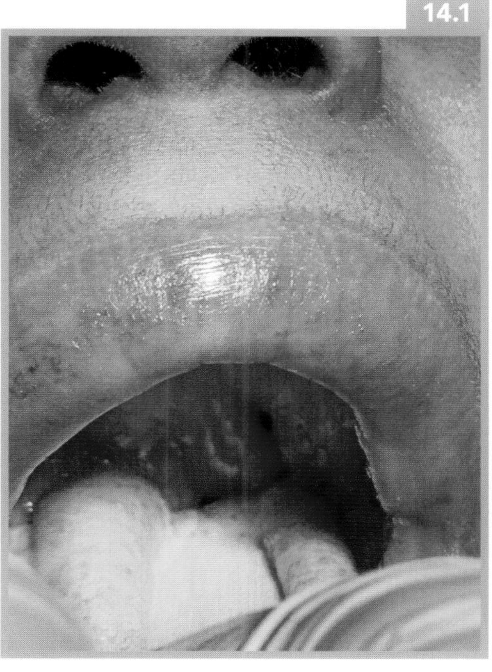

14.1

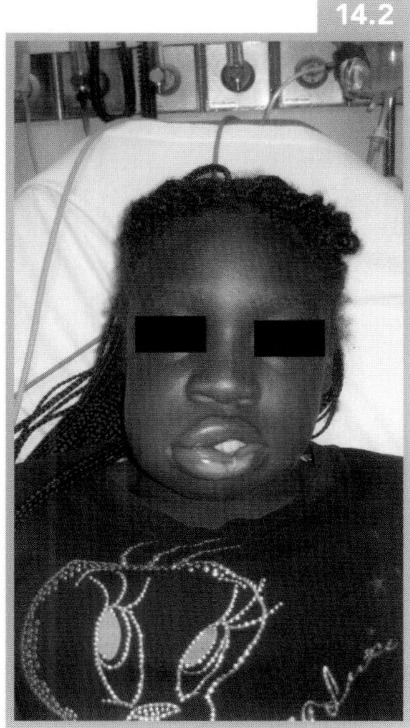

14.2

1. What is the diagnosis?
2. What specific medications could cause this condition?
3. Why is prompt action required?

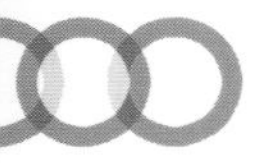

Answers

1. This patient has angioedema. Angioedema is a localized swelling due to extravasation of fluid into interstitial tissues. The cause may be idiopathic, food induced, infection induced, hereditary, allergic, or medication induced. It commonly occurs on the head, neck, hand, and gastrointestinal tract. No lab testing is required for diagnosis. Initial treatment includes airway and circulatory stabilization.

2. Non-histamine-induced angioedema may occur from therapy with angiotensin-converting enzyme (ACE) inhibitors, as in this patient. The ACE inhibitors most commonly prescribed to children include lisinopril, captopril, and enalapril. Angioedema can occur at any time during ACE inhibitor therapy. African American patients are more susceptible. Patients will need to be switched to another class of anti-hypertensive medications.

   In patients with no associated risk factors, the diagnosis of C1 esterase inhibitor deficiency should be considered. A history of minor trauma often precedes symptoms in these patients.

3. Prompt treatment is required to prevent airway obstruction. In contrast to histamine-induced allergic angioedema, which is treated with epinephrine, antihistamines, and steroids, non-histamine-induced angioedema does not respond to these traditional therapies. Patients with C1 esterase inhibitor deficiency are managed with infusion of recombinant C1 inhibitor. If unavailable and symptoms are progressing, FFP (fresh frozen plasma) can be given.

Keywords: medications, airway, life-threatening, drug reactions

Bibliography

Dykewicz MS. Cough and angioedema from angiotensin-converting enzyme inhibitors: New insights into mechanisms and management. *Curr Opin Allergy Clin Immunol* 2004;4:267.

Hoffman RJ, Wang VJ, Scarfone R. *Fleisher & Ludwig's 5-Minute Pediatric Emergency Medicine Consult.* Philadelphia: Wolters Kluwer Health/Lippincott Williams & Wilkins, 2012.

Nagarajan V, Patel A. ACE inhibitor related angioedema. *QJM* 2011;105(11):1129–9.

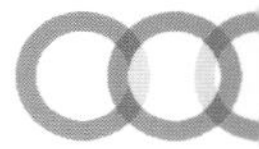

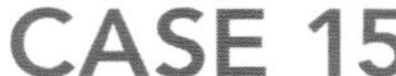

CASE 15

Barbara Pawel

Question

A 4-year-old male is brought to the emergency department with perioral burns and drooling after chewing on an extension cord.

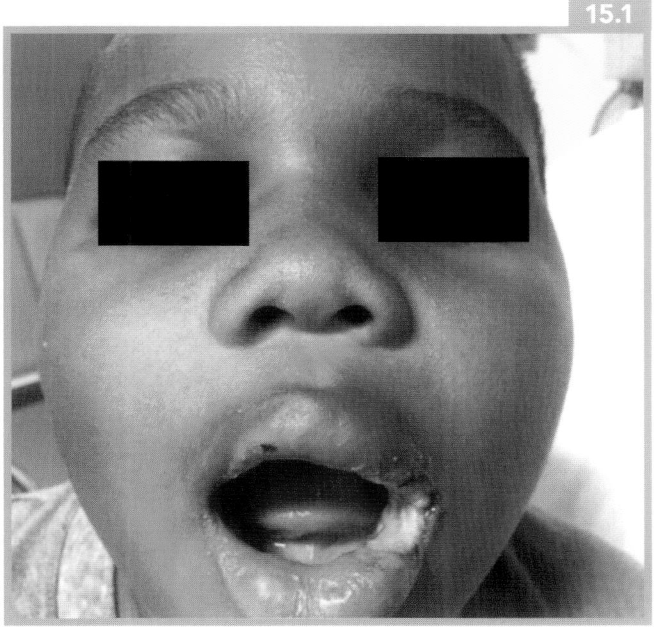

15.1

Name a serious delayed complication of oral commissure burns.

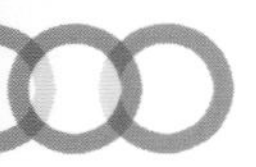

Answer

Delayed hemorrhage from the labial artery can occur anytime within the first 3 weeks when the eschar separates.

Oral burns caused by electrical trauma tend to occur during the teething period (3–36 months) from chewing on the female ends of live extension cords or exposed wires. Saliva acts as a medium to transport electrical current to the mucosa, causing intense heat and coagulation necrosis. Carefully inspect for burns, blisters, and charred skin, especially around the mouth. Destructive full thickness burns can extend to the tongue, floor of mouth, buccal mucosa, and labial vestibule. Edema and excessive drooling occurs within several hours. An eschar forms and later separates (1–3 weeks) with subsequent healing by secondary intention. An arterial hemorrhage can occur with eschar separation. Commissure injuries can lead to debilitating microstomia, which can affect speech, jaw and tongue movement, oral intake, oral hygiene, and cause facial distortion. Early reconstruction (commissuroplasty) and removable commissural splints are interventions to help prevent contractures.

Keywords: head and neck/ENT, environmental, pitfalls, oropharyngeal injury

Bibliography

Hashem FK, Al Khayal Z. Oral burn contractures in children. *Ann Plast Surg* 2003;51(5):468–71.

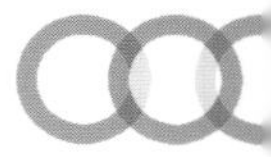

CASE 16

Barbara Pawel

Question

An 8-year-old child presents to the emergency department with wrist pain after falling on his outstretched hand. The images appear next.

16.1

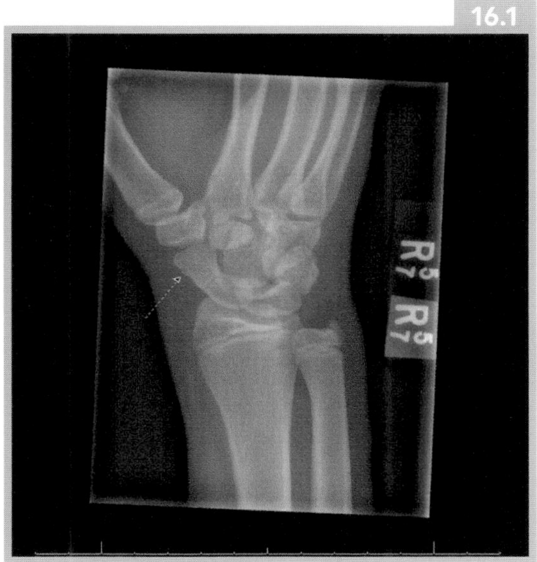

16.2

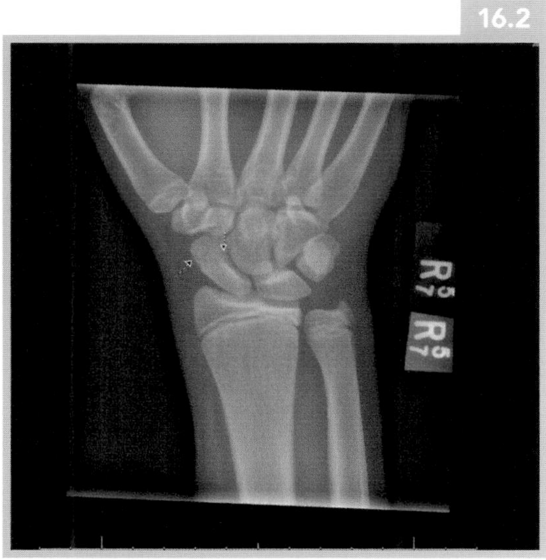

What complications are associated with scaphoid fractures and which types of scaphoid fractures are more likely to lead to these complications?

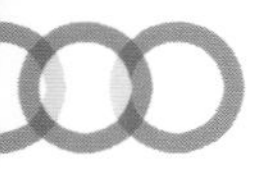

Answer

Proximal scaphoid fractures are more prone to interruption of the arterial blood supply, leading to avascular necrosis and nonunion.

The scaphoid is the most common carpal bone fractured in children. Symptoms include pain along the radial aspect of the wrist, decreased range of motion, and tenderness in the anatomical snuffbox. In young children, the scaphoid is covered by articular cartilage and a circumferential epiphyseal plate. This leads to subtle injuries, such as buckle fractures, with minimal x-ray findings. Due to the ossification sequence, the most common location for a fracture in children is the distal pole of the scaphoid. In these fractures, the blood supply usually remains intact so complications such as avascular necrosis and nonunion are less common. Adolescents are more likely to fracture the proximal pole or waist with a higher complication rate. Initial x-rays, including a scaphoid view, may be negative. If a scaphoid fracture is suspected, apply a thumb spica splint and the patient should have follow-up with an specialist. Early immobilization reduces nonunion rates.

Keywords: orthopedics, extremity injury, procedures, pitfalls

Bibliography

Ahmed I, Ashton F, Tay WK, Porter D et al. The pediatric fracture of the scaphoid in patients aged 13 years and under: An epidemiological study. *J Pediatr Orthop* 2014;34(2):150–4.

Gholson JJ, Bae DS, Zurakowski D, Waters PM et al. Scaphoid fractures in children and adolescents: Contemporary injury patterns and factors influencing time to union. *J Bone Joint Surg Am* 2011;93(13):1210–9.

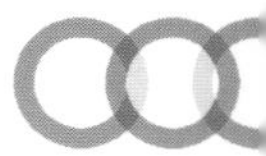

CASE 17

Emily Obringer

Questions

A 5-year-old girl presents to the emergency department with a 3-week history of left-sided neck and facial swelling. The area is slightly warm and minimally tender; however, the swelling is now limiting her neck range of motion. She does not have any pets but frequently visits her cousins, who just bought a kitten. On exam she's non-toxic-appearing, not drooling, and has no meningismus but has pain with rotation of her neck.

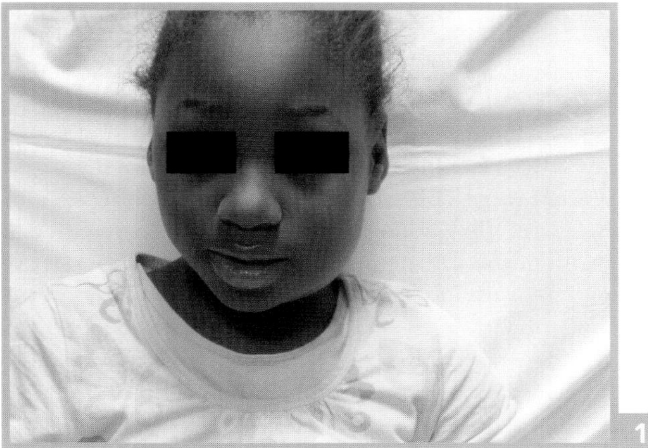

17.1

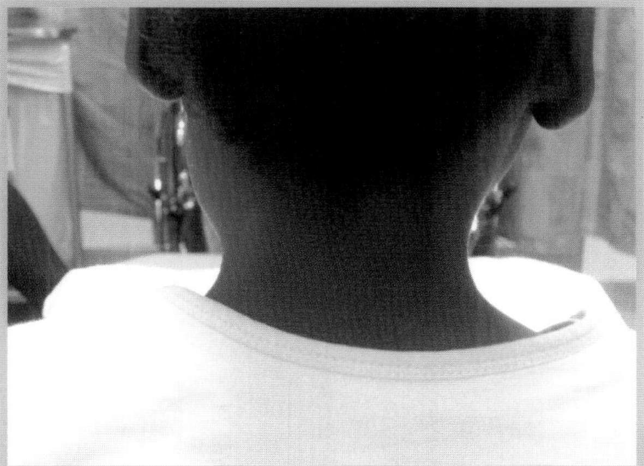

17.2

1. What additional infection-related questions should the clinician ask when investigating neck swelling?
2. What are the two most common infectious causes of subacute unilateral cervical lymphadenitis?

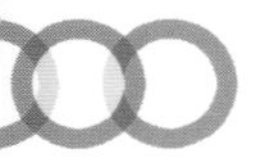

Answers

1. When investigating the etiology of neck swelling, particular attention should be given to properly identifying the specific location that is affected. The evaluation and management of cervical adenopathy, parotitis, superficial midline neck swelling, and deep neck infections are quite different. Examining the patient from behind may help to clarify the location. Exposure, travel, and immunization histories are essential, and an accurate description of length of symptoms can help guide the clinician.

2. The two most common infectious causes of subacute unilateral cervical lymphadenitis are cat scratch disease (due to *Bartonella henselae*) and non-tuberculous mycobacterial infection. Other infectious causes include tuberculosis, toxoplasmosis, and actinomycosis.

   Regional lymphadenopathy is the most common presentation of cat scratch disease and is typically seen in immunocompetent hosts with exposure to cats, especially kittens. A primary skin lesion usually appears 7 to 12 days after the scratch and is then followed by regional lymphadenopathy 5 to 50 days later (median, 12 days) (American Academy of Pediatrics, 2012). Serum antibody testing is frequently positive and may help solidify the diagnosis. The disease is frequently self-limited and resolves in 2 to 4 months. Treatment is usually symptom-based, but some experts recommend a 5-day course of azithromycin to speed recovery (American Academy of Pediatrics, 2012). Needle aspiration may relieve pain symptoms; however, incision and drainage should be avoided due to the potential development of fistulae.

   Non-tuberculous mycobacteria (NTM) account for 70%–95% of mycobacterial lymphadenitis in the United States, with *Mycobacterium avium complex* and *Mycobacterium scrofulaceum* causing the majority of cases (Gosche and Vick, 2006). Children less than 5 years old are most commonly affected. Gradual increase of the unilateral cervical node(s) is seen over the course of 2 to 3 weeks. Frequently, the skin overlying the infection becomes violaceous and thin. Fistulae may also form. For NTM infection, surgical excision is curative. However, if complete lymph node removal is not possible, then a multi-drug regimen may be required and drug choice should be based on culture (in acid-fast bacilli medium) and susceptibility results.

Keywords: infectious diseases, mass, airway, head and neck/ENT, skin and soft tissue infection

References

American Academy of Pediatrics. Cat scratch disease. In *Red Book: 2012 Report of the Committee on Infectious Diseases,* Pickering LK, Baker CJ, Kimberlin DW, Long SS, eds. Elk Grove Village, IL: American Academy of Pediatrics, 2012:269–71.

Gosche JR, Vick L. Acute, subacute, and chronic cervical lymphadenitis in children. *Sem Pediatr Surg* 2006;15:99–106.

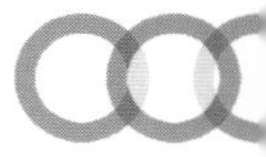

CASE 18

Emily Obringer

Question

A 7-year-old girl presents with a neck mass. Her mother reports that the swelling has increased over the last several days and is warm, red, and now oozing from the center. On exam, the patient has a tender, fluctuant mass of the midline neck, and a small amount of pus is able to be expressed.

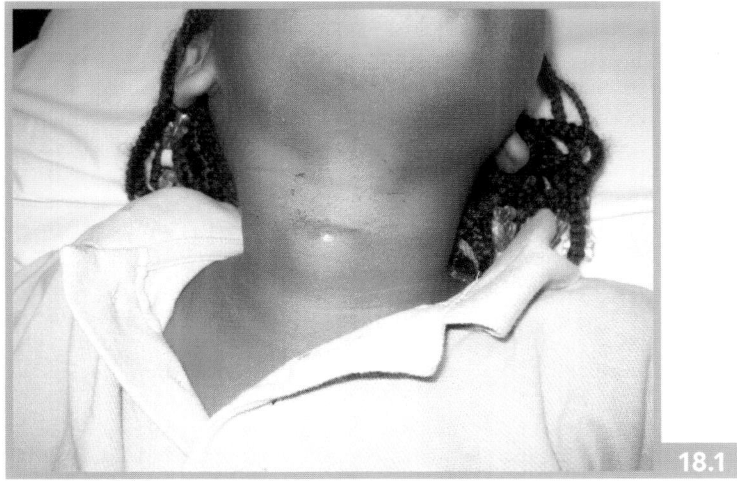

18.1

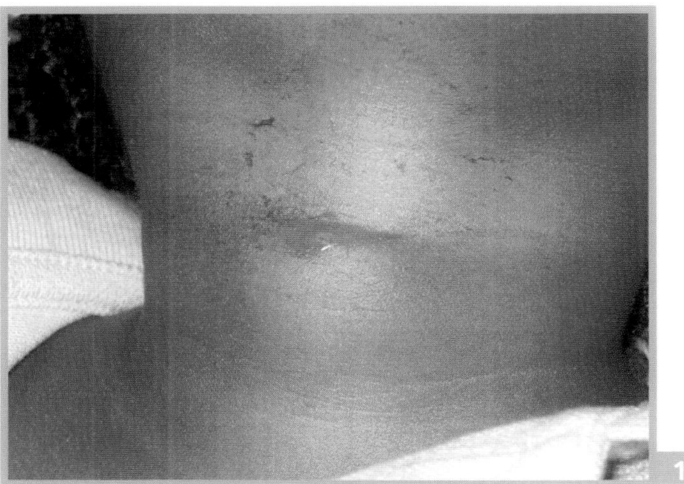

18.2

What is the most likely etiology of the mass?

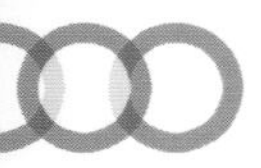

Answer

The differential diagnosis for a neck mass in a child is wide and includes developmental, infectious, and less likely neoplastic etiologies. Location, size, recent exposure history, onset and duration of symptoms, as well as associated symptoms such as fever may help narrow the differential. If the mass is hard and fixed, malignancy is more likely.

Diagnostic testing and initial management depend on the most likely diagnosis. If reactive lymphadenitis is suspected, laboratory testing is typically not indicated and empiric antibiotics may be initiated. If historical clues are present or the mass does not respond to antibiotics, infectious titers may be obtained, such as *Bartonella henselae*, Epstein-Barr virus, human immunodeficiency virus, and others. Ultrasonography is the preferred imaging method for a neck mass in a child. If a developmental or neoplastic etiology is suspected, the patient should be referred to a specialist.

Given the midline location of this child's neck mass, the most likely diagnosis is an infected thyroglossal duct cyst; alternatively, an infected dermoid cyst or branchial anomaly could be present. Thyroglossal duct cysts are congenital abnormalities resulting from the failed involution of the thyroglossal duct. They are typically located over the hyoid bone and may move vertically with swallowing. Classically, patients present before 10 years of age with a painless midline neck mass that fluctuates in size and has a tendency to become infected. In the case presented here, empiric antibiotics, ultrasonography, and referral to a specialist should be considered.

Keywords: head and neck/ENT, infection, congenital anomaly, skin and soft tissue infection

Bibliography

American College of Radiology. ACR Appropriateness Criteria. Neck mass/adenopathy. https://acsearch.acr.org/docs/69504/Narrative. Accessed May 24, 2017.

Meier JD, Grimmer JF. Evaluation and management of neck masses in children. *Am Fam Physician* 2014;89(5):353–8.

Simon LM, Magit AE. Impact of incision and drainage of infected thyroglossal duct cyst on recurrence after Sistrunk procedure. *Arch Otolaryngol Head Neck Surg* 2012;138(1):20–4.

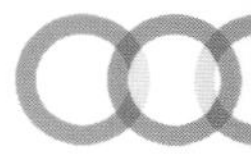

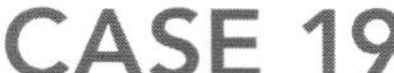

CASE 19

Emily Obringer

Questions

A child presents to the emergency department with severe, acute abdominal pain. The mother reports that the child passed this (see photo) in his stool several days ago.

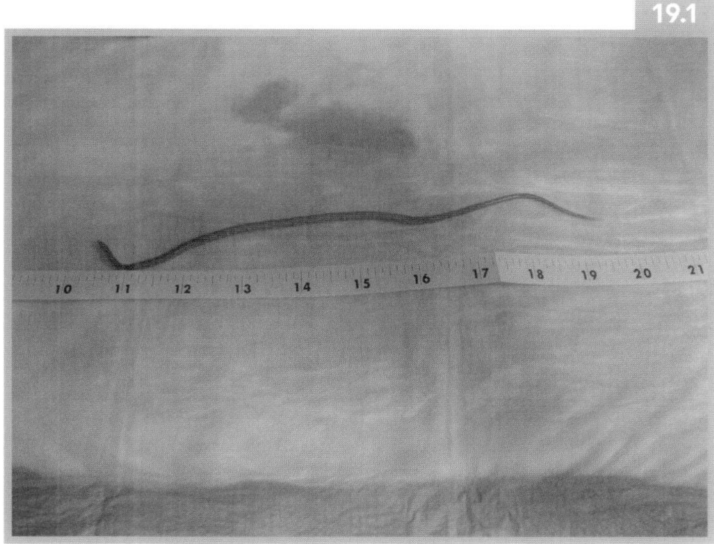

19.1

1. What potential complication of *Ascaris lumbricoides* (roundworm) infection do you suspect?
2. Name at least three antihelminthic agents that are effective against *Ascaris lumbricoides*.

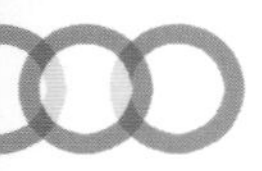

Answers

1. The child may be experiencing acute intestinal obstruction, a known complication of *Ascaris lumbricoides* infection associated with heavy worm burden.

   Ascaris lumbricoides is the most common helminthic infection worldwide (Bethony et al., 2006). Infections frequently occur in areas with inadequate sanitation measures and where human feces is used as fertilizer (American Academy of Pediatrics, 2015). Adult worms mature and multiply in the small intestines and, along with ova, can be passed into the stool. Diagnosis can typically be made with examination of a stool sample for ova or direct visualization of the adult worm. In cases of small bowel obstruction due to *Ascaris lumbricoides*, antihelminthic treatment, as well as conservative management for small bowel obstruction, including administration of intravenous fluids and nasogastric suctioning, is indicated. Occasionally, surgical intervention may be required to relieve obstruction.

2. *Ascaris lumbricoides* is most commonly treated with a benzimidazole, such as mebendazole or albendazole. Mebendazole can be given twice daily for 3 days, whereas albendazole is given as a one-time dose. Nitazoxanide and ivermectin can also be used.

Keywords: infectious diseases, gastrointestinal, abdominal pain

References

American Academy of Pediatrics. *Ascaris lumbricoides* infections. In *Red Book: 2015 Report of the Committee on Infectious Diseases*, 30th ed., Kimberlin DW, Brady MT, Jackson MA, Long SS, eds. Elk Grove Village, IL: *American Academy of Pediatrics* 2015:221–2.

Bethony J, Brooker S, Albonico M, Geiger SM, Loukas A, Diemert D, Hotez PJ. Soil-transmitted helminth infections: Ascariasis, trichuriasis, and hookworm. *Lancet* 2006;367:1521–32.

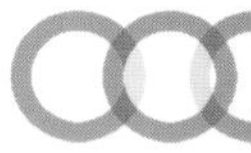

CASE 20

Michael Gottlieb

Questions

A 12-year-old boy presents to the emergency department with right knee pain after he fell onto his flexed knee while running. He endorses severe pain and is unable to ambulate after the injury. He denies any other injuries. He is neurologically intact and has good pulses distally. A series of radiographs was ordered and are displayed next.

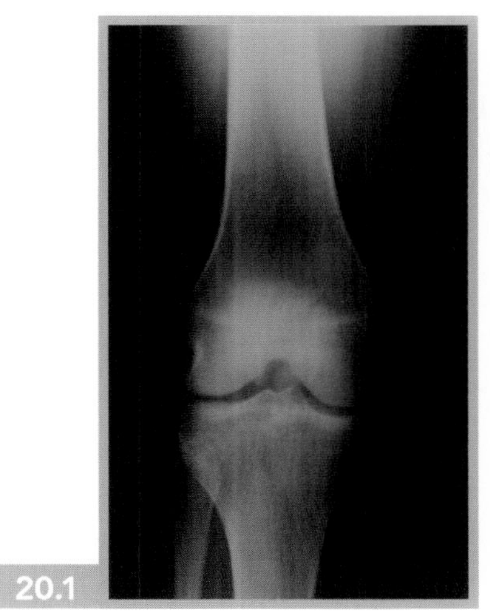

20.1

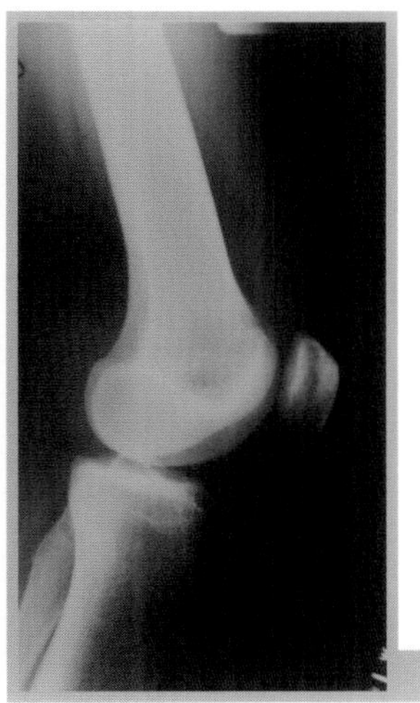

20.2

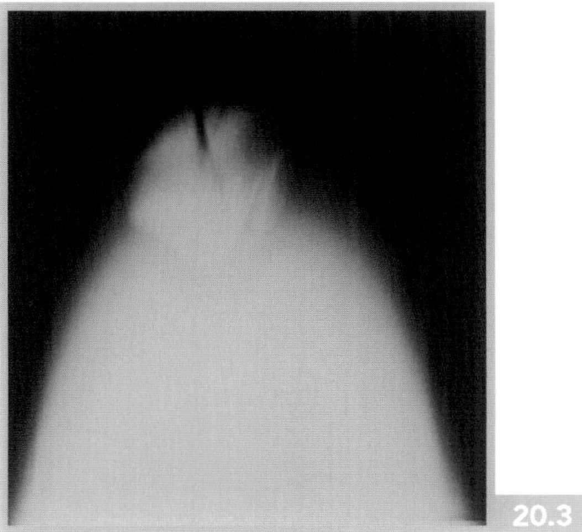

20.3

1. Why is it important to assess knee extension with this injury?
2. What are the indications for operative management?

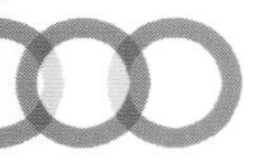

Answers

1. This patient is presenting with a patellar fracture. These typically present with patellar pain after direct trauma to the area and are best visualized with the sunrise or Merchant view on x-ray (see Image 20.3). Inability to perform a straight leg raise suggests failure of the extensor mechanism, which is one of the indications for operative management.

2. Most cases can be treated conservatively with a knee immobilizer and early weight-bearing as tolerated. However, there are several indications for operative reduction and internal fixation. These include open fractures, loss of extensor mechanism, or significant displacement of fracture fragments. Alternatively, vertical, non-displaced fractures with an intact extensor mechanism can be treated conservatively.

Keywords: orthopedics, extremity injury, blunt trauma

Bibliography

Melvin JS, Mehta S. Patellar fractures in adults. *J Am Acad Orthop Surg* April 2011;19(4):198–207.

Scolaro J, Bernstein J, Ahn J. Patellar fractures. *Clin Orthop Relat Res* April 2011;469(4):1213–5.

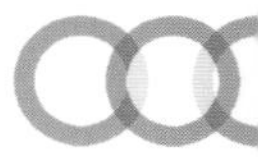

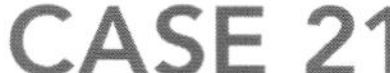

CASE 21

Alisa McQueen

Question

A toddler with eczema presents with this rash for 2 days. He has a low-grade fever and is fussier than usual. His rash is spreading despite topical steroids, which usually control his eczema flares.

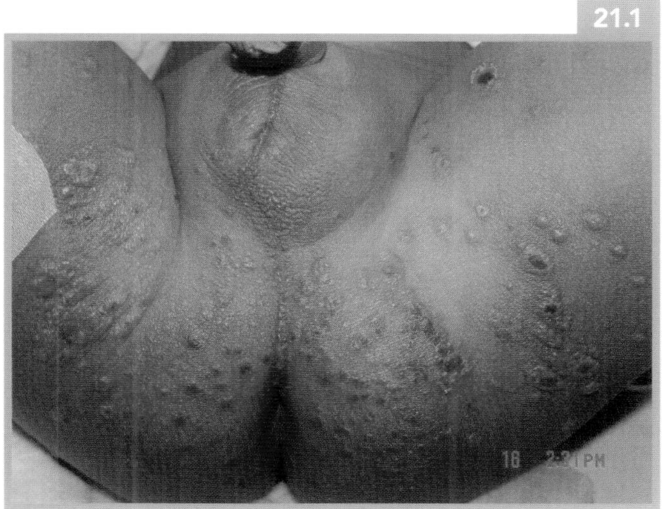

21.1

What is this condition and how should he be treated?

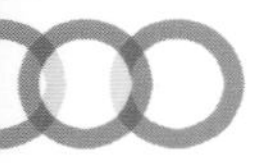

Answer

Close inspection of this rash reveals both tiny blisters and punched-out erosions suggestive of herpes simplex virus (HSV) infection. Children with atopic dermatitis are particularly susceptible to dissemination of herpes simplex infection, giving rise to eczema herpeticum, also known as Kaposi varicelliform eruption. Diagnosis is confirmed by identification of HSV from the lesions, either by Tzanck prep demonstrating multinucleated giant cells or isolation of HSV by viral culture, polymerase chain reaction, or direct fluorescent antibody testing. If the diagnosis is suspected, therapy with systemic acyclovir should be instituted immediately. Children who are ill-appearing, have mucosal involvement requiring parenteral hydration, or are immunosuppressed may require hospitalization. If the eyes are involved, prompt ophthalmologic consultation is prudent.

Keywords: dermatology, infectious diseases, fever, skin and soft tissue infection

Bibliography

Kress DW. Pediatric dermatology emergencies. *Curr Opin Pediatr* 2011;23(4):403–6.

Jen M, Chang MW. Eczema herpeticum and eczema vaccinatum in children. *Pediatr Ann* 2010;39(10):658–64.

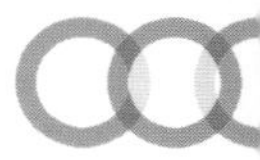

CASE 22

Emily Obringer

Question

An obese teenager presents with a chief complaint of painful bumps in her axilla that intermittently drain pus. She has been treated for similar symptoms in the past with a variety of antibiotics and topical creams. You suspect a diagnosis of hidradenitis suppurativa.

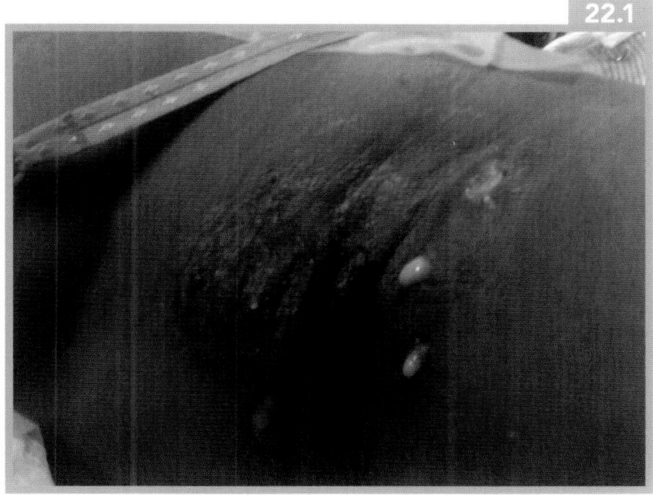

22.1

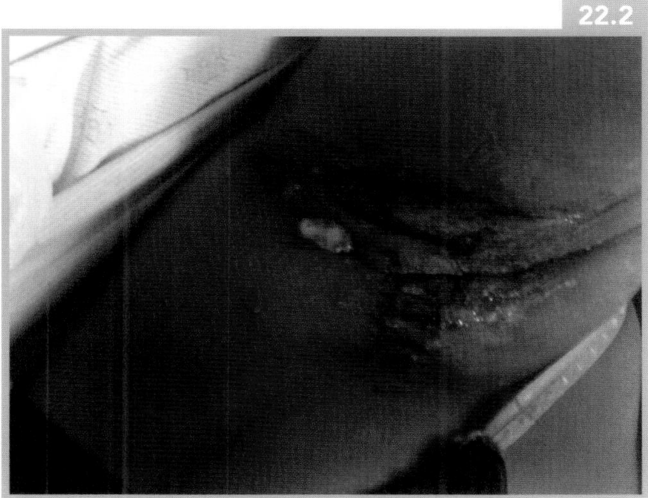

22.2

What are the most common pathogens found in abscesses associated with hidradenitis suppurativa?

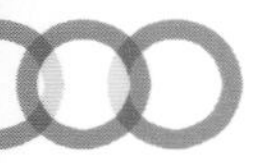

Answer

Hidradenitis suppurativa is a chronic inflammatory disease of apocrine-gland-bearing skin, as found in the axilla and groin. Cellulitis, abscesses, and sinus tract formation are common. Most infections are polymicrobial and include both aerobic and anaerobic species. Randomized controlled trials regarding effective treatments are limited; however, topical and oral antibiotics are a mainstay of therapy (Woodruff et al., 2015).

Keywords: dermatology, skin and soft tissue infection, mass

Reference

Woodruff CM, Charlie AM, Leslie KS. Hidradenitis suppurativa: A guide for the practicing physician. *Mayo Clin Proc* 2015;90(12):1679–93.

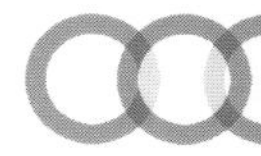

CASE 23

Michael Farnham and Timothy Ketterhagen

Questions

A mother brings her 7-year-old son to the emergency department with complaints of a sore throat and fever. He has had symptoms for the past 3 to 4 days. He is now developing a rash and his mother thinks his tongue appears more red than usual. He denies any cough, vomiting, diarrhea, or dysuria. Immunizations are up to date. No recent travel is reported. He has had a decreased appetite but has been drinking fluids well. No recent illnesses are reported.

Physical exam reveals a developmentally normal young boy who is in no apparent distress. Vital signs are normal, except for a fever. There is a diffuse fine papular rash with a sandpaper texture that blanches with pressure. Anterior cervical lymphadenopathy is present bilaterally. Tonsils are enlarged, erythematous, and an exudate is present. The tongue is red with prominent papillae. The cardiac and pulmonary exams are unremarkable. The physical exam is otherwise unremarkable.

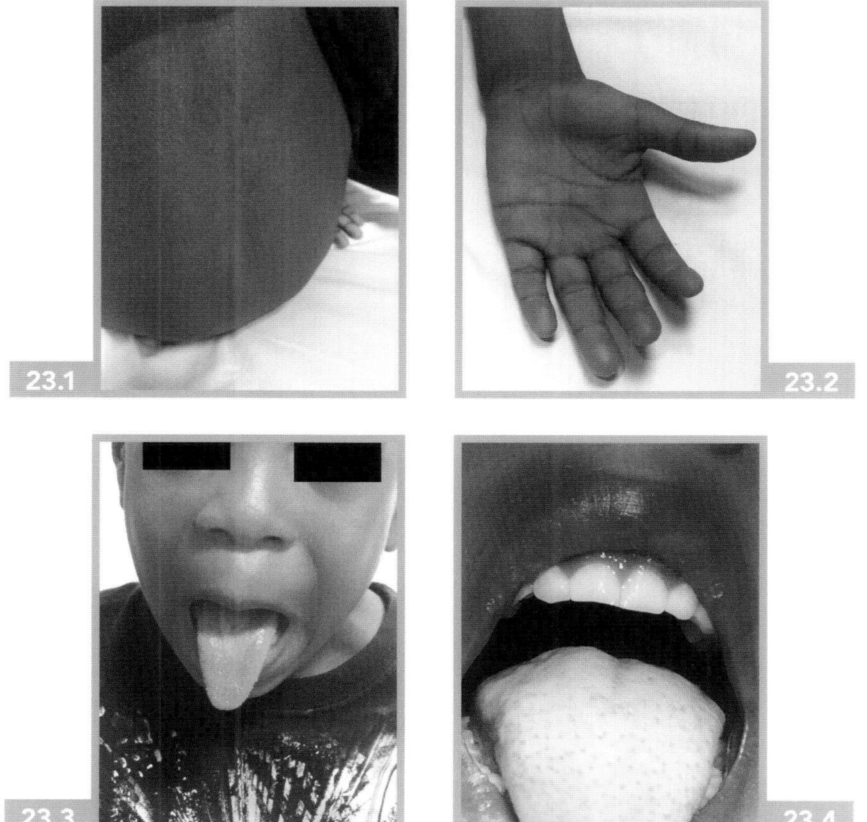

23.1 23.2 23.3 23.4

1. What is the most likely diagnosis and how would this diagnosis differ from other exanthems or vasculitis?
2. What are possible complications and sequelae for this illness?

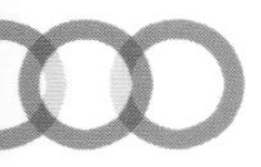

Answers

1. This child has scarlet fever, which is caused by an infection of group A beta-hemolytic streptococcus but may also be caused by *Staphylococcus aureus*. Scarlet fever may be differentiated from Kawasaki disease by the absence of ophthalmological symptoms and edema of the extremities. The rash will also likely desquamate during the course of disease. Pastia's lines, a sign of streptococcal infection, may also form in the skin creases. Epstein-Barr virus is a common mimicker that should be considered in cases of fever, malaise, and a papular rash. Scarlet fever is a clinical diagnosis, although confirmation of streptococcal pharyngitis may be obtained. Group A streptococcus is sensitive to penicillin, which is the first-line therapy; penicillin-allergic patients can be treated with clindamycin or azithromycin.

2. Most cases of scarlet fever resolve without complications with the appropriate treatment. However, certain serotypes of group A streptococci are rheumatogenic and may cause serious complications like rheumatic fever and glomerulonephritis. Other complications include peritonsillar abscess, pneumonia, septicemia, or meningitis.

Keywords: infectious diseases, dermatology, rash, fever

Bibliography

Dinkla K, Rohde M, Jansen WT, Kaplan EL, Chhatwal GS, Talay SR. Rheumatic fever–associated *Streptococcus pyogenes* isolates aggregate collagen. *J Clin Invest* 2003;111(12):1905–12.

Hoffman RJ, Wang VJ, Scarfone R. *Fleisher & Ludwig's 5-Minute Pediatric Emergency Medicine Consult.* Philadelphia: Wolters Kluwer Health/Lippincott Williams & Wilkins, 2012.

Pichichero ME. Complications of streptococcal tonsillopharyngitis. http://www.uptodate.com/contents/complications-of-streptococcal tonsillopharyngitis. Accessed April 28, 2016.

Zitelli BJ, Davis HW. *Atlas of Pediatric Physical Diagnosis*. 4th ed. St. Louis, MO: Mosby, 2002.

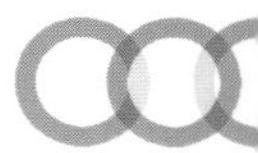

CASE 24

S. Margaret Paik

Questions

A 4-year-old girl presents to the emergency department with vaginal bleeding. She is urinating normally without pain, but there is blood on the toilet paper. There is no history of vomiting, diarrhea, abdominal pain, or change in her bowel habits. Her appetite has been normal. She has been well without fever or ill contacts. There is no history of trauma. The family does not have any concerns for sexual abuse.

On physical examination she is well-appearing. Her abdomen is soft and non-tender. She has a sexual maturity rating of 1. There is an erythematous, round "doughnut"-shaped lesion protruding from the urethra without active bleeding. It is slightly tender to palpation. The hymen appears unremarkable without lacerations or notches. No blood is seen in the introitus.

24.1

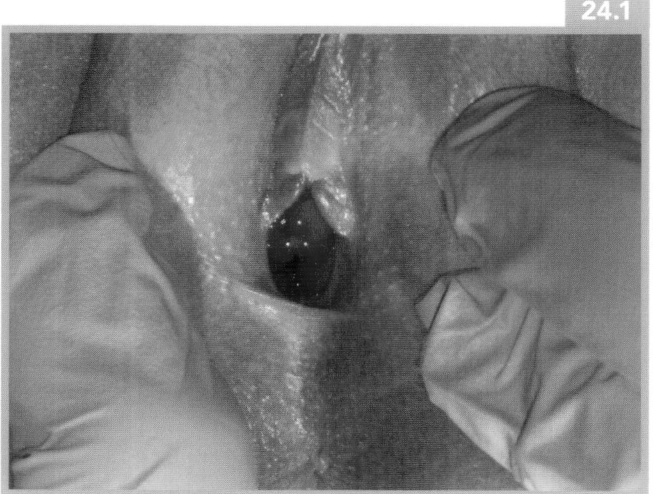

1. What is seen in the image?
2. What are the initial treatment options?

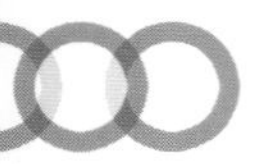

Answers

1. This patient has a prolapse of the urethra. A "doughnut" appearance is seen with complete circumferential urethral prolapse. Dysuria, bleeding, urinary hesitancy, or urinary frequency are the most common complaints, and are seen primarily in pre-pubertal black girls or post-menopausal white women. The differential diagnosis includes ureterocele, condyloma, and rhabdomyosarcoma. Sarcoma botryoides from the distal urethra can have a similar appearance.
2. Initial treatment options include topical estrogen cream and sitz baths. Urethral prolapse usually resolves within a few weeks. Necrosis is a rare complication and warrants surgical intervention. Other indications for operative management include persistence of the prolapse or significant bleeding.

Keywords: genitourinary, child abuse mimicker, mass, hematuria

Bibliography

Hillyer S, Mooppan U, Kim H, Gulmi F. Diagnosis and treatment of urethral prolapse in children: Experience with 34 cases. *Urology* 2009;73:1008–11.

Richardson D, Hajj S, Herbst A. Medical treatment of urethral prolapse in children. *Obstet Gynecol* 1982;59:69–74.

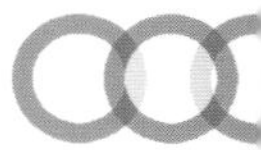

CASE 25

Timothy Ketterhagen

Questions

A 16-year-old female presents to the emergency department with abdominal pain. She states that she has had abdominal discomfort for the past week; however, the pain worsened in the last couple of days. She describes the pain as initially dull, but now sharp and worse in the lower abdomen. She reports that her last menstrual period was 3 months ago, but that she has "never been regular." She also reports that she feels "bloated," which she attributes to eating a lot of fast food, but it is worsening. She last stooled 5 days ago and states that it was "a little hard." The patient's appetite has decreased, but she denies any vomiting, cough, fever, rhinorrhea, dysuria, diarrhea, or rash. The patient denies any sexual activity and she has never been pregnant.

On physical exam, the patient is sick but not toxic in appearance and appears to be in moderate pain. Vital signs are normal. Heart and lung exam are unremarkable. Abdominal exam shows a distended abdomen with diffuse tenderness that is worse in the RLQ (right lower quadrant) as well as fullness in the periumbilical region. No rebound tenderness is found, but the patient is guarding when her RLQ is palpated. Bowel sounds are normal. GU (genitourinary) exam shows normal female genitalia, Tanner stage 5, no lesions, no vaginal discharge or bleeding. There is no CVA (costovertebral angle) tenderness.

25.1

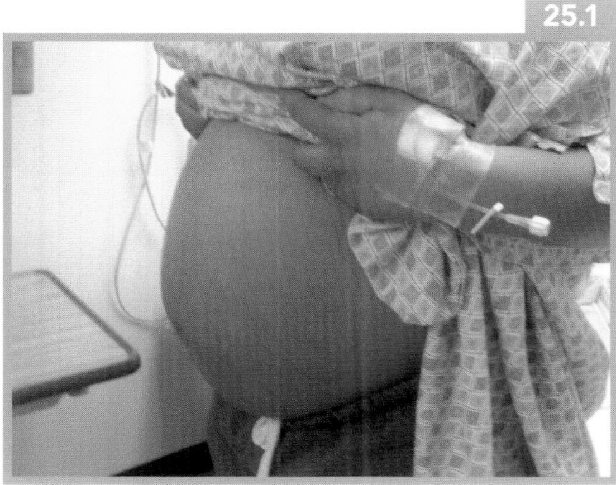

25.2

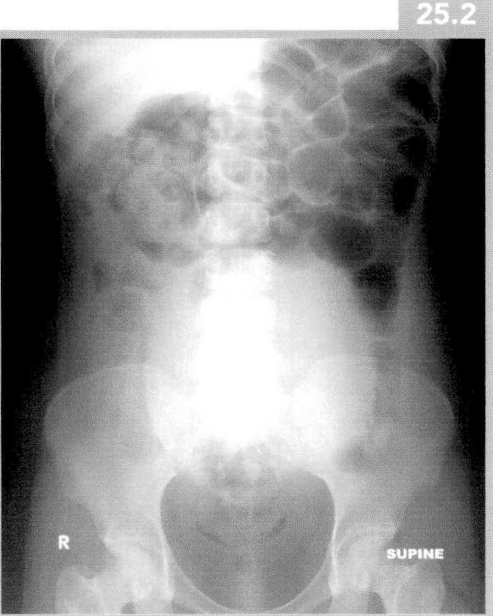

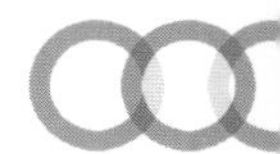

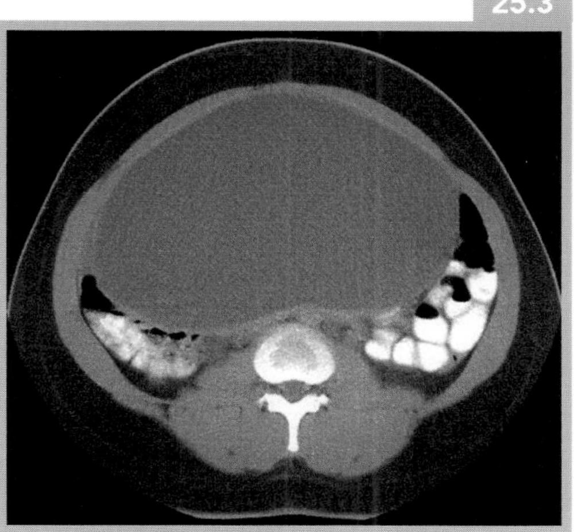
25.3

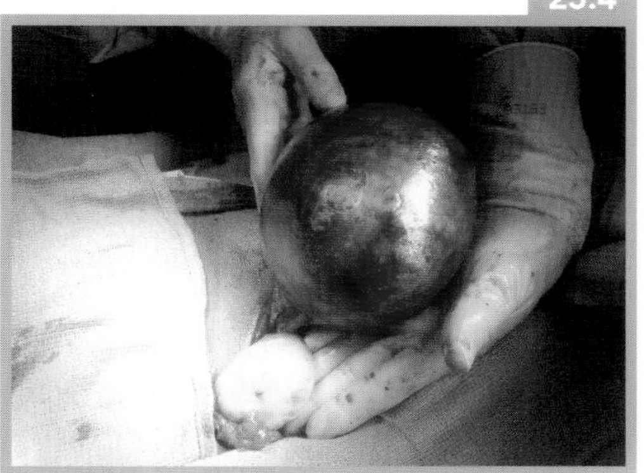
25.4

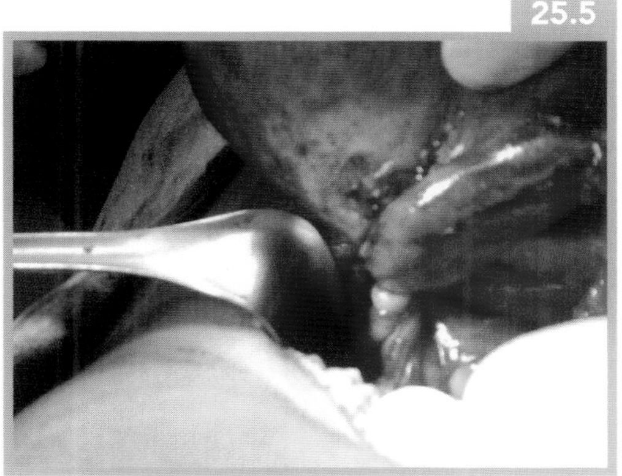
25.5

1. What is the diagnosis?
2. What workup is indicated in this patient?

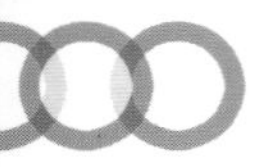

Answers

1. This patient has an ovarian cyst with torsion. Ovarian cysts are fluid-filled structures arising from the ovary. Ovarian cysts are seen in all age groups. Follicular cysts are thin-walled, and rupture easily with minimal bleeding. Corpus luteal cysts rupture just before menstruation begins and may result in severe bleeding. Most ovarian cysts are asymptomatic. Patients may present with a painless abdominal mass, increasing abdominal girth, or vague symptoms such as vomiting or constipation. Adolescents may present with pelvic pain, urinary complaints, or menstrual irregularities.
2. Workup may include pregnancy test, CBC (complete blood count), GC (gonorrhea)/chlamydia. Further testing may be required to rule out other pathology. Ultrasound is the preferred imaging modality with Doppler to assess blood flow if ovarian torsion is suspected. CT and MRI may also be used to visualize cysts.

The differential can be broad in a patient presenting with abdominal pain, but it is important to consider and rule out serious diagnoses. The differential includes, but is not limited to, ovarian torsion, ovarian cyst rupture, ovarian cyst torsion, pregnancy, ectopic pregnancy, endometriosis, tubo-ovarian abscess, pelvic inflammatory disease (PID), appendicitis, constipation, inflammatory bowel disease (IBD), dysmenorrhea, pancreatitis, cholecystitis, nephrolithiasis, and neoplasm. Surgical excision of the cyst may be indicated for severely symptomatic patients, cysts >5 cm and rapidly enlarging, solid cysts, or large cysts that persist for >3–4 months. The majority of ovarian cysts regress spontaneously within 4–8 weeks.

Keywords: gynecology, ultrasound, mass, abdominal pain, CT

Bibliography

Hoffman RJ, Wang VJ, Scarfone R. *Fleisher & Ludwig's 5-Minute Pediatric Emergency Medicine Consult.* Philadelphia: Wolters Kluwer Health/Lippincott Williams & Wilkins, 2012.

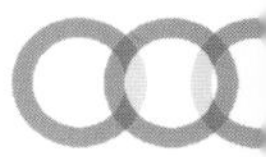

CASE 26

Victoria Rodriguez

Questions

A 10-year-old female presents to the emergency department with a new rash that she reports has been progressively spreading. She was seen in the emergency department with a sore throat about a month ago.

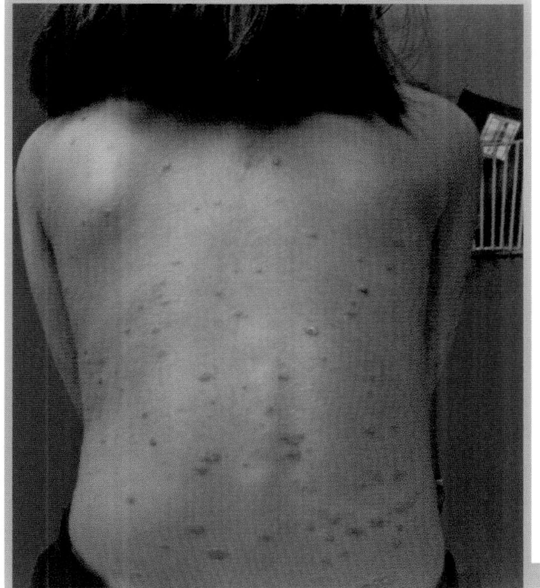

26.1

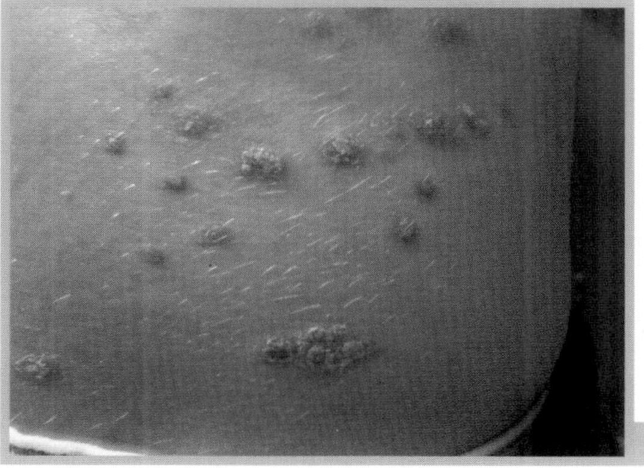

26.2

1. What is the diagnosis?
2. What infectious agent may trigger this (non-infectious) condition?
3. Which topical agent is one of the first-line treatment modalities for this condition?

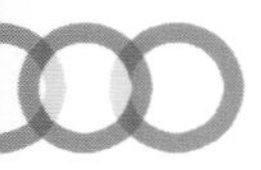

Answers

1. Guttate psoriasis presents with multiple small, erythematous, round or "droplike" papules and plaques with a silvery scale. The distribution is concentrated in the trunk, but lesions may appear on the extremities as well as the scalp. Unlike pityriasis rosea, guttate psoriasis does not follow skin lines, has a thicker scale, and a positive Auspitz sign (lifting the scale may reveal bleeding dermal capillaries).
2. Group A streptococcal infection has a well-recognized association with first-time guttate psoriasis outbreaks. The connection is unclear, but cross-reactivity of streptococcal and native antigens is suspected. Screening for group A streptococcus in asymptomatic patients is controversial; however, as studies on the benefits of antibiotic therapy have shown mixed results.
3. Topical steroids, in addition to UV (ultraviolet) phototherapy, are considered first-line treatments. Steroids may be prescribed at strengths similar to those used in eczema, although risks for skin thinning and systemic absorption should be considered in patients with diffuse skin lesions.

Keywords: dermatology, infectious diseases

Bibliography

Browning JC. An update on pityriasis rosea and other similar childhood exanthems. *Curr Opin Pediatrics* August 2009;21(4):481–5.

Krishnamurthy K, Walker A, Gropper CA, Hoffman C. To treat or not to treat? Management of guttate psoriasis and pityriasis rosea in patients with evidence of group A streptococcal infection. *J Drugs Dermatol* March 2010;9(3):241–50.

Silverberg NB. Pediatric psoriasis: An update. *Ther Clin Risk Manag* 2009;5:849–56.

Silverberg NB. Update on pediatric psoriasis. Part 1: Clinical features and demographics. *Cutis* September 2010;86(3):118–24.

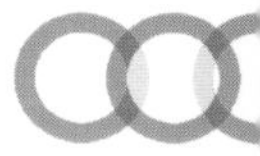

CASE 27

Emily Obringer

Question

An otherwise healthy toddler presents with a rash (see photos) after a recent viral illness. He is afebrile and well-appearing. You note on exam that the rash is symmetrical in distribution and localized to the extremities, buttocks, and face. The torso is largely spared.

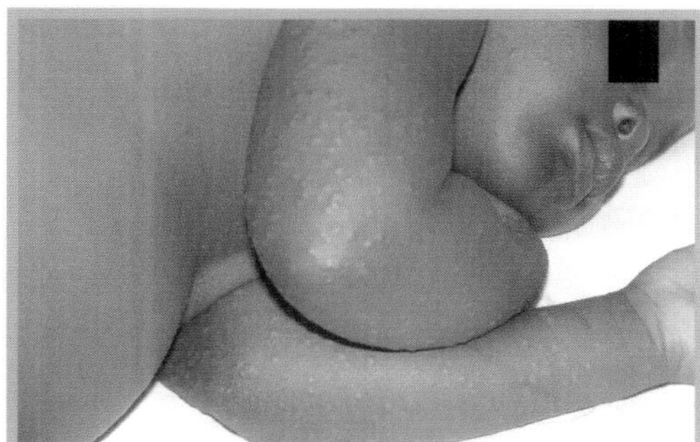

27.1

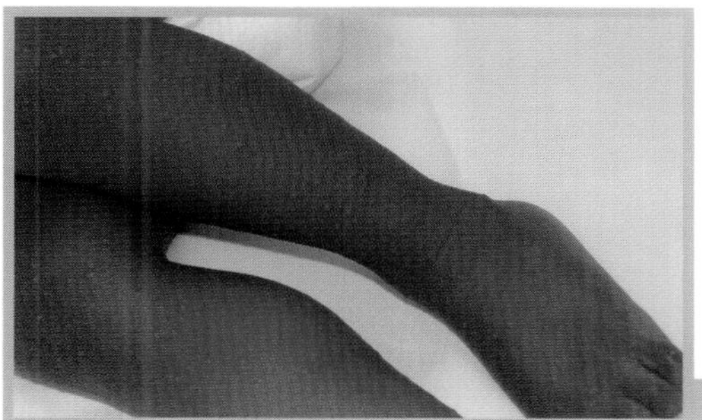

27.2

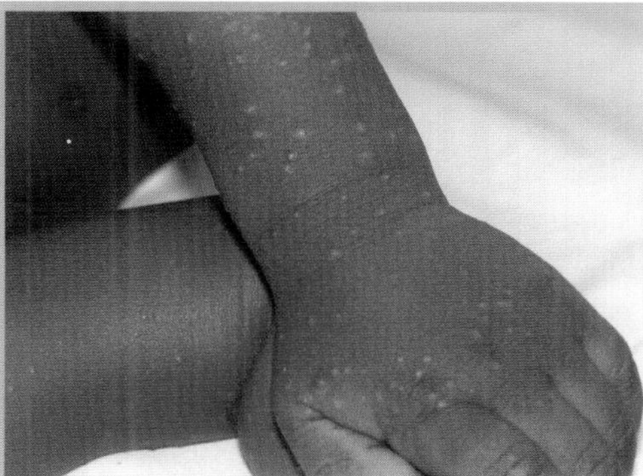

27.3

What is the diagnosis?

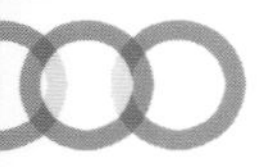

Answer

Gianotti-Crosti syndrome or papular acrodermatitis of childhood is a self-limited skin reaction usually preceded by a viral infection. Common infectious agents associated with the syndrome include Epstein-Barr virus and hepatitis B virus, as well as a variety of other common viral pathogens (Lauren and Garzon, 2012). Immunizations have also been linked to development of Gianotti-Crosti syndrome. The rash is characterized by monomorphic, erythematous papules distributed on the extensor surfaces of the arms and legs, the buttocks, and the face. Treatment is supportive and lesions may last for 3 to 6 weeks (Lauren and Garzon, 2012).

Keywords: infectious diseases, dermatology

Reference

Lauren CT, Garzon MC. Papules, nodules, and ulcers. In *Principles and Practice of Pediatric Infectious Diseases*, 4th ed., Long SS, Pickering LK, Prober CG, eds. Edinburgh: Elsevier-Saunders, 2012:449–54.

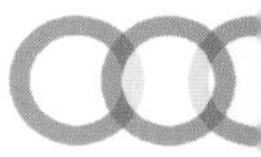

CASE 28

Emily Obringer

Questions

A 5-year-old girl presents with a rash to the lower extremities and buttocks, as well as colicky abdominal pain. She is afebrile and you note palpable purpura to pressure-dependent areas of the body. When she does not have abdominal pain, she is comfortable and interactive. She recently had an upper respiratory tract infection.

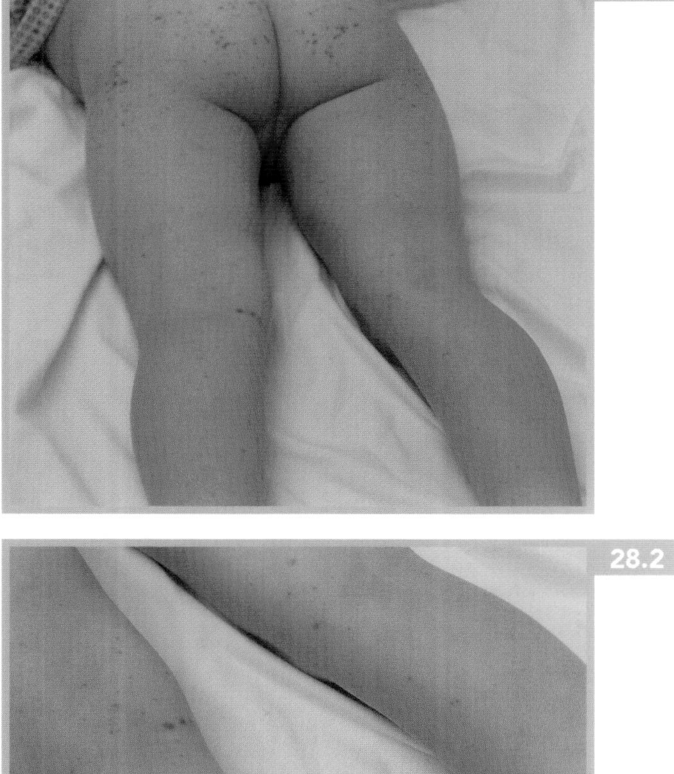

28.1

28.2

1. You are suspicious that this child may have Henoch-Schönlein purpura (HSP). What other physical exam finding is frequently present?
2. Although HSP is largely a clinical diagnosis, what is the single most important laboratory test to obtain?

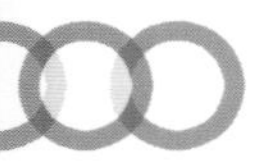

Answers

1. Henoch-Schönlein purpura (HSP) is the most common vasculitis of childhood. The peak incidence occurs from 4 to 6 years of age, and there is a 2:1 male predominance. In addition to palpable purpura and abdominal pain, joint pain and swelling are common physical exam findings in this systemic disease. Joint symptoms are frequently migratory and typically occur in the large joints of the lower extremities (Reid-Adam, 2014). Although the cause is poorly understood and is likely multifactorial, HSP is frequently preceded by an upper respiratory tract infection (Reid-Adam, 2014). Typically, the illness is self-limited and resolves on average in 4 weeks (Saulsbury, 2010).
2. A urine analysis is a recommended component of the workup for HSP and is important in patient prognosis. Nephritis occurs in 40%–50% of patients with HSP and is the most commonly associated long-term morbidity (Saulsbury, 2010). Renal dysfunction can be present initially or can develop over the course of several months. The disease spectrum is broad and includes microscopic hematuria and microscopic proteinuria to gross hematuria and even nephrotic syndrome. The severity of nephritis correlates with progression to chronic renal disease. Patients should be followed up with urine analyses and blood pressure screening for several months to monitor for subclinical disease. A biopsy may be indicated when there is concern for nephritic or nephrotic disease. IgA immune complex deposition is the typical finding on histology (Reid-Adam, 2014).

Keywords: renal/nephrology, dermatology, rheumatology, hematuria, infectious diseases

References

Reid-Adam J. Henoch-Schönlein purpura. *Pediatr Rev* 2014;35(10):447–9.
Saulsbury F. Henoch-Schönlein purpura. *Curr Opin Rheumatol* 2010;22:598–602.

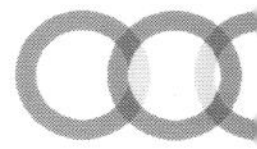

CASE 29

Emily Obringer

Question

A preschooler presents with abnormal nail findings one month after a viral illness that consisted of oral ulcers and a rash. She has a normal diet and is otherwise healthy. There is no history of trauma to the nail bed.

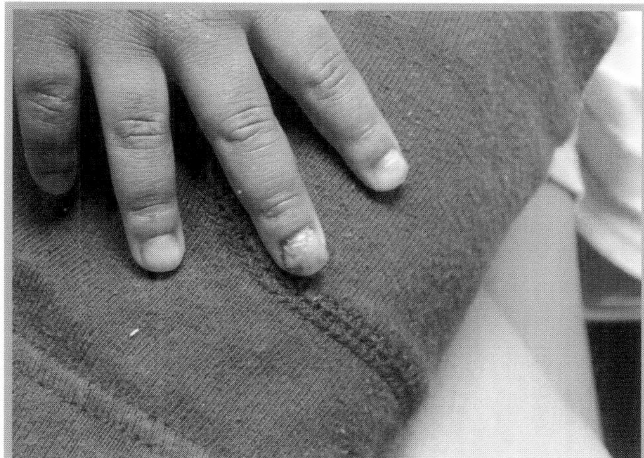

29.1

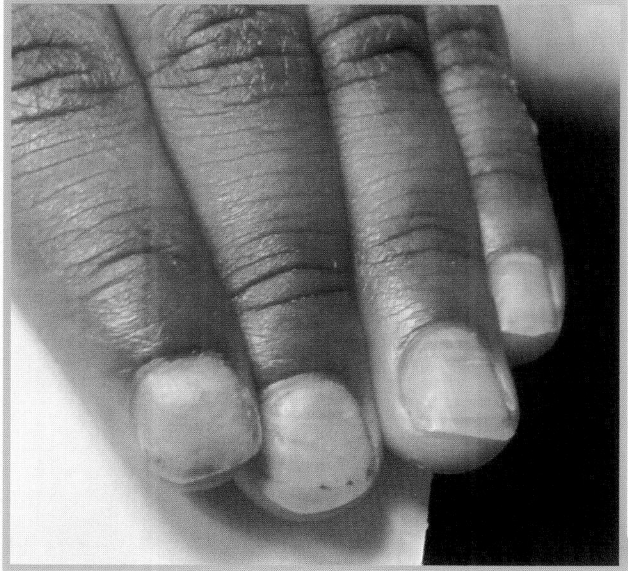

29.2

What was the likely preceding viral illness?

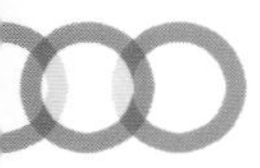

Answer

Hand, foot, and mouth disease is a common viral illness caused by coxsackie A16 and enterovirus D71, as well as other species in the *Enterovirus* genus. The typical disease presentation includes fever, painful oral ulcers, and a rash that frequently involves the palms and soles. Onychomadesis, or shedding of the nails, has been reported as a complication of the illness, typically presenting about 4 weeks after initial symptoms resolve (Bracho et al., 2011; Wei et al., 2010). Subsequent nail growth is normal.

Keywords: infectious diseases, dermatology

References

Bracho MA, Gonzalez-Candelas F, Valero A, Cordoba J, Salazar A. Enterovirus co-infections and onychomadesis after hand, foot, and mouth disease, Spain, 2008. *Emerg Infect Dis* 2011;17(12):2223–31.

Wei SH, Huang YP, Liu MC, Tsou TP et al. An outbreak of coxsackievirus A6 hand, foot, and mouth disease associated with onychomadesis in Taiwan, 2010. *BMC Infect Dis* 2011;11:346.

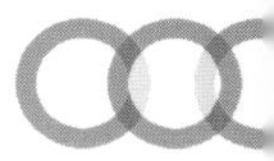

CASE 30

Michael Farnham and Timothy Ketterhagen

Questions

A mother brings her 8-month-old son into the emergency department with a complaint of pain in the left ear. Mother states that the patient has been rubbing his left ear for the past few days and today she noticed that the left ear appears different from the right. He was recently treated for a left acute otitis media 1 week ago. He has had fevers for the past 2 to 3 days and has been fussier than usual. He has had mild rhinorrhea, but otherwise no cough, vomiting, diarrhea, or rash. No sick contacts are reported and immunizations are up to date. He has been tolerating feeds and urinating a normal amount.

On physical exam, he is fussy but not ill-appearing. Nasal congestion is present. There is proptosis of the left ear and the left tympanic membrane is erythematous, dull, and bulging. The patient cries when the left ear and mastoid process are palpated. There is minimal overlying erythema and warmth. Cardiac and pulmonary exam are normal. The physical exam is otherwise unremarkable.

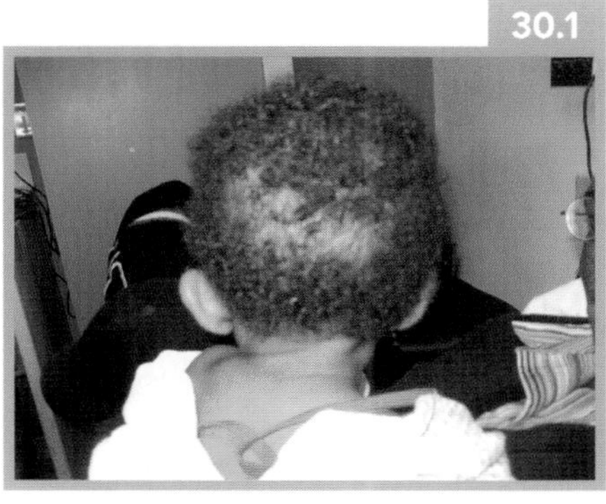

30.1

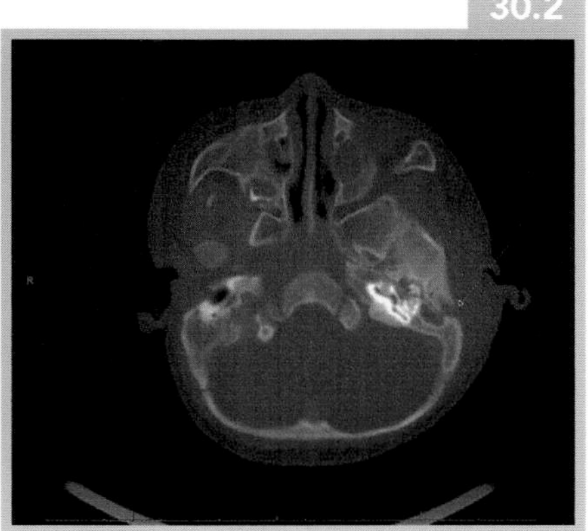

30.2

1. What is the diagnosis, and what pathogens are responsible?
2. Why is prompt intervention required, and what possible complications may occur?

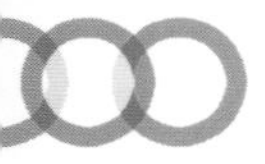

Answers

1. This child has mastoiditis, an infection in the mastoid cavity. It is most commonly caused by *Streptococcus pneumoniae* as well as *Streptococcus pyogenes* and *Haemophilus influenzae. Staphylococcus aureus* may also be associated with mastoiditis. Gram-negative bacteria that can cause mastoiditis include *Pseudomonas aeruginosa* and *Moraxella catarrhalis.* Patients will often present after an episode of acute otitis media with fever, pain behind the ear, asymmetry of the ears, and hearing loss. Some patients may develop an abscess on the skin overlying the mastoid bone.

2. Workup may include CBC (complete blood count), inflammatory markers, and blood culture. A temporal bone CT scan should be obtained when mastoiditis is suspected. Prompt intervention with an intravenous broad-spectrum antibiotic is important, along with the drainage of pus from the middle ear and/or mastoid cavity. Complications of mastoiditis include osteomyelitis, nerve palsy, hearing loss, and intracranial extension due to the proximity to the temporal bone. Therefore, prompt intervention is required.

Keywords: head and neck/ENT, infection, do not miss, fever

Bibliography

Bluestone CD, Klein KO. Intratemporal complications and sequelae of otitis media. In *Pediatric Otolaryngology*, 4th ed., Bluestone CD, Alper CM, Stool SE, Arjmand EM, Casselbrant ML, eds. Philadelphia: Saunders, 2003:687.

Hoffman RJ, Wang VJ, Scarfone R. *Fleisher & Ludwig's 5-Minute Pediatric Emergency Medicine Consult.* Philadelphia: Wolters Kluwer Health/Lippincott Williams & Wilkins, 2012.

Luntz M, Brodsky A, Nusem S, Kronenberg J et al. Acute mastoiditis—The antibiotic era: A multicenter study. *Int J Pediatr Otorhinolaryngol* 2001;57:1.

Mitchell RB, Pereira KD. *Pediatric Otolaryngology for the Clinician.* Dordrecht: Humana Press, 2009:231–2.

Wald ER. Acute mastoiditis in children: Clinical features and diagnosis. http://www.uptodate.com/contents/acute-mastoiditis-in-children-clinical-features-and-diagnosis? Accessed April 28, 2016.

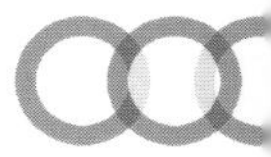

CASE 31

Emily Obringer

Question

A 3-year-old boy presents with a rash and 6 days of fever. His mother reports that he has been more fussy than usual and has not wanted to eat or drink. On exam you note bilateral nonexudative conjunctivitis, an enlarged cervical lymph node, and erythematous and edematous hands, feet, and lips. The rash is seen in the following.

31.1

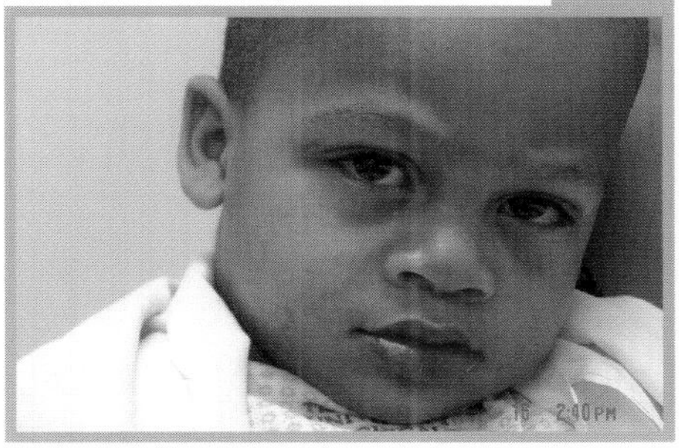

31.2

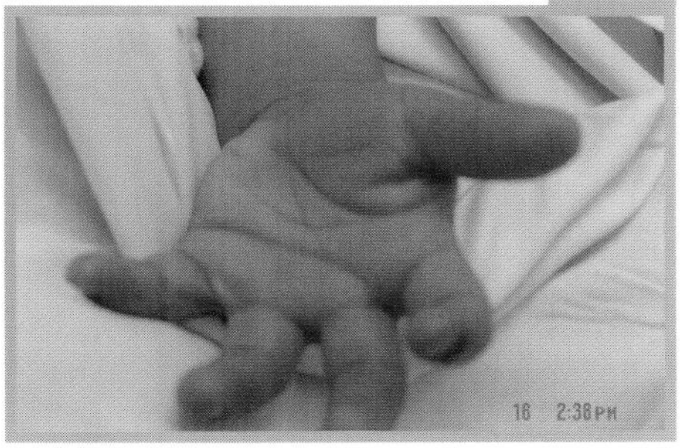

31.3

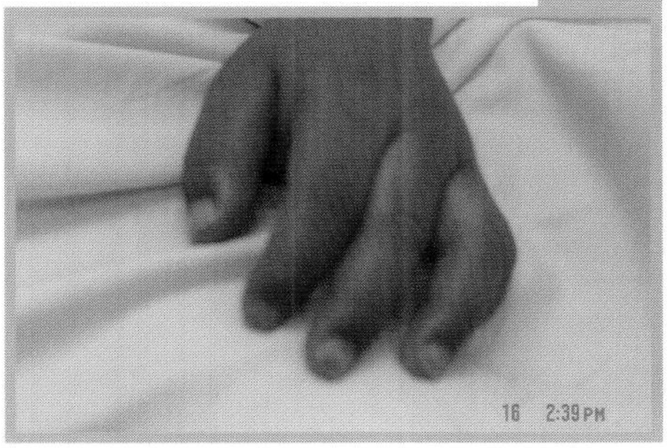

31.4

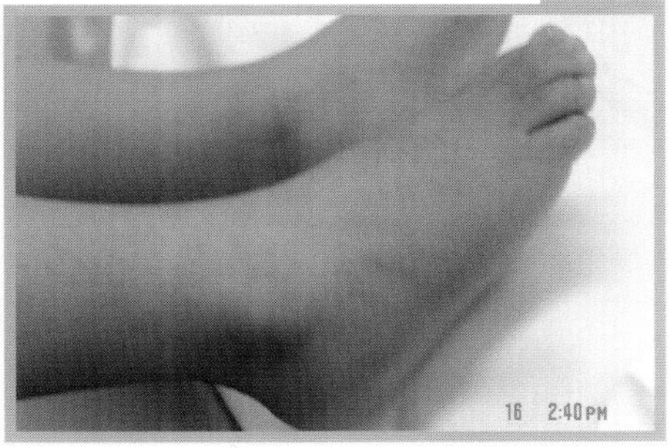

31.5

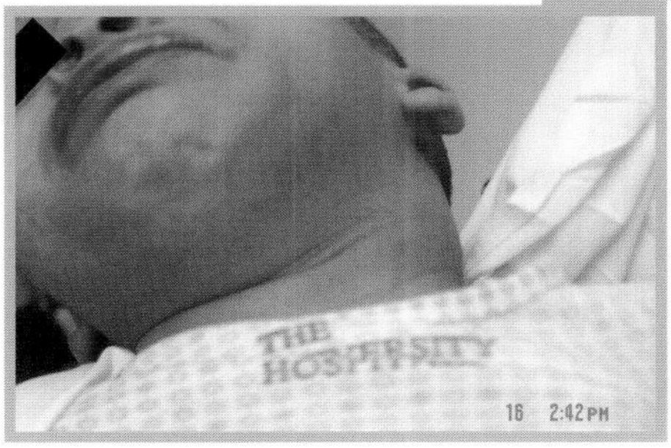

31.6

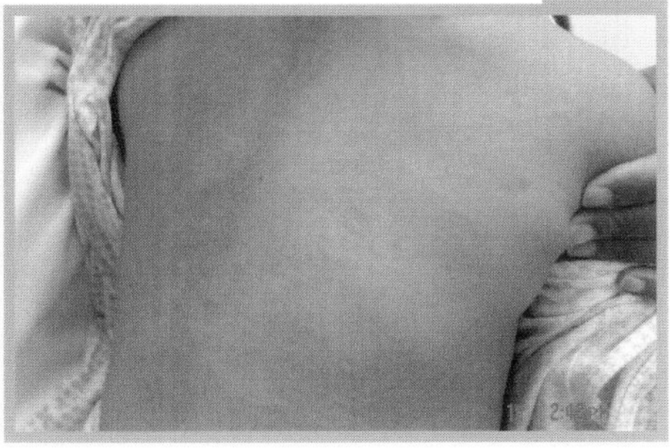

You suspect this child has Kawasaki disease. What else is in the differential diagnosis?

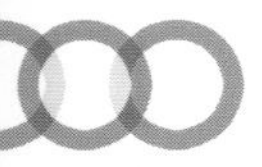

Answer

Kawasaki disease (KD) is an inflammatory process that is most commonly seen in children <5 years old and is characterized by high fever lasting greater than 5 days, rash, limbic-sparing conjunctival injection, erythema of the palms and soles, oral changes, and unilateral cervical lymphadenopathy measuring >1.5 cm in diameter. Coronary artery aneurysms are the most feared complication of the disease and the risk can be mitigated by prompt initiation of treatment with intravenous immunoglobulin.

As there are no diagnostic tests for KD and the clinical findings are not specific, the clinician must rule out other disease processes. Measles should be considered in an unimmunized infant or child who presents with fever, rash, cough, coryza, and conjunctivitis. Airborne precautions should be initiated if measles is suspected. A diagnosis of adenovirus infection in a child with signs and symptoms of KD is particularly challenging as the two diseases have similar clinical features. A patient with exudative pharyngitis and exudative conjunctivitis and a positive nasopharyngeal sample for adenovirus is unlikely to have KD. Alternatively, erythema of the palms and soles, strawberry tongue, and a desquamating groin rash is unlikely to be related to adenovirus infection.

Keywords: infectious diseases, do not miss, fever, rash

Bibliography

American Academy of Pediatrics. Measles. In *Red Book: 2015 Report of the Committee on Infectious Diseases*, Kimberlin DW, Brady MT, Jackson MA, Long SS, eds. Elk Grove Village, IL: American Academy of Pediatrics, 2015:535–47.

McCrindle BW, Rowley AH, Newburger JW, Burns JC et al. Diagnosis, treatment, and long-term management of Kawasaki disease: A scientific statement for health professionals from the American Heart Association. *Circulation* 2017;135(17):e927–99.

Rowley AH, Shulman ST. Editorial commentary: Missing the forest for the trees; Respiratory viral assays in patients with Kawasaki disease. *Clin Infect Dis* 2013;56:65–6.

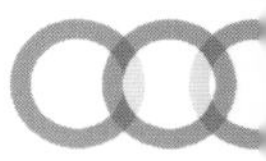

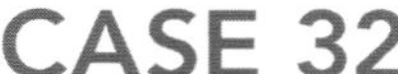

CASE 32

Emily Obringer

Questions

A 6-year-old girl presents with low-grade fever, mild respiratory symptoms, and left-sided facial swelling for the past 2 days.

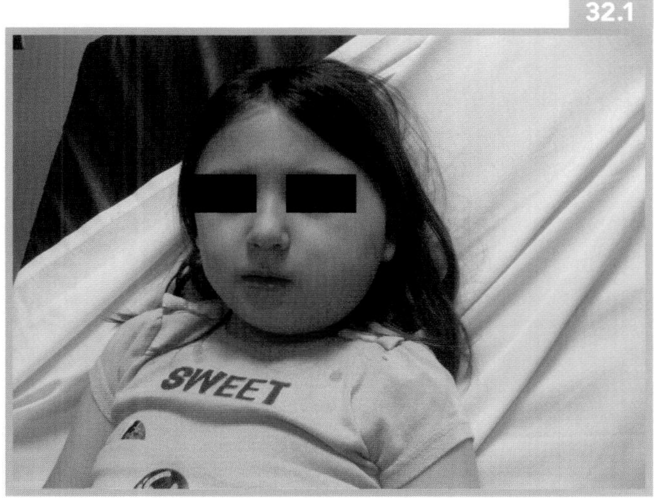

1. In addition to mumps, what other vaccine-preventable viral disease can cause parotitis?
2. What isolation precautions should be implemented when mumps is suspected?

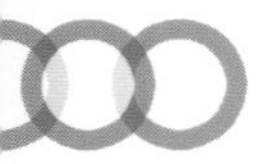

Answers

1. Mumps is the most common cause of viral parotitis (Gutierrez, 2012). Although unvaccinated individuals are at greatest risk of contracting the disease, outbreaks are known to occur among vaccinated individuals, especially older adolescents and young adults (Barskey et al., 2009). Parotitis is the most common manifestation of mumps; however, about one-third of patients do not have clinically evident salivary gland swelling and may have only mild respiratory symptoms (American Academy of Pediatrics, 2015). When present, parotitis is usually unilateral initially but can become bilateral in up to 70% of cases (Gutierrez, 2012).

   Another vaccine-preventable disease that is associated with parotitis is influenza, specifically influenza A (Krilov and Swenson, 1985). Other viruses associated with parotitis include parainfluenza, Epstein-Barr virus, cytomegalovirus, coxsackievirus A, and echovirus (Gutierrez, 2012). HIV infection may be associated with parotitis, but this usually manifests as chronic, bilateral parotid swelling.

2. Mumps is spread through contact with infected respiratory tract secretions. In addition to standard precautions, droplet precautions should be implemented in any case of suspected mumps (American Academy of Pediatrics, 2015). (Note: As mentioned earlier, other viral diseases may present in a similar manner to mumps and additional precautions, such as contact isolation, may therefore be indicated while awaiting diagnostic testing.)

Keywords: infectious diseases, mimickers, infection, fever

References

American Academy of Pediatrics. Mumps. In *Red Book: 2015 Report of the Committee on Infectious Diseases*, 30th ed., Kimberlin DW, Brady MT, Jackson MA, Long SS, eds. Elk Grove Village, IL: American Academy of Pediatrics, 2015.

Barskey AE, Glasser JW, LeBaron CW. Mumps resurgences in the United States: A historical perspective on unexpected elements. *Vaccine* 2009;27(44):6186–95.

Gutierrez K. Mumps virus. In *Principles and Practice of Pediatric Infectious Diseases*, 4th ed., Long SS, Pickering LK, Prober CG, eds. Philadelphia: Elsevier-Saunders, 2012:1125–9.

Krilov LR, Swenson P. Acute parotitis associated with influenza A infection. *J Infect Dis* 1985;152(4):853.

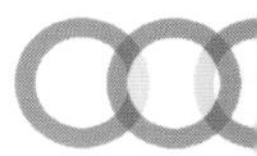

CASE 33

Nina Mbadiwe

Question

A healthy 3-year-old boy is brought to the emergency department by his mother because she is concerned about a lesion on his eyelid that has been growing over the past 3 months. It has now begun to intermittently bleed.

On exam he is well-appearing. He has a solitary pedunculated 1 cm mildly erythematous lesion on his left upper eyelid with minimal yellow crusting. There is no active bleeding.

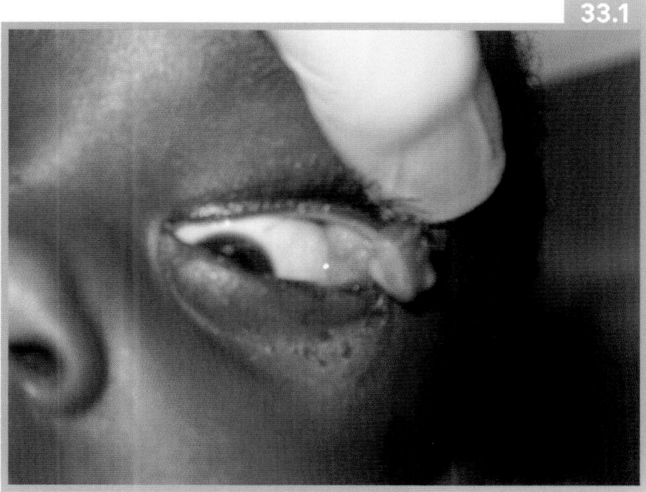
33.1

What is the next step in the management of this case?

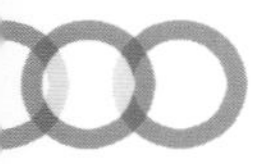

Answer

Pyogenic granuloma is also known histologically as lobular capillary hemangioma. It is one of the most common vascular tumors in infants and children. It is benign and can occur on the skin or mucous membranes. The average age of diagnosis is 6–10 years old.

Diagnosis is based upon a papule that bleeds easily and has developed over a few days to weeks. The lesion usually starts as a small red papule that grows rapidly over weeks to months then stabilizes. Spontaneous regression is rare.

In most cases there is no apparent cause, although it is thought that prior trauma at the site, certain medications, and a history of capillary vascular malformations might be possible triggers.

Treatment is usually required because of frequent ulceration and bleeding. A subspecialty referral would be indicated to discuss treatment options including simple curettage with electrocautery, excision, laser surgery, cryotherapy, or topical/intralesional therapies.

Keywords: dermatology, head and neck/ENT, ophthalmology, mass

Bibliography

Goldsmith LA, Katz SI, Gilchrest BS, Paller AS, Leffell DJ, Wolff K. *Fitzpatrick's Dermatology in General Medicine*. 8th ed. New York: McGraw-Hill, 2012.

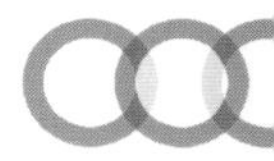

CASE 34

Alisa McQueen

Question

A teenager has been bothered by a lump in her knee for some time. Generally it is not painful, but by the end of the day it becomes sore from rubbing against her other leg. She is otherwise healthy with no other complaints. On examination she has a firm, fixed protuberance above her left knee which is non-tender. The knee joint itself is normal; the overlying skin is normal, and her distal neurovascular exam is also normal.

Her right knee is shown next:

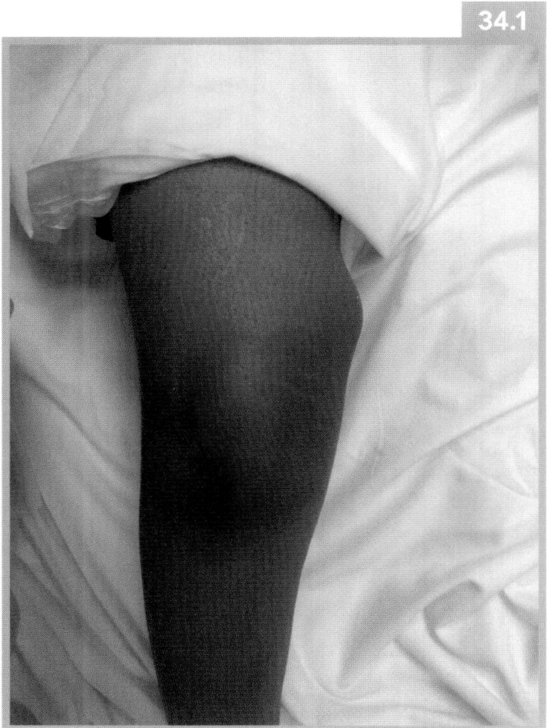
34.1

What would be your next step in making a diagnosis?

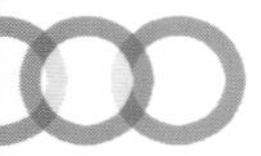

Answer

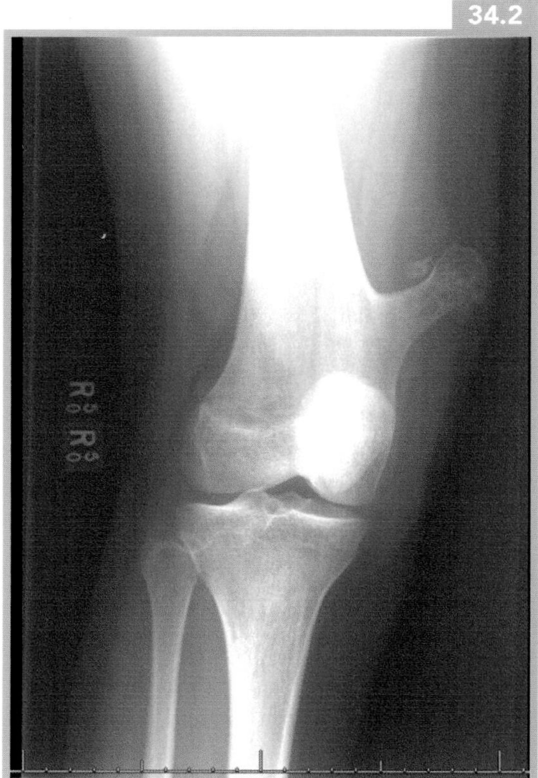

An x-ray reveals a bone spur arising from the metaphysis of the femur with well-defined borders and no radiographic evidence of bone destruction or soft tissue infiltration. The appearance and location are most consistent with an osteochondroma.

A benign bone tumor, also known as an osteocartilaginous exostosis, arises from the cortex of long bones (femur and humerus are the most common) and continues to grow with the child until the growth plates have fused. When the size or location causes troublesome symptoms, local excision may be performed. Because there is a small risk of malignant transformation, lesions that are not excised should be monitored with serial examinations and radiographs.

Keywords: orthopedics, congenital anomaly, benign, mass

Bibliography

Springfield DS, Gebhardt MC. Bone and soft tissue tumors. In *Lovell and Winter's Pediatric Orthopaedics*, 6th ed., Morrissy RT, Weinstein SL, eds. Philadelphia: Lippincott Williams & Wilkins, 2006:493.

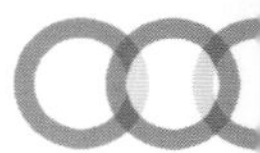

CASE 35

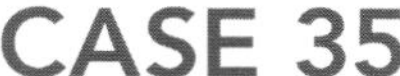

Nina Mbadiwe

Question

A 7-year-old boy presents to the emergency department with insidious development of a limp with intermittent bilateral groin pain. He has had no fever, weight loss, or systemic symptoms. Neither he nor his parents recall any trauma.

On exam he is afebrile and in no acute distress but appears slightly uncomfortable secondary to pain. He has an antalgic gait with decreased hip motion (on abduction and internal rotation); otherwise his exam is normal.

What imaging is needed to establish the diagnosis?

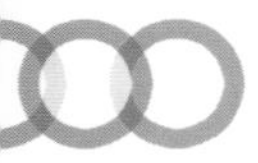

Answer

Legg-Calvé-Perthes disease results in idiopathic avascular necrosis of the hip (proximal femoral epiphysis). The etiology is unknown. It usually occurs in children between the ages of 3 and 12 and affects boys more than girls (4:1 ratio). Patients typically present with a limp and might also have groin, anterior thigh, or knee pain. Initial radiographs (anterior-posterior and frog leg views) may be normal. Later in the course of the disease, radiographs usually show increased density and deformity (flattening or fragmentation) of the femoral head.

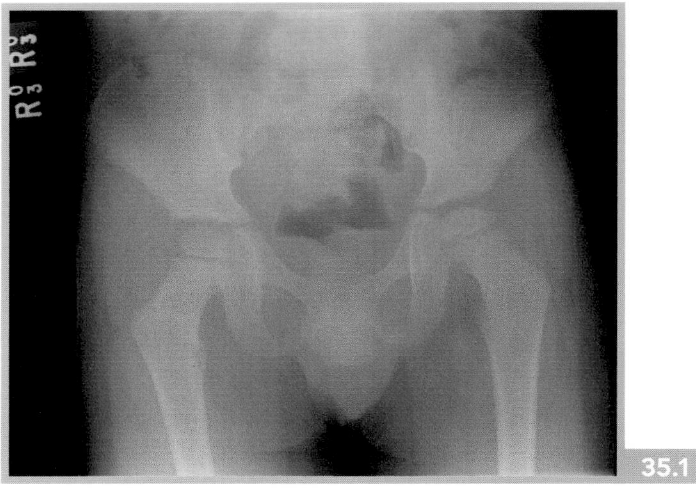
35.1

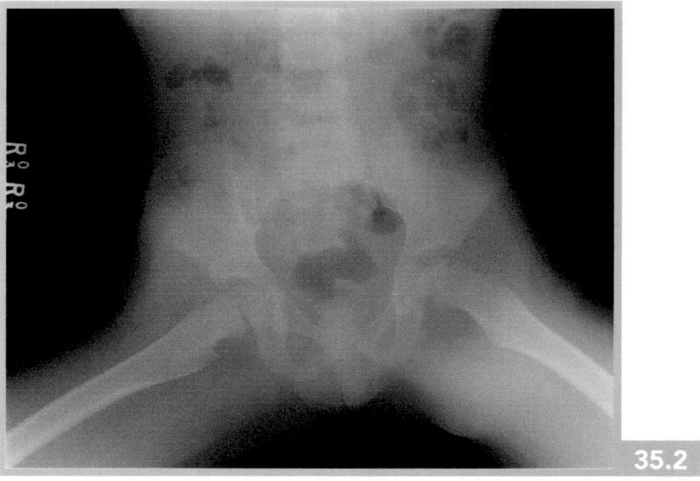
35.2

Keywords: orthopedics, limp

Bibliography

Weinstein SL. Legg-Calvé-Perthes syndrome. In *Lovell and Winter's Pediatric Orthopaedics*, 6th ed., Morrissy RT, Weinstein SL, eds. Lippincott, Williams, and Wilkins, 2006.

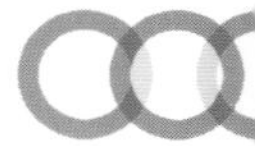

CASE 36

Nina Mbadiwe

Question

A 13-year-old otherwise healthy girl presents to the emergency department with 2 days of right leg and knee pain, which started after she fell off of her bike. She denies numbness, paresthesia, or other injuries.

On exam she is afebrile and in no acute distress. She has tenderness to palpation with minimal swelling just proximal to the right knee. There is no warmth or erythema of the area. Radiographs of the leg demonstrate a pathological fracture.

36.1

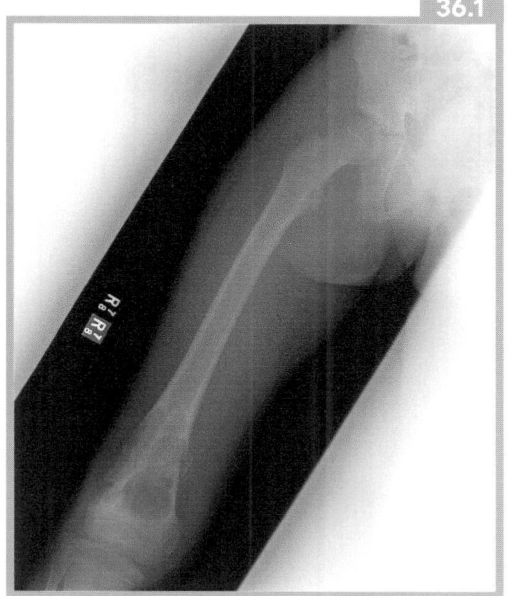

36.2

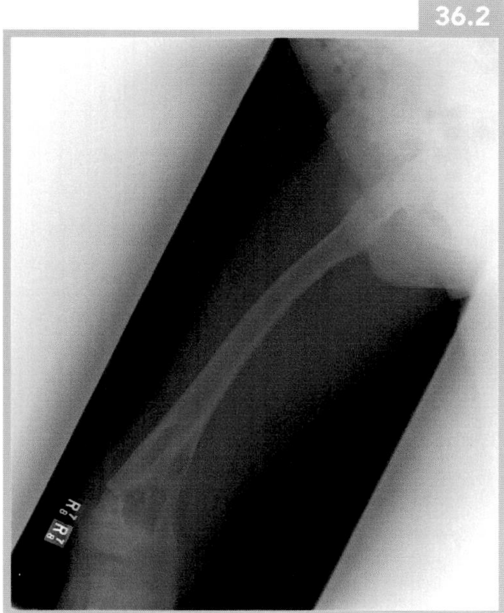

What is the differential diagnosis for a pathologic fracture?

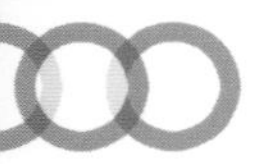

Answer

A pathologic fracture is the result of bone that is weak secondary to an underlying disease process such as rickets, bone tumors, juvenile osteoporosis, chronic renal insufficiency, osteogenesis imperfecta, unicameral bone cysts, aneurysmal bone cysts, or non-ossifying fibromas. It usually occurs as a result of minor trauma; therefore, subtle pathologic fractures may go undetected. The proximal femur and humerus are the most frequent sites for pathologic fractures.

Keywords: orthopedics, extremity injury

Bibliography

Ortiz EJ, Isler MH, Navia JE, Canosa R. Pathologic fractures in children. *Clin Orthop Relat Res* 2005;116.

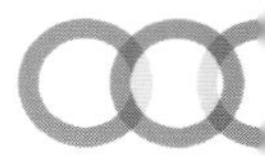

CASE 37

Timothy Ketterhagen

Question

A mother brings her 6-year-old son to the emergency department due to a concern for a missing tooth. The patient was reportedly playing tag with his sister 15 minutes prior to arrival when he fell and hit his mouth on the corner of a table. The patient did not lose consciousness and has been acting appropriately since the incident. Mother brought the patient's tooth with her to the emergency department. Patient is complaining of minimal mouth pain but denies any other injuries.

Physical exam shows an alert and interactive boy. Examination of the oral cavity shows absence of the upper right central incisor with minimal blood in the socket. No other oral injury is noted. The rest of the physical exam is unremarkable. The injury is shown next.

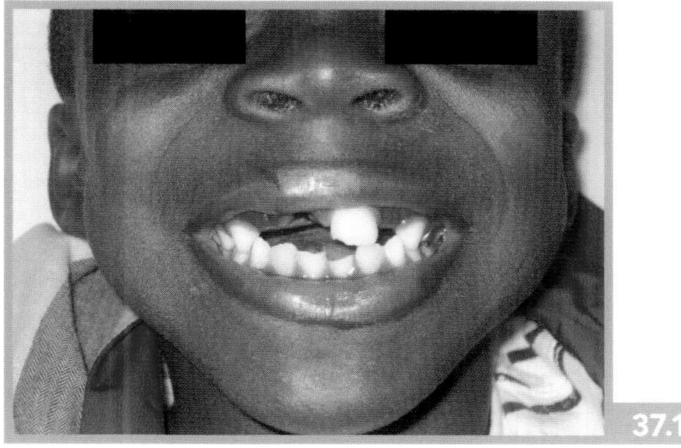

37.1

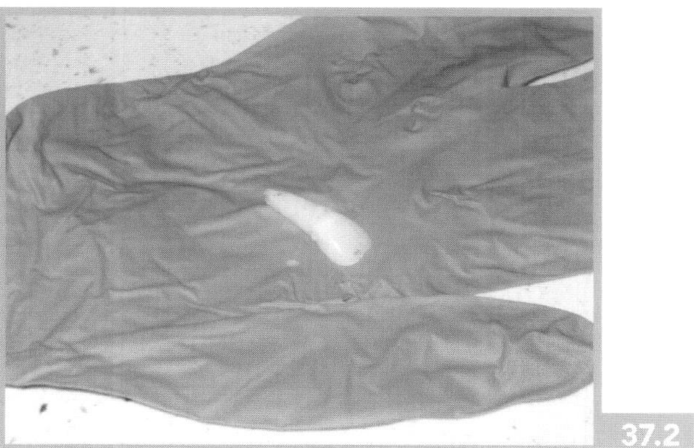

37.2

What factors should be considered to determine whether the tooth should be reimplanted?

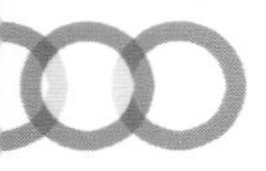

Answer

Avulsion is the term used to describe complete displacement of a tooth from the socket. Aspiration, intrusion, and fracture must be considered. Initial control of bleeding should be performed.

The factors that should be considered prior to reimplantation of an avulsed tooth include whether the tooth is primary or permanent, care prior to reimplantation, and time since tooth displacement. Primary teeth should not be replaced. Replacement of a permanent tooth has the best prognosis if it is reimplanted within 15–30 minutes of the injury. Prior to reimplantation, the tooth can be rinsed gently, but scrubbing should be avoided and handling should be minimized. If the tooth is not replaced immediately, the tooth can be preserved in a balanced salt solution, milk, or less effectively in saline or saliva. The tooth should be inserted into a previously irrigated socket in its normal position. Adequate analgesia or anesthesia should be provided. Dental consultation is required for splinting and further management.

Keywords: head and neck/ENT, dental injury, oropharyngeal injury

Bibliography

Fleisher GR, Ludwig S, eds. *Textbook of Pediatric Emergency Medicine.* 6th ed. Philadelphia: Lippincott Williams & Wilkins, 2010.

Hoffman RJ, Wang VJ, Scarfone R. *Fleisher & Ludwig's 5-Minute Pediatric Emergency Medicine Consult.* Philadelphia: Wolters Kluwer Health/Lippincott Williams & Wilkins, 2012.

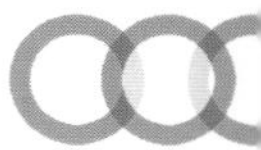

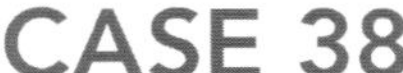

CASE 38

Leah Finkel

Question

A 5-year-old boy with no past medical history presents after falling with a pencil in his mouth. He was running in school, tripped, and landed on it. On exam he is in moderate pain with some mild blood oozing from inside his mouth. There are no signs of respiratory distress.

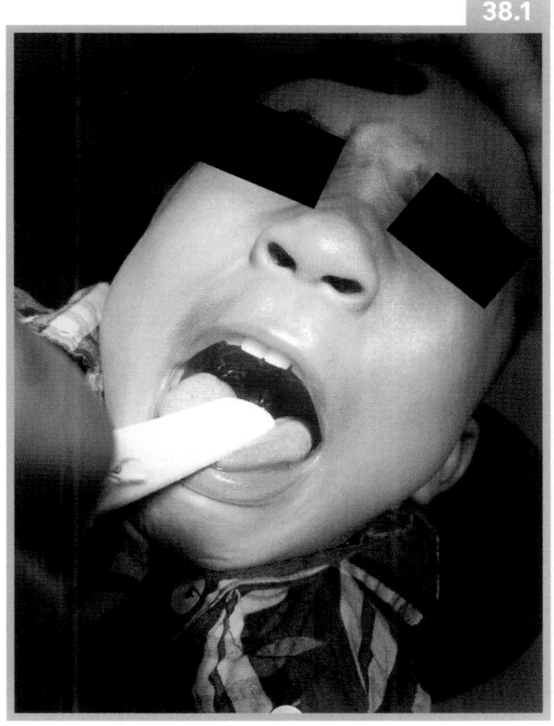

38.1

What do you see on examination and how would you manage this?

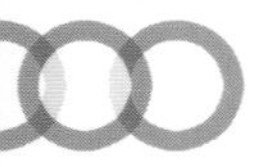

Answer

This is a case of uvular trauma.

Penetrating injuries of the oropharynx occur with some frequency in children. Initial evaluation should focus on the mechanism of injury, location of injury, wound characteristics, and the child's neurologic status. Minor oropharyngeal injuries typically heal spontaneously, but a small number of them can result in significant complications including deep neck infections or carotid artery bleeding. Furthermore, injury to the internal carotid artery may lead to thrombus formation as well as a dissecting aneurysm or pseudoaneurysm that may lead to neurologic sequelae including stroke. Any concern for neurovascular damage should be evaluated with CT angiography or angiogram.

The majority of oropharyngeal injuries can be treated conservatively, including wounds through the hard palate. Wounds that may require intervention are ones in which there is a large avulsion flap, through-and-through wounds, or wounds with a potential retained foreign body. Consider the use of prophylactic antibiotics to prevent infection, in particular for patients requiring admission or those who have deeper and larger injuries. Oral injuries also require tetanus prophylaxis.

Keyword: head and neck/ENT, oropharyngeal injury, penetrating trauma

Bibliography

Kupietzky A. Clinical guidelines for treatment of impalement injuries of the oropharynx in children. *Pediatr Dent* 2000;22:3.

Hellman J, Schott SR, Gootee MJ. Impalement injuries of the palate in children: Review of 131 cases. *Int J Otorhinolaryngol* 1993;22:6.

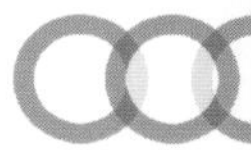

CASE 39

Michael Gottlieb

Questions

A 5-year-old boy presents to the emergency department with his parents complaining of left eye pain for the past 2 days. He endorsed some preceding viral symptoms, but stated the pain began today after rubbing his left eye. His visual acuity is 20/20 bilaterally, but he does endorse some haziness at the superior aspect of his left visual field. He has no conjunctival injection or pain with extraocular movement. Fluorescein staining is performed and demonstrated in the following.

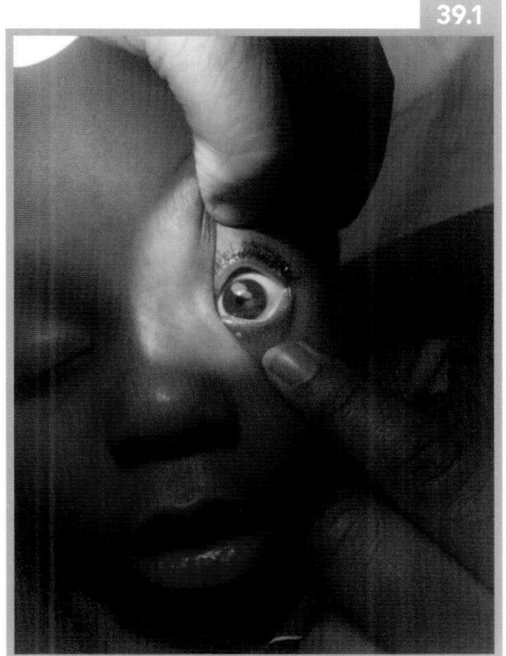

39.1

1. What is the difference between a corneal abrasion and a corneal ulcer?
2. What infection is commonly associated with prolonged contact lens use?

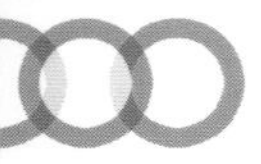

Answers

1. A corneal abrasion occurs when the corneal epithelium is damaged, and can result from direct trauma or prolonged contact lens use. Symptoms include foreign body sensation, pruritus, and pain. Photophobia may also occur if there is an associated iritis. A corneal ulcer is an infected corneal abrasion. This may occur due to bacteria from the external environment or may be the precipitating etiology, as in cases of viral or fungal keratitis. The latter can be differentiated by the presence of conjunctival injection, purulent discharge, elevation of the ulcer edges from inflammation, or the presence of dendritic lesions.
2. Prolonged contact lens use increases the risk of *Pseudomonas aeruginosa*. This is a more dangerous pathogen and is resistant to many of the standard ophthalmologic antibiotics. Therefore, any patient presenting with a corneal abrasion from prolonged contact lens use should receive an antibiotic with antipseudomonal coverage, such as ciprofloxacin, ofloxacin, or gentamicin.

Keywords: ophthalmology, foreign body, infection

Bibliography

Ahmed F, House RJ, Feldman BH. Corneal abrasions and corneal foreign bodies. *Prim Care* September 2015;42(3):363–75.

Wipperman JL, Dorsch JN. Evaluation and management of corneal abrasions. *Am Fam Physician* January 2013;15;87(2):114–20.

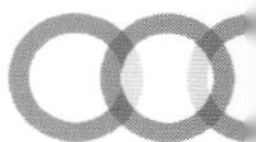

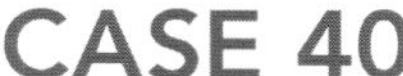

CASE 40

Michael Gottlieb

Questions

A 12-year-old boy is brought to the emergency department by ambulance with confusion and a severe headache after falling off of a ladder. He is able to speak but is using inappropriate words and cannot form sentences. He localizes pain in all extremities and his eyes open to verbal command. He is taken for a CT scan and the image is demonstrated next (Image 40.1).

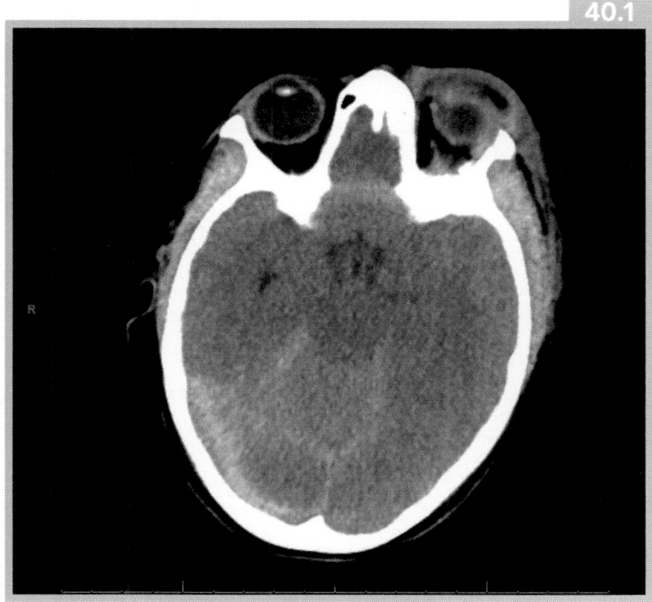

40.1

1. What is his Glasgow Coma Scale score based upon the given information?
2. What type of hemorrhage is present on his CT scan?

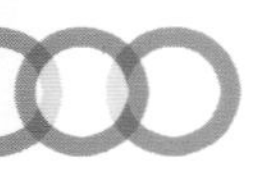

Answers

1. The Glasgow Coma Scale (GCS) score is an assessment of mental status that may be indicative of injury severity and is valuable when communicating with consultants. The GCS score consists of three components (eye opening, verbal response, and motor function), with a maximal score of 15 (Table 40.1). This patient's GCS score is 11 (3E, 3V, 5M).

Table 40.1 Glasgow Coma Scale (GCS)

	Adult/Older Child	Younger Child/Infant
Eye Opening		
4	Spontaneous	Spontaneous
3	To command	To voice
2	To pain	To pain
1	None	None
Verbal		
5	Coherent	Smiles
4	Confused	Cries but consolable
3	Inappropriate words	Persistent crying and screaming
2	Incomprehensible sounds	Grunting, agitated
1	None	None
Motor		
6	Obeys commands	Spontaneous movement
5	Localizes pain	Localizes pain
4	Withdraws from pain	Withdraws from pain
3	Flexes to pain (decorticate posturing)	Flexes to pain (decorticate posturing)
2	Extends to pain (decerebrate posturing)	Extends to pain (decerebrate posturing)
1	None	None

2. This patient has a subdural hematoma. A subdural hematoma is typically caused by tearing of the cerebral bridging veins. The onset of symptoms is more gradual and appears crescentic on CT. The hematoma is able to cross suture lines but cannot cross dural reflections (i.e. the tentorium cerebelli or the falx cerebri). Conversely, epidural hematomas are caused by injury to cerebral arteries, most commonly the middle meningeal artery. They appear biconvex on CT and are able to cross dural reflections but cannot cross suture lines.

Keywords: neurosurgery, altered mental status, headache, do not miss, blunt trauma

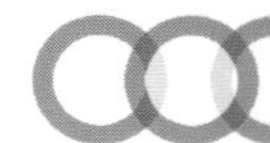

Bibliography

Rosman NP, Oppenheimer EY, O'Connor JF. Emergency management of pediatric head injuries. *Emerg Med Clin North Am* April 1983;1(1):141–74.

Wright DW, Merck LH. Head trauma. In *Tintinalli's Emergency Medicine: A Comprehensive Study Guide*, Tintinalli JE, Stapczynski J, Ma O, Yealy DM, Meckler GD, Cline DM, eds. New York: McGraw-Hill, 2016.

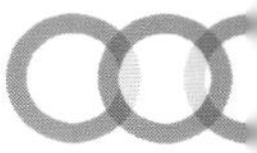

CASE 41

Michael Gottlieb

Questions

A 10-year-old boy with no significant past medical history is brought to the emergency department with shortness of breath after a motor vehicle crash. On arrival he developed progressively worsening shortness of breath and hypoxia, and was found to have significantly decreased breath sounds on the left side. He was intubated and a chest tube was placed. His chest x-ray and abdominal CT are shown next.

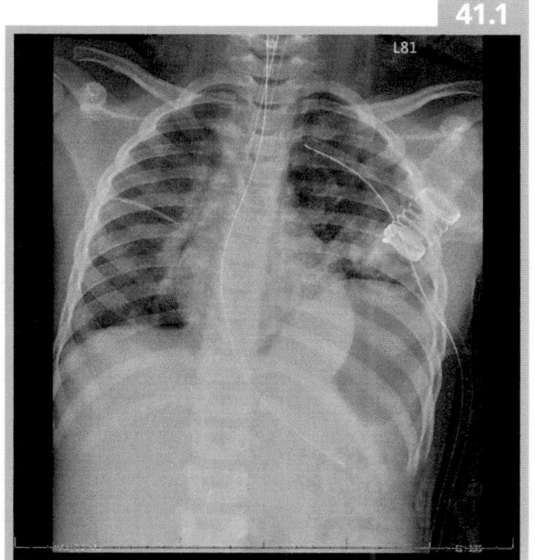

41.1

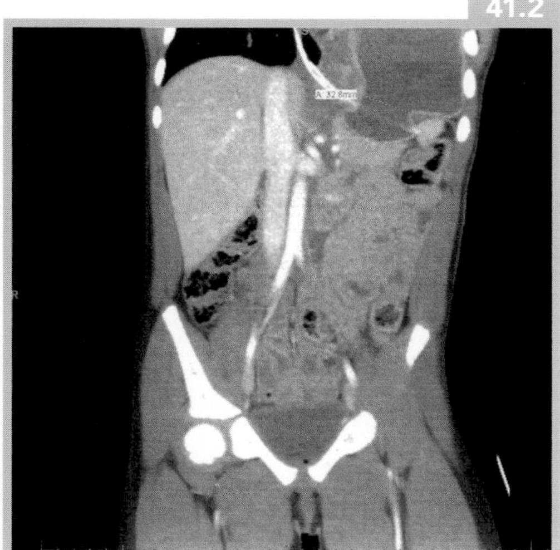

41.2

1. What is the most sensitive modality to identify a traumatic diaphragmatic rupture? On which side of the body is it more common?
2. What is the treatment of a traumatic diaphragmatic hernia?

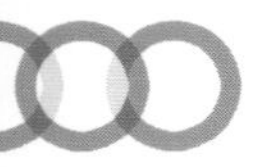

Answers

1. Chest radiography has the lowest sensitivity for diagnosing diaphragmatic rupture. Computed tomography (CT) has improved sensitivity compared with chest radiography, but can still miss a significant number of cases. While laparoscopy has been suggested to identify most cases, video-assisted thoracoscopy has been demonstrated to have the highest sensitivity. Diaphragmatic ruptures are significantly more common on the left side than the right due to the protective nature of the liver on the right.

2. Most symptomatic cases require surgical intervention. Since the diaphragm is both constantly moving and under continuous tension from the abdominal contents, diaphragmatic tears generally will not heal on their own. As the tear widens, the abdominal contents increasingly herniate into the chest cavity due to the increased intra-abdominal pressure in comparison with the intrathoracic pressure. This can lead to a chronic cough, shortness of breath, orthopnea, and even intestinal injury if the organ becomes strangulated within the hernia.

Keywords: blunt trauma, respiratory distress, life-threatening, do not miss, acute abdomen

Bibliography

Rashid F, Chakrabarty MM, Singh Y, Iftikhar SY. A review on delayed presentation of diaphragmatic rupture. *World J Emerg Surg* August 2009;21(4):32.

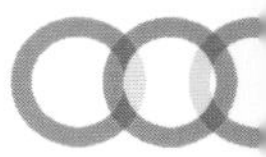

CASE 42

Emily Obringer

Questions

A 5-year-old girl was bitten on the hand by the family dog. Both the dog and the child are fully vaccinated. The dog has been acting normally. The wound was cleaned at home and a dressing applied. She now presents 2 days later with pain and swelling.

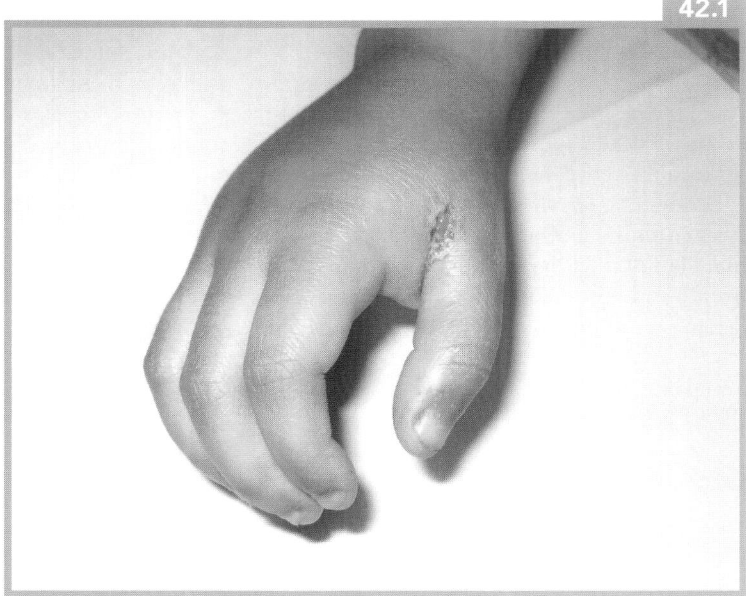
42.1

1. In which clinical scenarios should a patient with a dog bite wound be prescribed antimicrobials?
2. In which clinical scenarios is rabies prophylaxis indicated after dog bite injury?

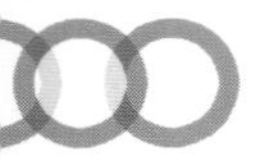

Answers

1. Dog bite wounds become infected in only about 10%–15% of cases and are frequently polymicrobial (American Academy of Pediatrics, 2009). The most common organisms are *Pasteurella* species, *Staphylococcus aureus*, *Streptococcus* species, and anaerobes (Talan et al., 1999). A typical empiric antimicrobial regimen is oral amoxicillin-clavulanate. The physician should note that this regimen does not cover methicillin-resistant *S. aureus* (MRSA), and when this organism is isolated from a bite wound culture, additional or alternative coverage may be indicated.

   In selected clinical scenarios, dog bite wounds warrant antimicrobial use. These include severe and crush injuries; puncture wounds; certain locations, such as the face, hand, foot, and genital area; immunocompromised patients; and when the wound looks infected (American Academy of Pediatrics, 2009). The duration of treatment is based on the severity and location of the injury.

2. Depending on geographic location, rabid dogs may be rare or common (Centers for Disease Control and Prevention, 2014). Therefore, assessing the risk of rabies is important for all dog bite injuries. If the dog appears rabid or is unable to be located and quarantined for a period of 10 days, the patient should begin rabies post-exposure prophylaxis. In addition, if during the 10-day quarantine period, the dog shows signs of rabies, then the patient should initiate rabies prophylaxis. When indicated, active and passive immunization is recommended. For previously unimmunized patients, rabies vaccine is given on the first day of post-exposure prophylaxis, and then again on days 3, 7, and 14 (American Academy of Pediatrics, 2009). In addition, rabies immune globulin (RIG) should be used concomitantly with the first dose of rabies vaccine. Half of the RIG should be infiltrated directly into the dog bite wound with the rest administered intramuscularly in a site (or multiple sites, if necessary) distant from where the rabies vaccine was administered (American Academy of Pediatrics, 2009).

Keywords: animal bite, bite wound, infectious diseases, hand injury, skin and soft tissue infection

References

American Academy of Pediatrics. Bite wounds. In *Red Book: 2009 Report of the Committee on Infectious Diseases*, 28th ed., Pickering LK, Baker CJ, Kimberlin DW, Long SS, eds. Elk Grove Village, IL: American Academy of Pediatrics, 2009:187–91.

Centers for Disease Control and Prevention (CDC). Reported cases of rabies in cats and dogs, by county, 2014. http://www.cdc.gov/rabies/resources/publications/2014-surveillance/2014-cats-and-dogs.html#dogs. Last modified April 29, 2016.

Talan DA, Citron DM, Abrahamian FM, Moran GJ, Goldstein EJC. Bacteriologic analysis of infected dog and cat bites. *NEJM* 1999;350:85–92.

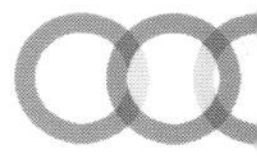

CASE 43

Timothy Ketterhagen

Question

A father brings his 18-month-old daughter to the emergency department for evaluation after she stepped on a fishhook. She was running on a pier at the family lake house when she felt a sharp pain in her left foot. No other injuries were reported.

On exam, the girl is alert and playful. A fishhook is seen embedded in the posterior aspect of the lateral left foot. No active bleeding observed. No neurovascular deficits are noted. Physical exam is otherwise unremarkable. The injury is shown in the following images.

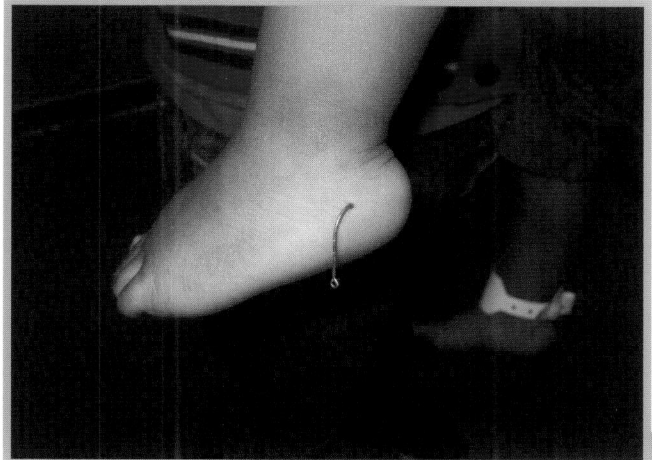

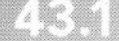

43.1

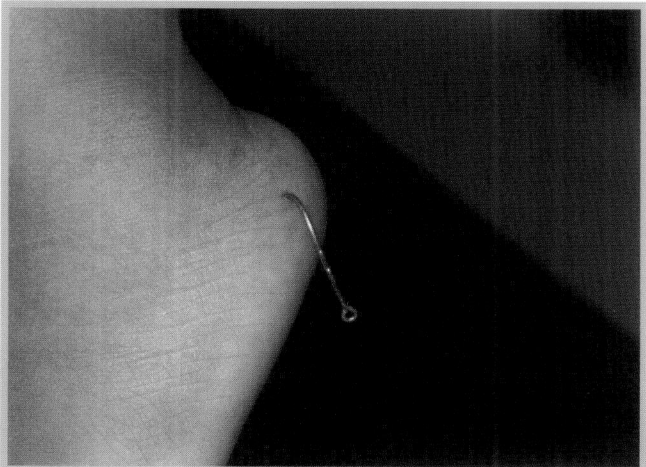

43.2

What techniques might be used to remove the fishhook?

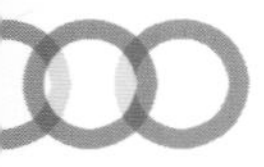

Answer

Most fishhook injuries are superficial. However, neurologic and vascular status should be assessed. Injuries that involve bones and tendons require careful evaluation. Imaging is generally not required. Injuries that involve the eye require immediate ophthalmologic evaluation. Tetanus status should be addressed and prophylactic antibiotics are generally not indicated.

There are several techniques that can be utilized to remove a superficial fishhook. Wound cleansing and local anesthesia should be implemented in all cases.

1. *Retrograde*: Apply downward pressure to the proximal end of the hook. Then back the hook out along the path of entry. Stop if resistance occurs. This method should not be used if the hook is known to have a barb at the end. (Low success rate)
2. *String*: Secure string to the midpoint of the bend of the hook. Apply downward pressure to the proximal end of the hook. Pull sharply on the string to release the barb and then remove the hook through the entry wound. (Can be attempted for deep-lying hooks)
3. *Needle cover*: Insert an 18-gauge or larger needle along the entrance wound parallel to the shank of the hook. Point the bevel of the needle toward the inside of the curve of the hook. Advance the needle until the needle catches on the barb of the hook. Then pull the fishhook out through the wound opening while the needle is still engaged with the barb. (Effective for larger hooks and superficial injuries)
4. *Advance-and-cut*: Using pliers or a needle driver, apply downward force along the curve of the hook, advancing the barb out through the skin. After the barb has been pushed through the skin, cut off the barb. The remaining hook can then be withdrawn through the entry wound. (Almost always successful)

Keywords: procedures, foreign body

Bibliography

Fleisher GR, Ludwig S, eds. *Textbook of Pediatric Emergency Medicine*. 6th ed. Philadelphia: Lippincott Williams & Wilkins, 2010.

Gammons M, Jackson E. Fishhook removal. *Am Fam Physician* 2001;63:2231–7.

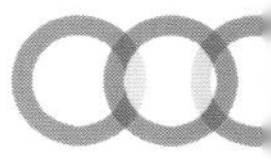

CASE 44

Diana Yan

Question

A 7-year-old male with a history of egg allergy presents to the emergency department after accidently sticking himself with his own EpiPen® (epinephrine autoinjector). He is complaining of pain and his father reports that his thumb has been cold and pale. He denies systemic symptoms including palpitations, sweating, or shakiness. Before this event, he had been feeling well. Past medical history is significant for mild persistent asthma and egg allergy. Other than the autoinjector, he takes an inhaled corticosteroid twice a day and albuterol as needed.

Physical exam shows a crying, but otherwise alert, active, and well-appearing child. Exam is significant for a pale, cold, right thumb with capillary refill greater than 3 seconds. There is pain with palpation of the thumb and the needle is stuck in the right thumb. He is still able to move his thumb, but sensation is decreased distally.

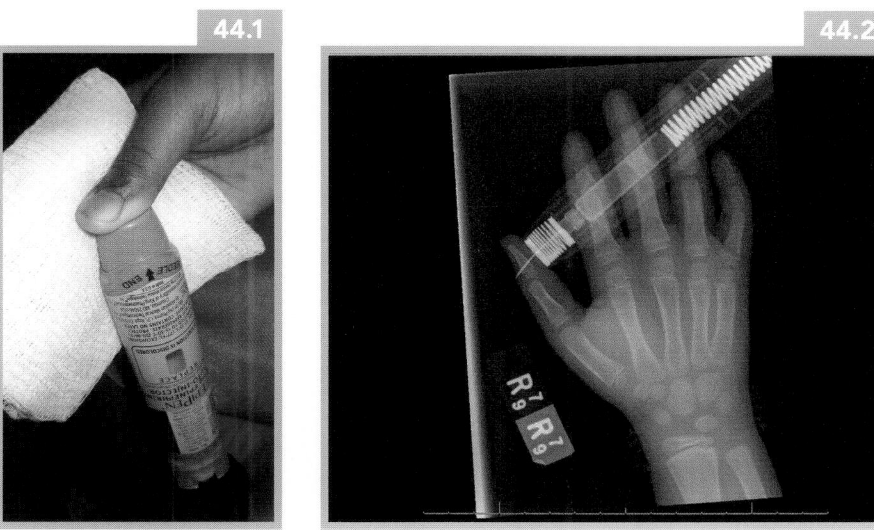

What is the appropriate management for the ischemic digit after epinephrine injection?

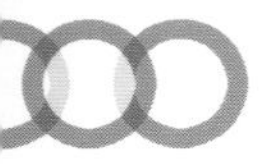

Answer

Supportive care. Accidental discharge of epinephrine autoinjectors is a common event and rarely requires intervention. A retrospective analysis of the Texas Poison Control Network database found 127 patients over 6 years who had injected epinephrine accidently into their digits and showed that there were no cases of clinically significant systemic effects nor any vascular-related comorbidities. None of these patients needed admission to the hospital or surgical consult or intervention. About 58% of patients had resolution of their symptoms within 2 hours, whereas 10% of patients had no symptoms to begin with. Most clinicians observed their patients, whereas 29 patients were treated with topical nitroglycerin paste, local phentolamine injection, local terbutaline, or a combination of the three. Warm soaks alone were also used in 32% of cases. In all of these cases (from observation to medical therapy), there was complete resolution of symptoms without any complications. Because of this, it is recommended to observe patients for at least 2 hours and to consider medical therapy at that time if there are still persistent symptoms of ischemia.

Keywords: penetrating trauma, medications, hand injury

Bibliography

Muck AE, Beharta VS, Borys DJ, Morgan DL. Six years of epinephrine digital injections: Absence of significant local or systemic effects. *Ann Emerg Med* 2010;56:270–4.

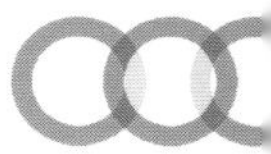

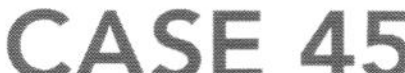

CASE 45

Diana Yan

Question

A 9-year-old female with a history of tree nut allergy presents to the emergency department after the school nurse injected the patient's epinephrine autoinjector into the patient's left thigh. The patient developed urticaria and difficulty breathing after eating brownies during a classroom party. Since the epinephrine injection, the patient's symptoms have improved, but the autoinjector remains embedded in her thigh. There is no other significant past medical history or other medications.

Physical exam shows an alert, awake, and active girl who is very worried about anyone touching her left thigh. There is pain when the epinephrine autoinjector is moved but no surrounding erythema or drainage in the left thigh. Strength is 5/5 in the extremity. Sensation is intact. Capillary refill is less than 2 seconds.

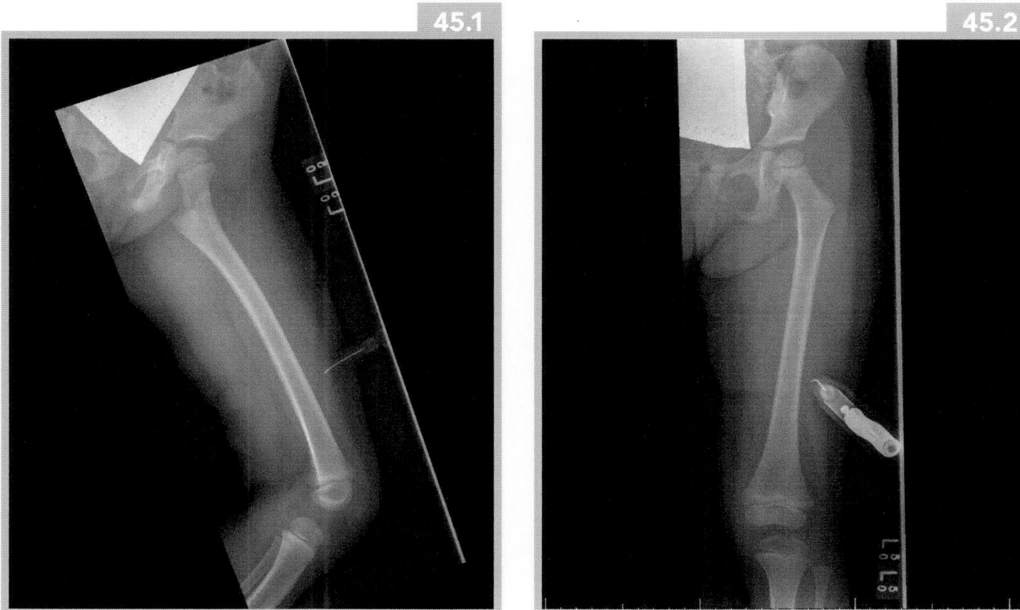

45.1 45.2

What complications can come from use of an epinephrine autoinjector?

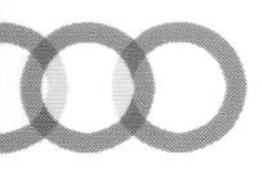

Answer

Laceration and embedded needle. This patient had anaphylaxis after ingestion of a known food allergen. Anaphylaxis is defined as having more than one system involved. Systems include skin/soft tissue (hives), respiratory (shortness of breath or wheezing), gastrointestinal (vomiting), central nervous system (confusion or altered mental status), and cardiovascular (hypotension). The patient's anaphylactic symptoms resolved after getting the appropriate treatment of epinephrine. In this case, the needle bent and likely caused a laceration. These lacerations can be significant and require multiple sutures to repair. Children are particularly at risk for this complication as they do not usually cooperate with painful intramuscular (IM) injections. Suggestions to decrease this risk include:

1. Immobilize the child's leg.
2. Hold the epinephrine autoinjector to the leg and inject rather than using the "swing and push" method.
3. Hold the needle in place for only 2 seconds, at most, instead of the company's suggestion of 10 seconds, if not all of the medicine is deployed within 0.2 seconds.

All of these suggestions are to create a more controlled environment so that there is a lower risk of injury and bent or embedded needles. In the case of embedded needles, the bone usually heals well and there are no complications. The most severe complication from this situation would be osteomyelitis. If the needle penetrates a digit, other concerns can be whitlow and impaired nail growth (if the needle goes through the nail bed). In a case study, amoxicillin-clavulanic acid was prescribed as a prophylactic antibiotic.

Keywords: penetrating trauma, extremity injury, medications, procedures

Bibliography

Brown JC, Tuuri RE, Akhter S, Guerra LD et al. Lacerations and embedded needles caused by epinephrine autoinjector use in children. *Ann Emerg Med* 2016;67:307–15.

Schintler MV, Arbab E, Aberer W, Spendel S, Scharnagl E. Accidental perforating bone injury using the EpiPen autoinjection device. *Allergy* 2005;60:259–60.

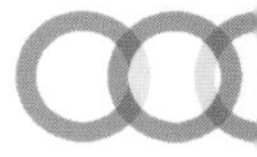

CASE 46

Timothy Ketterhagen

Question

A father brings his 14-year-old son to the emergency department after he injured his right hand. The patient punched a wall because he was upset. The patient is only complaining of pain in his right hand. He has no other complaints.

Physical exam shows a well-appearing young man. There is swelling along the ulnar aspect of the right hand. The patient is also unable to fully make a fist due to pain. The skin appears to be intact. No neurovascular deficits are noted; however, with flexion of the fingers, rotational deformity of the fifth digit is observed (shown here). The physical exam is otherwise unremarkable.

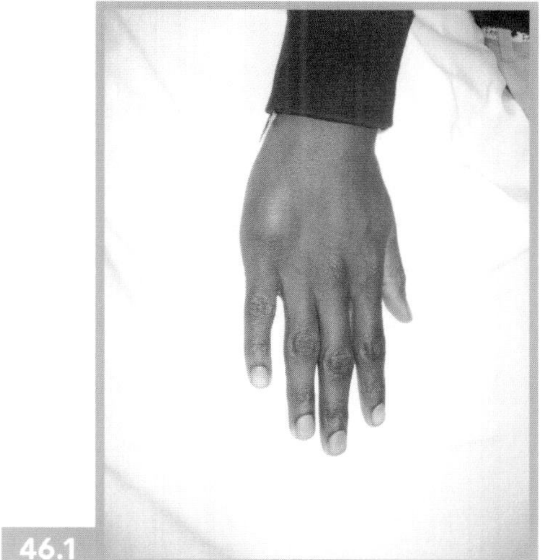

46.1

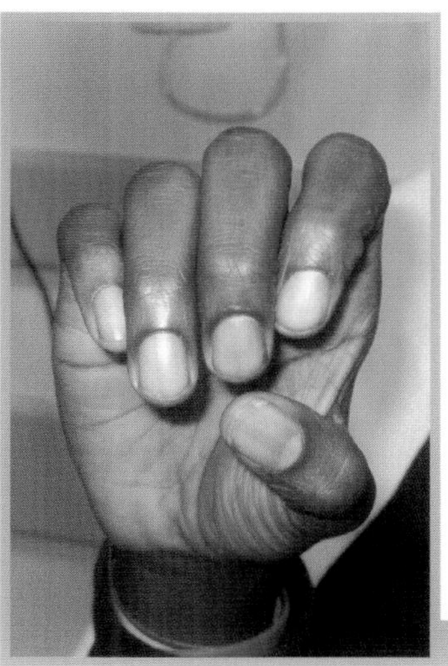

46.2

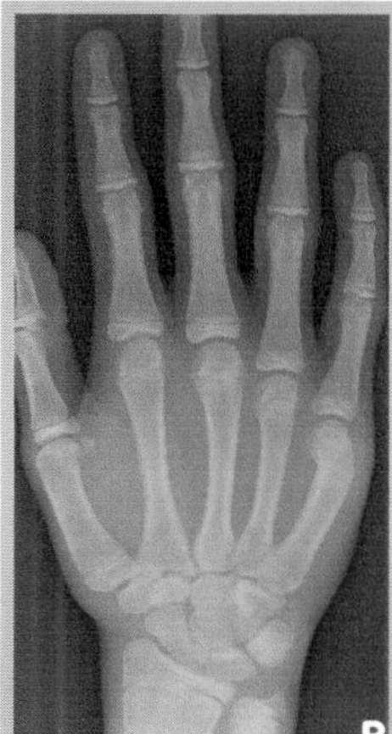

46.3

What do the above images display?

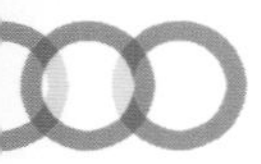

Answer

There is a transverse fracture to the neck of the fifth metacarpal. This type of fracture is referred to as a "boxer's fracture."

The most common metacarpal fracture occurs at the neck of the bone. The majority of fractures involve the fifth metacarpal. It is important to inspect the injuries for any skin trauma that might indicate an open fracture. Commonly used is the "10°, 20°, 30°, 40° rule" for metacarpal fractures. This refers to acceptable angulation of 10° for the second metacarpal progressing through each subsequent metacarpal to 40° of angulation for the fifth metacarpal. For fractures that exceed the tolerable amount of angulation, closed reduction is generally all that is required. Long-term function is preserved in the majority of cases despite a considerable amount of angulation of the fracture.

Keywords: extremity injury, blunt trauma, orthopedics, hand injury

Bibliography

Fleisher GR, Ludwig S, eds. *Textbook of Pediatric Emergency Medicine*. 6th ed. Philadelphia: Lippincott Williams & Wilkins, 2010.

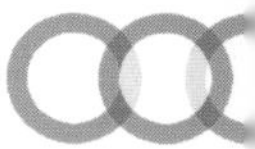

CASE 47

Michael Gottlieb

Questions

A 14-year-old boy with no significant past medical history presents with a splinter to his left third and fourth fingers sustained while helping his father move some wood in the backyard. He has no other injuries and his immunizations are up to date. His exam demonstrates a visible foreign body in both fingers. He is neurovascularly intact distally.

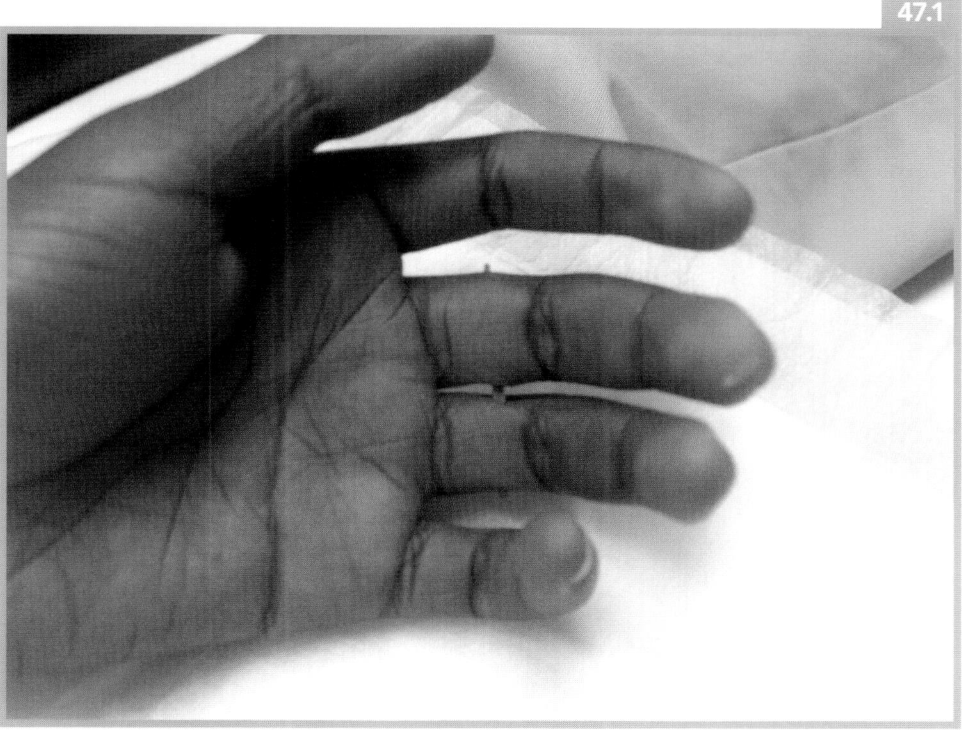

47.1

1. What imaging modalities are available to help identify foreign bodies?
2. Is antibiotic prophylaxis required after removal of foreign bodies?

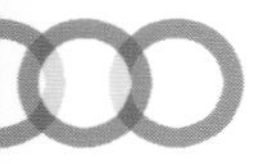

Answers

1. Although it is important to thoroughly inspect the area for retained foreign bodies, most experts recommend the addition of formal imaging to confirm that no foreign bodies are missed. The most common imaging modality is radiography. This may identify many retained foreign bodies and is ideal for those that are radiopaque (e.g. bones, teeth, metal, gravel). Ultrasound may also be used to visualize foreign bodies and is particularly valuable for those that are radiolucent (e.g. wood) or very small. Ultrasound may also be used to assist with localization and removal in real time. Computed tomography may be used in patients with a high suspicion for retained foreign body when alternate imaging is negative, but should be used sparingly due to the significant increase in radiation.
2. Infection rates are very low after successful removal of foreign bodies and, generally, prophylactic antibiotics are not indicated. The most common cause for subsequent infection is due to missed foreign bodies (especially organic foreign bodies), emphasizing the importance of identifying and removing these on the initial visit. The exception to this is with human bite wounds or bite wounds to the hand, as these may benefit from prophylactic antibiotics. It is also important to ensure that the tetanus status is up to date and provide tetanus prophylaxis if indicated.

Keywords: foreign body, penetrating trauma, hand injury, ultrasound

Bibliography

Halaas GW. Management of foreign bodies in the skin. *Am Fam Physician* September 1, 2007;76(5):683–8.

Lammers RL, Magill T. Detection and management of foreign bodies in soft tissue. *Emerg Med Clin North Am* November 1992;10(4):767–81.

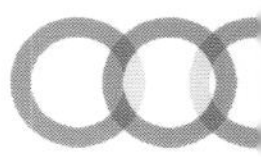

CASE 48

Michael Gottlieb

Questions

A 17-year-old girl presents with left fifth-digit pain. She was playing softball when the ball struck her finger, causing instant pain and a visible deformity. She denies any other injuries. There are no open wounds. She is neurologically intact and has good capillary refill distally. The radiographs are displayed next.

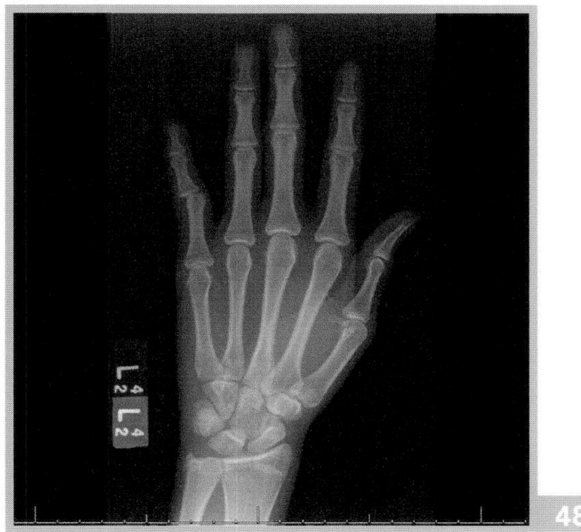

48.1

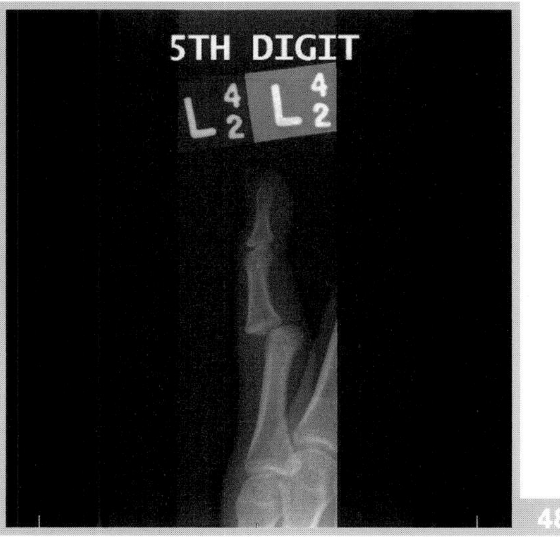

48.2

1. How is the reduction performed?
2. After the reduction, how is the finger stabilized?

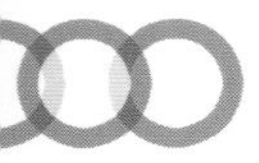

Answers

1. This patient has a dorsal dislocation of the fifth proximal interphalangeal joint (PIPJ). Reduction is performed by gently applying distal traction to the injured finger, while applying volar-directed pressure to the middle phalanx. The goal is to first separate the digits and then slide the dislocated digit back into place. Reduction is usually obvious on clinical examination and can be confirmed with a post-reduction radiograph.
2. Traditionally, the dislocated finger is splinted in 30° of flexion for one week, followed by buddy taping for another 1–2 weeks with early range of motion exercises. Prolonged immobility may lead to joint stiffness.

Keywords: hand injury, procedures, orthopedics

Bibliography

Borchers JR, Best TM. Common finger fractures and dislocations. *Am Fam Physician* April 15, 2012;85(8):805–10.

Leggit JC, Meko CJ. Acute finger injuries: Part II. Fractures, dislocations, and thumb injuries. *Am Fam Physician* March 1 2006;73(5):827–34.

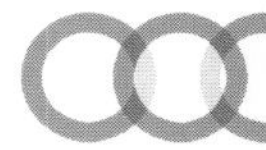

CASE 49

Diana Yan

Question

A healthy 6-year-old girl presents to the emergency department after falling while playing at an art museum about an hour ago. She reportedly tripped and fell on her outstretched arm. After falling, she immediately started to cry and her mother noticed a deformity of her right forearm. Her mother has seen her move her fingers, but she is refusing to move her arm, complaining of pain in the right forearm. The event was witnessed and there was no head trauma and loss of consciousness.

Physical exam shows an alert and awake girl who is calm if she stays in her mother's lap. There is a gross deformity of her right forearm. She can move her fingers well and has sensation in her fingers. Her hand is well perfused with capillary refill <2 seconds.

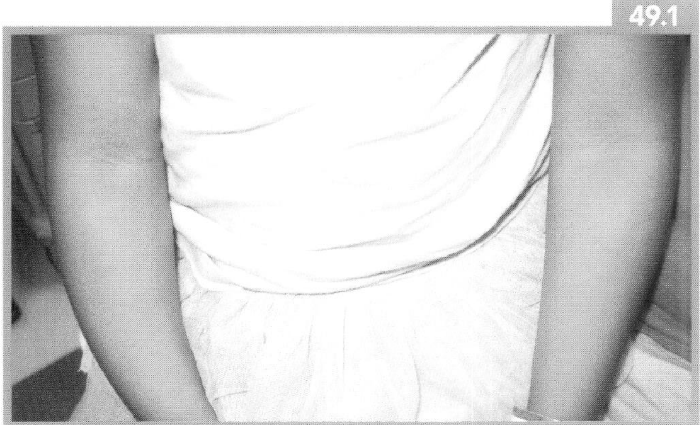

49.1

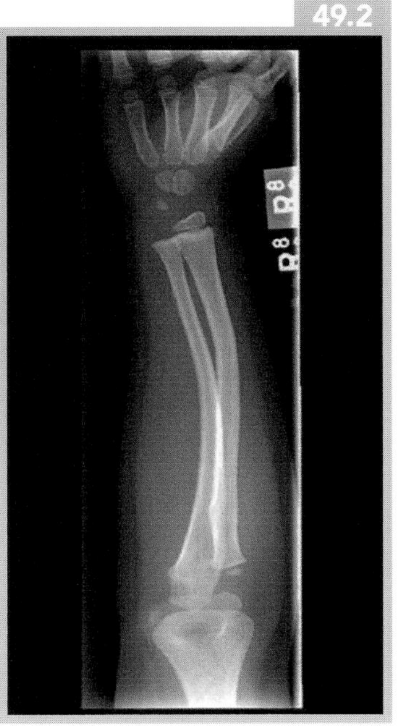

49.2

What is this type of fracture called and what is the most appropriate treatment?

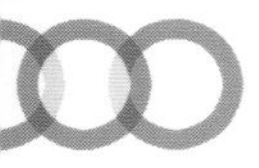

Answer

This is a greenstick fracture, which is ideally treated with closed reduction. Greenstick fractures tend to occur in children aged 5–14 years, when the bones are softer and more flexible. They are considered incomplete fractures as the bone bends and the fractures do not transverse the outer cortex of the bone. This plastic deformity usually occurs due to a torsional injury and is managed through closed reduction and cast immobilization. After initial casting, serial clinical and radiographic studies are recommended.

With the recent attention toward decreasing radiation exposure in children, several studies have re-examined how many post-reduction radiographs are needed and have explored other imaging modalities. In one retrospective study of 109 patients aged 2–15 years with forearm greenstick fractures, it was shown that pediatric greenstick fractures rarely needed to be manipulated after initial closed reduction. In the study, the authors proposed only getting two post-reduction films: one at week 2 and another at week 6. Others have explored the role of ultrasound in the diagnosis of distal forearm fractures as a way to further reduce radiation exposure. Herren et al. (2015) showed in a prospective study of 201 patients aged 4–11 years with distal forearm fractures (32% were greenstick fractures) that ultrasound had a 99.5% specificity and sensitivity in the diagnosis of distal forearm fractures. Ultrasound diagnosis of fracture includes the detection of a periosteal hematoma or detachment of the periosteum/cortical gap or bulge. It is also able to detect soft tissue injury, which x-ray cannot.

Keywords: orthopedics, extremity injury, procedures, ultrasound

Bibliography

Herren C, Sobottke R, Ringe MJ, Visel D, Graf M, Müller D, Siewe J. Ultrasound-guided diagnosis of fractures of the distal forearm in children. *Orthop Traumatol: Surg Res* 2015;101:501–5.

Ting BL, Kalish LA, Waters PM, Bae DS. Reducing cost and radiation exposure during the treatment of pediatric greenstick fractures of the forearm. *J Pediatr Orthop* 2016;36:816–20.

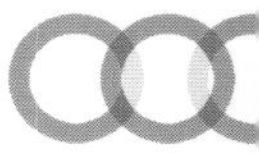

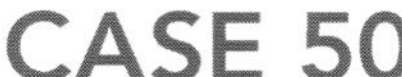

CASE 50

Michael Gottlieb

Questions

A 14-year-old boy presents to the emergency department with left knee pain after a sudden turn while playing soccer. He immediately fell to the ground and has not been ambulatory since. He denies any other injuries. He is neurologically intact and has good pulses distally. A radiograph was obtained at triage and is displayed next.

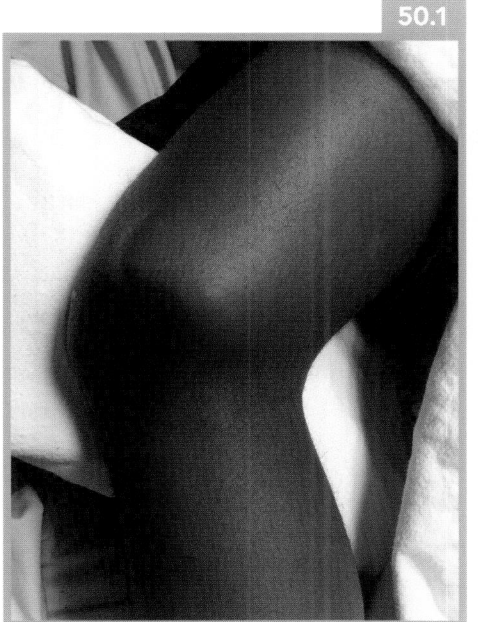

50.1

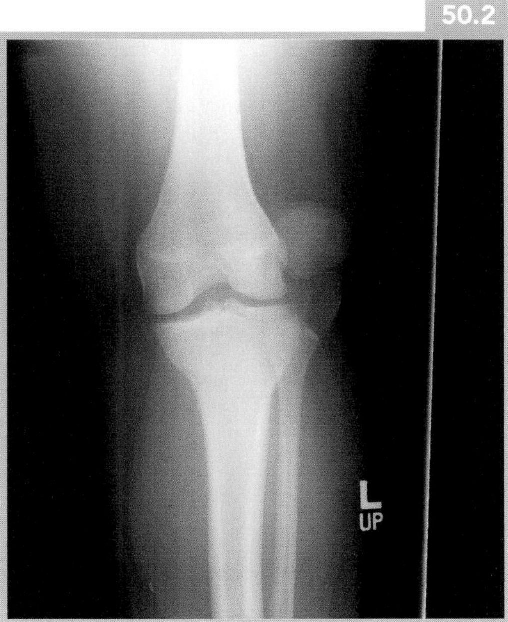

50.2

1. What is the diagnosis and treatment for this condition?
2. How is the reduction performed?

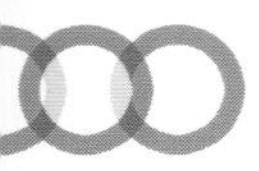

Answers

1. This patient is presenting with an acute patellar dislocation. This classically occurs with either direct trauma to the patella or a sudden twisting movement of the lower leg, and is more common in children due to the increased ligamentous laxity. This is a clinical diagnosis and requires rapid reduction, and many practitioners perform this reduction without radiographic confirmation. After discharge, patients should be referred to an orthopedic surgeon or sports medicine specialist for follow-up.

2. Reduction is performed by gentle knee extension with anteromedial or anterolateral pressure for lateral or medial dislocations, respectively. Although the reduction is fairly rapid and easy to perform, it is important to provide adequate analgesia for patient comfort and cooperation.

Keywords: extremity injury, orthopedics, procedures

Bibliography

Krause EA, Lin CW, Ortega HW, Reid SR. Pediatric lateral patellar dislocation: Is there a role for plain radiography in the emergency department? *J Emerg Med* June 2013;44(6):1126–31.

Lu DW, Wang EE, Self WH, Kharasch M. Patellar dislocation reduction. *Acad Emerg Med* February 2010;17(2):226.

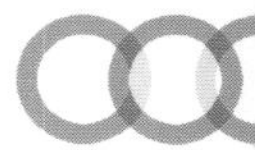

CASE 51

Michael Gottlieb

Questions

An 11-year-old boy presents with left hip pain after a motor vehicle collision. He was the restrained front passenger and denies head trauma or loss of consciousness. On exam, his left hip is shortened and internally rotated. His sensation, strength, pulses, and capillary refill are normal distally. A radiograph is obtained and presented next.

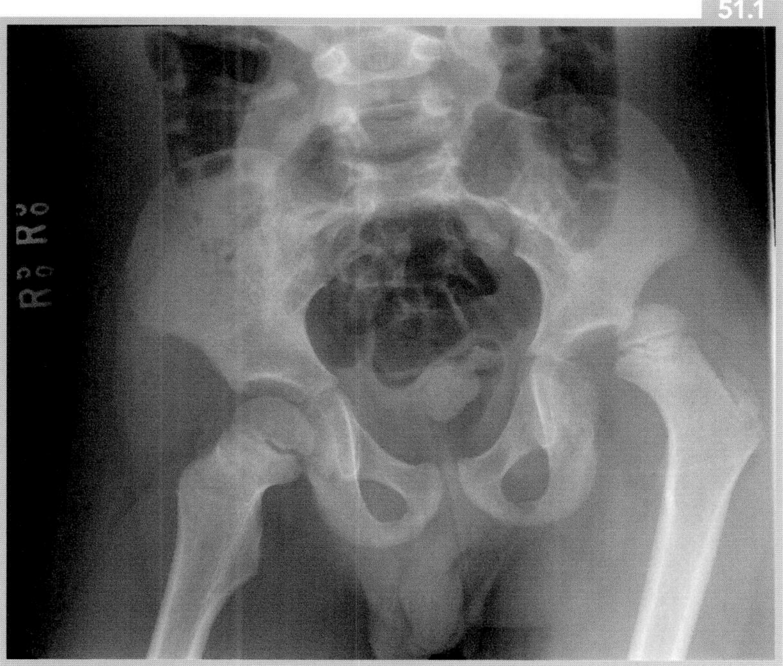

51.1

1. What are some potential complications of this injury?
2. What are some reduction techniques for this injury?

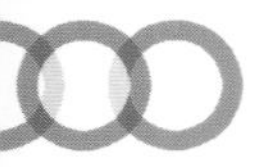

Answers

1. This patient is presenting with a hip dislocation. Clinically, these can be distinguished from femur fractures by noting that femur fractures present with the leg shortened and in external rotation, whereas hip dislocations present with the leg shortened and in internal rotation. Dislocations can be associated with sciatic or femoral nerve injuries, as well as an increased risk of early osteoarthritis. Early reduction is essential, as prolonged time spent dislocated increases the risk of avascular necrosis of the femoral head. This complication is more common in children with open physes, as in this case.

2. Unless a fracture is identified, reduction should be promptly performed in the emergency department to reduce the risk of avascular necrosis. Children with open physes should be managed in consultation with an orthopedic surgeon. The Allis technique involves the provider standing on the bed with the patient's hip and knee flexed. The provider lifts upward, while gently internally and externally rotating at the hip joint. A newer technique (referred to as the "Captain Morgan technique") involves the provider placing his or her knee underneath the supine patient's flexed knee and lifting up with the provider's calf while gently internally and externally rotating at the hip joint. This latter technique is preferable as it reduces the potential risk of injury to the provider.

Keywords: orthopedics, extremity injury, pitfalls, procedures

Bibliography

Stein MJ, Kang C, Ball V. Emergency department evaluation and treatment of acute hip and thigh pain. *Emerg Med Clin North Am* 2015 May;33(2):327–43.

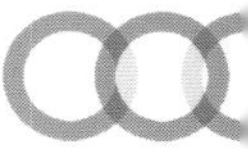

CASE 52

Kevin R. Schwartz

Question

A toddler with no significant past medical history loses her mitten while in freezing weather with her mother. The missing mitten was not noticed for several minutes. Hours later, her mother notes swollen fingers and brings her to the emergency department.

On exam, her vital signs are normal. She is awake and alert, and her exam is significant for the hand findings shown here, after active rewarming of the hands is completed.

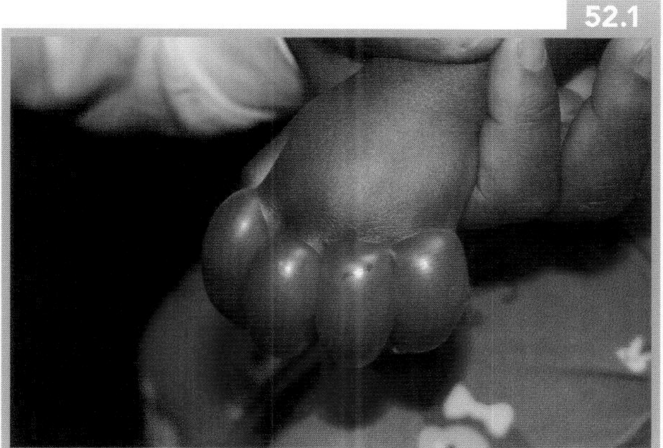

52.1

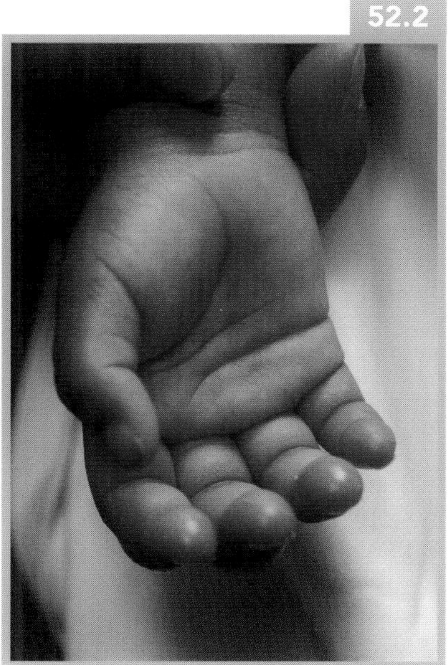

52.2

What are the recommendations for rewarming of frostbitten extremities? What additional treatments should be considered acutely and, when is surgical intervention required?

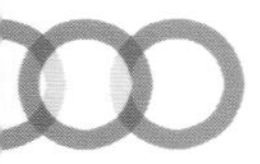

Answer

This patient has frostbite. Frostbite damages tissue by two mechanisms: (a) direct cellular damage from extracellular ice crystal formation with cell membrane damage causing intracellular dehydration and (b) epidermal ischemia as a consequence of inflammatory mediator release, endothelial injury, and emboli in the microvasculature causing progressive microvascular thrombosis and hypoxia to affected tissues.

Frostbite can be classified into four degrees:

1. First degree—characterized by a numb central whitish plaque with surrounding skin erythema
2. Second degree—characterized by blisters with milky or clear fluid and surrounding erythema
3. Third degree—characterized by hemorrhagic blisters over nonperfused skin with severe edema
4. Fourth degree—characterized by hard, woody, blue-gray, insensate tissue

First- and second-degree frostbite are considered superficial and, with proper care, likely to heal without tissue loss, whereas prognosis for third- and fourth-degree injuries is less favorable.

Management of frostbite in the field involves taking precautions to avoid warming/refreezing of the affected area and avoiding mechanical trauma to affected skin, both of which significantly increase tissue damage. In the emergency department, rapid rewarming using a water bath with a mild antibacterial agent added (povidone-iodine or chlorhexidine) at 38°–40°C is recommended. The extremity should be immersed until thawing is complete, usually between 15 and 30 minutes. Opiates are often required to control discomfort during rewarming. NSAIDs (usually ibuprofen) should be initiated for pain control and anti-inflammatory properties. Prophylactic antibiotics are controversial and not recommended as a standard approach.

There is emerging evidence that tissue plasminogen activator (TPA) administration can potentially decrease tissue damage and significantly lower subsequent amputation rates in severe frostbite. TPA should be considered in cases of severe frostbite which have occurred within 24 hours of presentation, have not undergone a freeze–thaw cycle, and where no other contraindications to TPA (e.g. bleeding, neurologic impairment) exist. Centers without capacity for TPA should consider transfer to a facility at which it can be administered.

Early amputation should be avoided unless overwhelming infection or wet gangrene is present. In general, most guidelines recommend allowing tissue to fully mummify (sometimes taking 1–3 months) prior to undertaking surgical debridement/amputation and closure. MRA (magnetic resonance angiography) and bone scan have emerged as modalities for helping to determine prognosis for limb salvage and may be used in surgical planning.

Keywords: environmental injuries, hand injury, medications, dermatology

Bibliography

Handford C, Thomas O, Imray CH. Frostbite. *Emerg Med Clin N Am* 2017;35:281–99.
Hutchison RL. Frostbite of the hand. *J Hand Surg Am* 2014;39:1863–8.

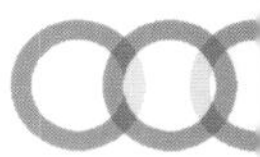

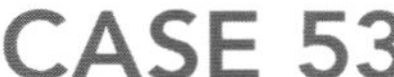

CASE 53

Alisa McQueen

Question

An almost 2-year-old, otherwise healthy, is in the emergency department with a rash on his cheeks.

He's afebrile, playful, looks well, and, indeed, has a bright red indurated but non-tender rash on his cheeks, captured in the following photograph.

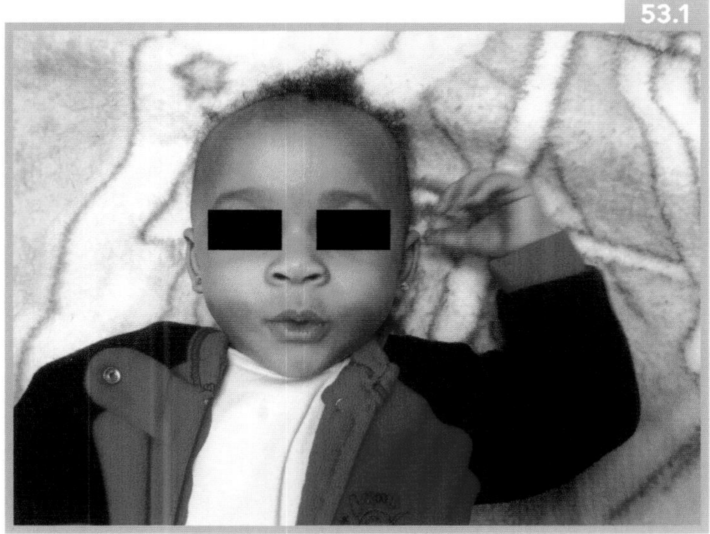

53.1

What historical question can you ask his family that will lead you to the diagnosis?

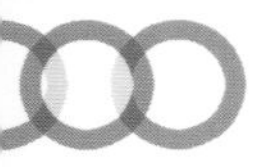

Answer

This is cold panniculitis, also called "popsicle panniculitis" thought to be due to subcutaneous fat necrosis in response to prolonged cold exposure. The erythema and induration typically appears 24–48 hours after exposure. This toddler had been sucking on a popsicle the day before. Cold panniculitis occurs only in the young, whose subcutaneous fat has a higher concentration of saturated fatty acids which crystalize with cold temperature. No treatment is required, and no skin scarring is expected; however, children who develop the condition are prone to recurrence.

Keywords: head and neck/ENT, dermatology, mimickers, environmental injuries

Bibliography

Day S, Klein BL. Popsicle panniculitis. *Pediatr Emerg Care* 1992;8(2):91–3.

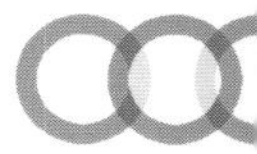

CASE 54

Veena Ramaiah

Question

A 3-year-old presents with blood in underwear and a laceration in her genitourinary area. Patient told her mom that she was playing with her 7- and 5-year-old brothers and they were sliding down a pole (a rod from a window shade) they had set up from the bed to the floor. There were hard plastic blocks on the ground near the end of the pole. Mom thinks her daughter slid onto the hard blocks causing the laceration.

The patient is able to tolerate an exam in the supine frog-leg position. On exam, there is a perineal laceration that seems to extend up to the distal posterior vaginal wall. There is bleeding from the laceration but not from the inside of the vagina as far as you can tell.

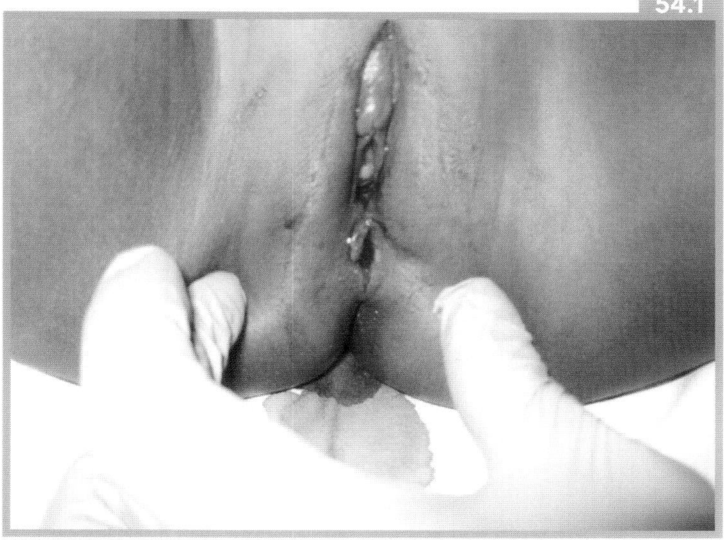

54.1

Is this a plausible explanation? What is your next step? How would you manage this laceration?

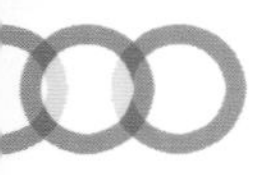

Answer

Genital lacerations are indicative of trauma to the genital area. It is plausible that this occurred from the child straddling an object forcefully—either impaling herself on the rod or falling forcefully on a hard object as it is primarily an external injury.

The concern of sexual abuse always exists with any genital injury. In order to increase the reliability of the history, the child should be interviewed separate from the caretakers, if verbal, to ask the events of the history.

This child was interviewed and reported getting hurt when she slid down the rod and fell. During a screening of sexual abuse history, she denied anyone hurting her or touching her.

Medically, an exam under sedation was arranged to ensure no intravaginal laceration, no extension into the rectum, and to repair the laceration.

In general, straddle injuries in females result in external injury. Most children fall forward so injury is often seen to the anterior structures such as the clitoris, the labia majora, and the fold between the labia majora and minora. Girls can also fall directly onto their perineum as in this case. Again the injury is primarily external and does not involve the hymenal tissue or the more internal structures.

Injuries from sexual abuse or assault are very uncommon overall—80%–90% of exams are normal—however, when they are present, they usually involve the posterior rim of the hymen (4 o'clock–8 o'clock) or the posterior fourchette.

Keywords: child abuse mimickers, genitourinary, blunt trauma

Bibliography

Adams JA, Kellogg ND, Farst KJ, Harper NS, Palusci VJ, Frasier LD, Levitt CJ, Shapiro RA, Moles RL, Starling SP. Updated guidelines for the medical assessment and care of children who may have been sexually abused. *J Pediatr Adolesc Gynecol* April 2016;29(2):81–7.

Saxena AK, Steiner M, Höllwarth ME. Straddle injuries in female children and adolescents: 10-year accident and management analysis. *Indian J Pediatr* August 2014;81(8):766–9.

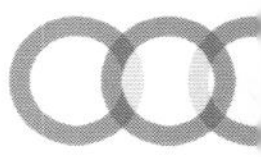

CASE 55

Kevin R. Schwartz

Question

A 13-year-old female with a seizure disorder was started on lamotrigine 2 weeks ago for seizure control. She presents to the emergency department with complaint of fever and rash. On exam, the patient is uncomfortable appearing with vital signs significant for fever to 38.4°C, HR 120, and skin findings as pictured.

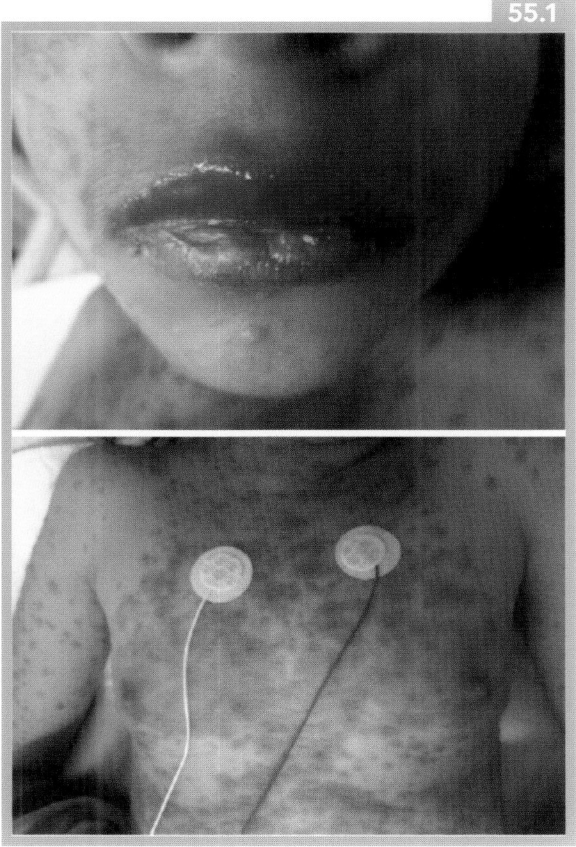

55.1

What is the diagnosis and with which medications is it most likely associated?

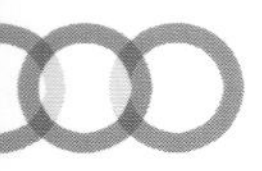

Answer

This is a case of Stevens-Johnson syndrome (SJS). SJS is classically characterized by a rash consisting of erythematous macules with dark, purpuric centers which progress to bullae and eventually begin to slough. The rash often starts on the face and chest as pictured here and spreads thereafter. Mucocutaneous involvement of the mouth/lips (shown here), eyes and/or urogenital system is present in >90% of cases. SJS exists on a continuum with toxic epidermal necrolysis (TEN) where the former involves <10% of total body surface area (TBSA) skin detachment and the latter >30%.

The medications commonly used in pediatrics which are most associated with SJS include several antiepileptics (lamotrigine, carbamazepine, phenobarbital, and phenytoin) and the antibiotic trimethoprim-sulfamethoxazole. Many other drugs have also been associated with SJS, though less commonly, including beta-lactam antibiotics, cephalosporins, flouroquinolones, and a number of NSAIDs.

The most crucial aspects of treatment are withdrawal of the causative agent and assiduous supportive wound care, often in a burn center. IVIG (intravenous immunoglobulin) steroids and other immunosuppressant agents have been trialed, with evidence for their benefit not yet clearly established. Mortality is as high as 10% in SJS and 30% in TEN.

Keywords: drug reactions, do not miss, dermatology

Bibliography

Ferrandiz-Pulido C, Garcia-Patos V. A review of causes of Stevens-Johnson syndrome and toxic epidermal necrolysis in children. *Arch Dis Child* 2013;98(12):998–1003.

Mockenhaupt M, Viboud C, Dunant A. Stevens-Johnson syndrome and toxic epidermal necrolysis: Assessment of medication risks with emphasis on recently marketed drugs. The EuroSCAR-study. *J Invest Dermatol* 2008;128(1):35–42.

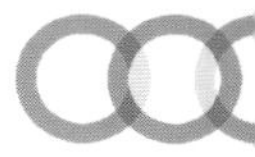

CASE 56

Lauren Allister

Question

A 19-year-old male college student arrives in the emergency department having felt unwell for 1 day with subjective fevers, malaise, and a small area of rash initially localized to his left elbow. He has noted that the rash has begun to spread down his arm over the past few hours.

On exam, the patient is awake, alert, and conversant. His vitals on arrival are T 100°F, HR 130, BP 133/60, RR 20, O_2 100% RA. His physical exam is notable for a tired but non-toxic appearance, some mild neck and muscle pains, and the rash on his left upper extremity, shown here.

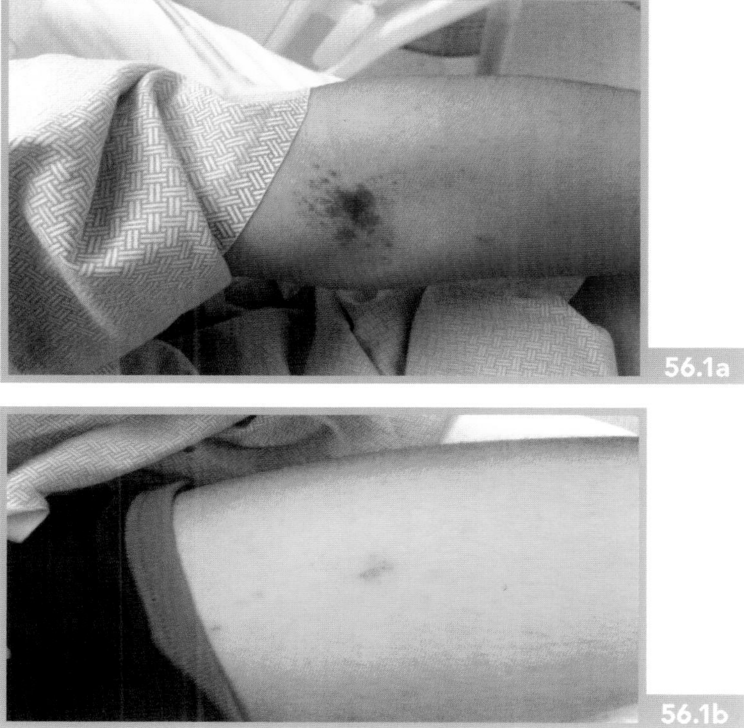

56.1a

56.1b

Is this patient's rash of concern? What are the next immediate steps in the evaluation of this patient?

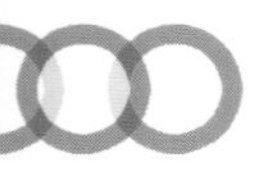

Answer

Any patient with the acute onset of a febrile illness with a petechial rash and meningococcal illness should be on a differential diagnosis. This patient's rash, in conjunction with the patient's age, his residence in a college dormitory, and other constitutional symptoms, is concerning for an evolving *Neisseria meningitidis* infection.

Neisseria meningitidis is a common cause of community-acquired bacterial meningitis in children and adults. *Neisseria meningitidis* is carried in the nasal passages and is spread through inhalation of aerosolized particles, making living in close quarters (such as college dormitories) an ideal environment for disease spread. *Neisseria meningitidis* can produce a range of clinical symptoms, from fever and bacteremia to fulminant disease with death possible within hours of onset.

Prompt recognition and rapid initiation of antibiotics are the cornerstones of care for *Neisseria meningitidis* infection. Identification is key in initiating treatment to prevent long-term sequelae, which include limb loss, hearing loss, skin scarring, neurologic deficits, and death. The overall case fatality is approximately 10%–15% and is as high as 25%–30% in patients with meningococcemia (Cohn and MacNeil, 2015). Once *Neisseria meningitidis* is suspected, antibiotics should be administered within 30 minutes (Tunkel et al., 2010).

Of note, this patient had received one of the available meningococcal vaccines prior to his college matriculation. While most commercially available vaccines cover against the serotypes Y and C, which make up the majority of *Neisseria meningitidis* infections, this patient's organism was serotype B.

Keywords: infectious diseases, life-threatening, do not miss

References

Cohn A, MacNeil J. The changing epidemiology of meningococcal disease. *Infect Dis Clin North Am* December 2015;29(4):667–77.

Tunkel AR, van de Beek D, Scheld WM. Acute meningitis. In *Principles and Practice of Infectious Diseases*, 7th ed., Mandell GL, Bennett JE, Dolin R, eds. Philadelphia: Churchill Livingstone, 2010:1189.

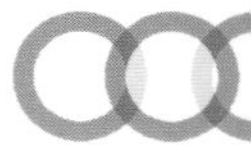

CASE 57

Kevin R. Schwartz

Question

A 17-year-old boy from Massachusetts presents in late summer to the emergency department with the rash pictured here. He has no other complaints. On exam he has several erythematous, flat lesions shown here. He's otherwise well-appearing with no tachycardia, work of breathing, joint pain, or swelling. An EKG is obtained and is pictured here.

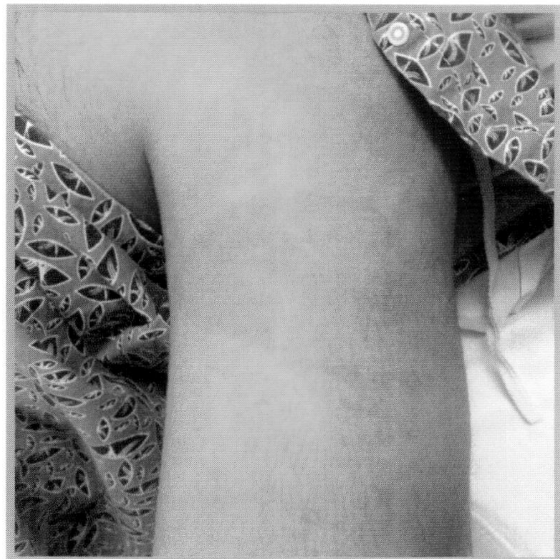

57.1

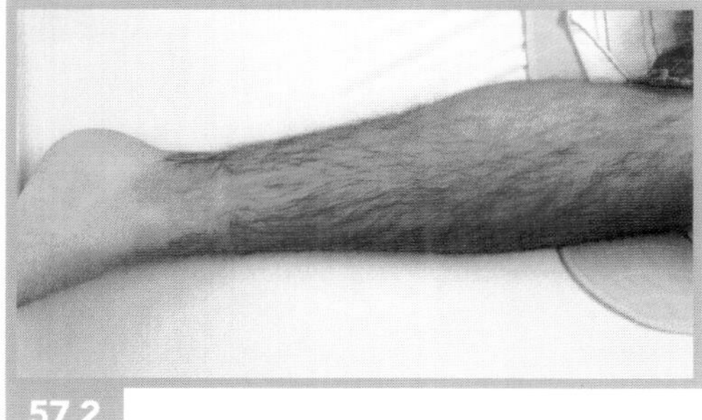

57.2

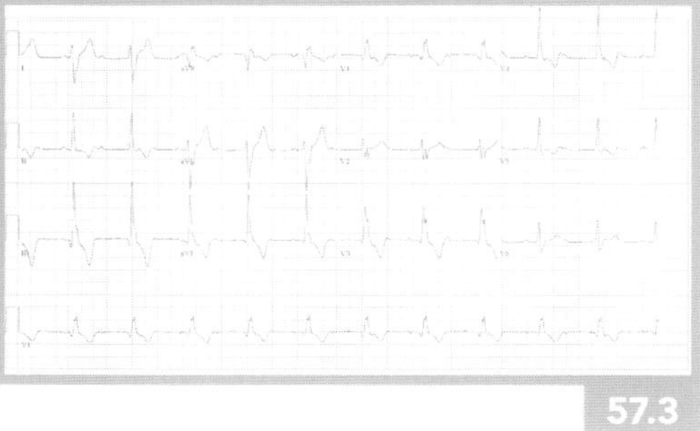

57.3

What are the cardiac manifestations of this diagnosis and during which stage of illness do they occur?

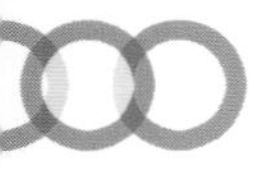

Answer

The patient has Lyme disease, as characterized by the classic erythema migrans lesions on his skin. Lyme disease, a bacterial infection caused by the spirochete *Borrelia burgdorferi* (United States), *Borrelia afzelii*, and *Borrelia garinii* (Europe and Asia), is transmitted through the bite of the *Ixodes* deer tick and has three stages:

1. Early localized disease—This is characterized by an erythema migrans rash at the site of a tick bite, generally within 2 weeks of the bite and may be accompanied by fever, headache, fatigue, arthralgias, and myalgias. Serologic testing for disease is often negative at this stage. (See also Case 79.)
2. Early disseminated disease—This stage is characterized by multiple erythema migrans rashes as well as the systemic signs pictured occurring weeks to months after the initial tick bite. Meningitis, cranial nerve palsies (especially CN VII), and carditis (usually characterized by atrioventricular [AV] block) may occur in this stage of illness.
3. Late disease—Occurs weeks to months after untreated initial infection. This is characterized by arthritis (>90% involving the knee). Fever is uncommon at this stage.

Lyme carditis seen in early disseminated Lyme disease causing AV block may progress from first-degree to second- and third-degree AV block (as pictured here) rapidly and unpredictably. For patients with first-degree heart block and a PR interval >300 ms or second- or third-degree AV block, inpatient management is recommended.

Keywords: dermatology, rash, cardiology

Bibliography

Kimberlin D, Brady MT, Jackson MA, Long SS et al. *Red Book: Report of the Committee on Infectious Diseases.* 30th ed. Elk Grove Village, IL: American Academy of Pediatrics, 2015.

Robinson ML, Kobayashi T, Higgins Y, Calkins H, Melia MT. Lyme carditis. *Infect Dis Clin North Am* 2015;29(2):255–68.

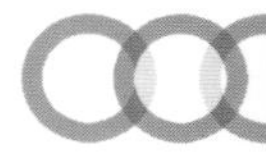

CASE 58

Lauren Allister

Question

A 14-year-old African American female with a history of eczema presents to the emergency department with pain, swelling, and purulent discharge from her scalp. One month prior to presentation, she had a hair weave placed at a salon. She had some initial pain after placement which subsided, but over the past week increasing pain and pruritus. A family member removed the weave yesterday and noted swelling and a foul-smelling discharge.

On exam, she is awake and alert but uncomfortable. Her exam is notable for the appearance of her scalp, shown in the photograph.

58.1

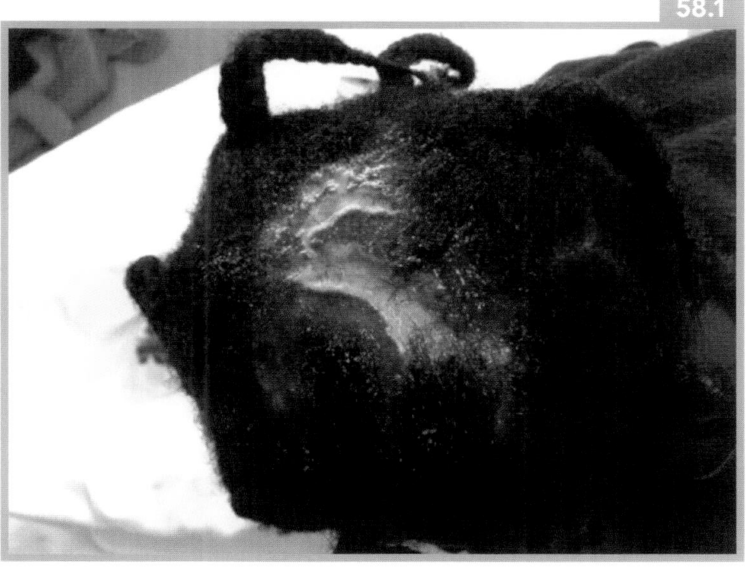

What is the explanation for this dramatic presentation? How should she be treated and what are the long-term outcomes?

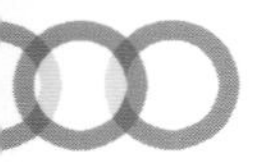

Answer

This patient's history and exam is consistent with dissecting cellulitis of the scalp (DCS). This dermatologic condition is predominantly seen with specific hair grooming practices, such as the use of chemical relaxers, heat straightening, tight braiding, and weaving, which can cause scalp irritation and follicular damage.

The pathogenesis of DCS involves initial follicular occlusion followed by a combination of infection and traumatic forces driving formation of inflammatory pustules, fluctuant cysts and abscesses, suppurative nodules, and draining sinus tracts. Medical therapy is considered the first-line treatment and includes topical antibiotics, intralesional steroids, oral antibiotics, isotretinoin as monotherapy or in combination with rifampin, and oral prednisone. Other principles of care include optimizing wound care and educating patients about possible sequelae of these grooming practices. Long-term consequences include disfigurement, permanent hair loss, emotional distress, and decreased quality of life.

Keywords: dermatology, skin and soft tissue infections

Bibliography

Madu P, Kundu RV. Follicular and scarring disorders in skin of color: Presentation and management. *Am J Clin Dermatol* August 2014;15(4):307–21.

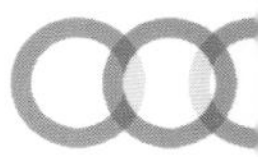

CASE 59

Kevin R. Schwartz

Question

A 5-year-old boy presents to the emergency department with fever, vomiting, and alteration in consciousness. He returned from a trip to Nigeria visiting family 2 weeks previously. On exam he is somnolent, pale, with a palpable liver. A peripheral blood smear is sent and is pictured here.

59.1

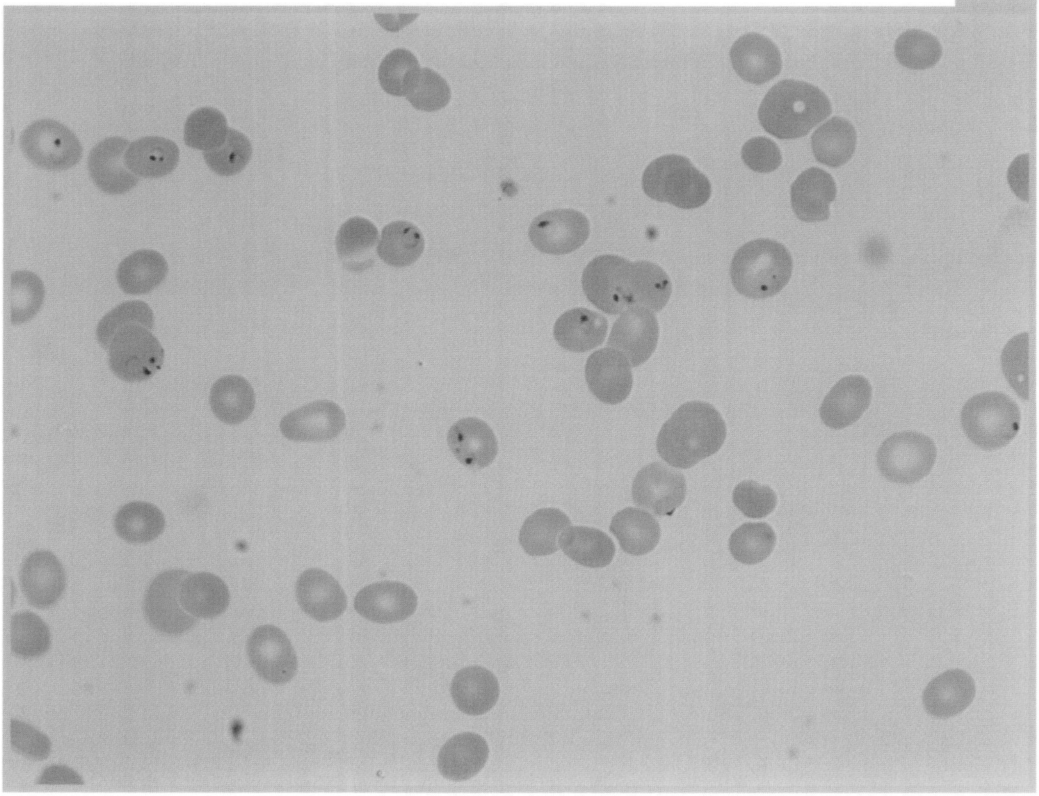

What is the diagnosis, in whom should it be considered, and what are the treatment priorities in the emergency department?

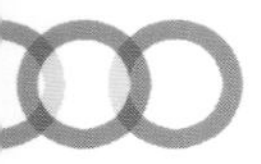

Answer

The pictured blood smear demonstrates intracellular parasites within the red blood cells. Given the patient's recent travel to West Africa, malaria is the most likely diagnosis. The patient's significantly altered mental status suggests cerebral malaria. Cerebral malaria is defined by impaired consciousness, delirium, and/or seizures in the setting of known or suspected malaria infection. Without treatment, cerebral malaria is nearly always fatal.

Plasmodium falciparum represents the most lethal form of malaria and is most often associated with cerebral malaria. The incubation period is generally 12–14 days and almost all cases will present within 30 days of exposure. This diagnosis should be considered in any traveler from a malaria-endemic area presenting with fever within 30 days of their return.

Prompt parenteral anti-malarial therapy should be initiated for severe malaria with either artesunate or, if this is unavailable, quinine or quinidine. Respiratory support ranging from supplemental oxygen to mechanical ventilation may be required. Hypoglycemia is common and should be assessed for and treated. Seizures occur in a majority of cases and should be treated with benzodiazepines. Anemia is a common associated symptom and should be addressed with PRBCs (packed red blood cells) transfusion, in general for Hb <7 gm/dL.

Keywords: infectious diseases, do not miss, fever

Bibliography

White NJ, Pukrittayakamee S, Hien TT. Malaria. *Lancet* 2014;383(9918):723–35.

World Health Organization. *Guidelines for the Treatment of Malaria*. 3rd ed. Geneva: WHO, 2015.

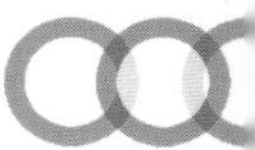

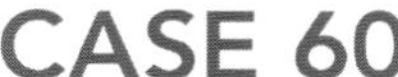

CASE 60

Kevin R. Schwartz

Question

A 5-year-old girl presents with fever, back pain, and difficulty walking. On exam, she is febrile, tachycardic, and uncomfortable appearing. Her neurologic exam is notable for reduced strength in both lower extremities and hyperreflexic deep tendon patellar reflexes.

What is the differential diagnosis for back pain with fever in a child, and what testing and imaging are indicated in the emergency department?

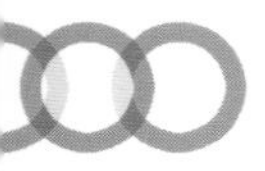

Answer

While back pain is a common complaint in adults, it is an uncommon symptom in children, especially younger children. Careful consideration should be given to a child with this complaint.

In a child with back pain and fever, discitis, vertebral osteomyelitis, and epidural abscess should be considered. Other diagnoses such as pneumonias and pyelonephritis may also present with back pain, but focal pain over the vertebral column is uncommon with these diagnoses.

Patients with discitis frequently may recover without antibiotics and often has an indolent course. Vertebral osteomyelitis presents in a similar fashion to osteomyelitis elsewhere.

It is critical to maintain a high index of suspicion for epidural abscess. Early surgical decompression may be necessary to preserving neurologic function. The classic presentation for epidural abscess is the triad of spinal pain, fever, and neurologic deficits; however, all three features are not always initially present.

For all of the aforementioned diagnoses, MRI is the imaging modality of choice and, when spinal epidural abscess is suspected, should be undertaken expeditiously. Labs including CBC (complete blood count), blood culture, chemistries, and inflammatory markers should be sent. Empiric antibiotic therapy including MRSA coverage should be initiated.

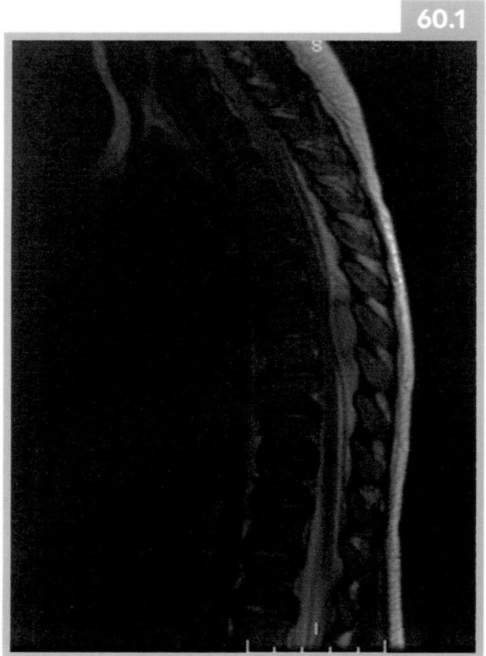
60.1

Keywords: infectious diseases, fever, neurosurgery, do not miss, MRI

Bibliography

Hawkins M, Bolton M. Pediatric spinal epidural abscess: A 9-year institutional review and review of the literature. *Pediatrics* 2013;132(6):e1680–5.

Payne WK, Ogilvie JW. Back pain in children and adolescents. *Pediatr Clin North Am* 1996;43(4):899–917.

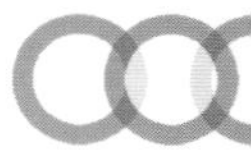

CASE 61

S. Margaret Paik

Questions

A 13-year-old boy is brought in by paramedics after falling onto his right knee during basketball practice. He is unable to fully extend his right knee or bear weight, and prefers to keep his right leg in flexion. A "gap" is noted in the middle of the patella and the patella appears to be high riding. Anteroposterior and lateral knee radiographs are shown next.

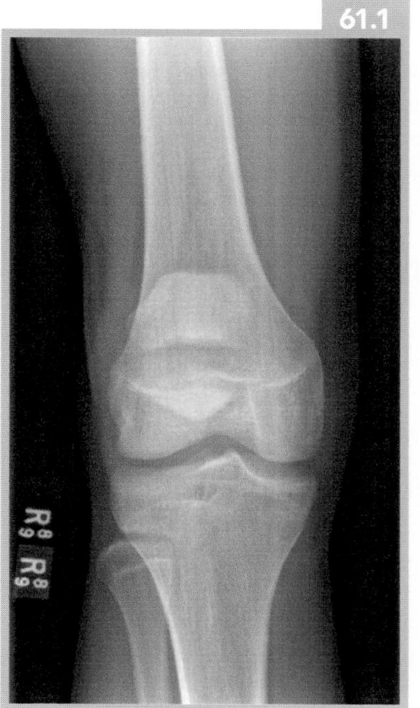

61.1

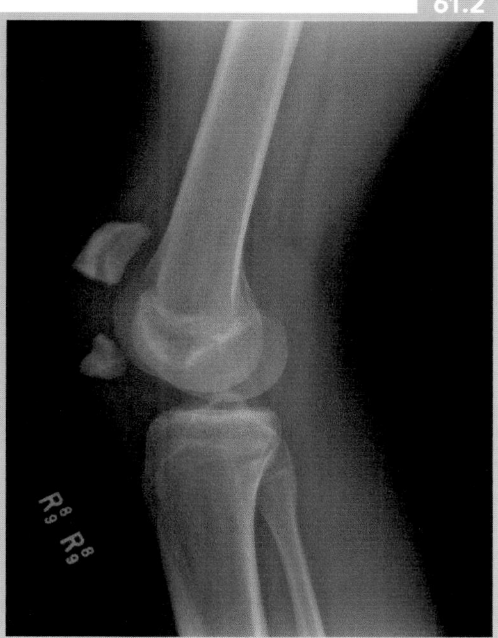

61.2

1. What are the two major mechanisms of injury?
2. How are fractures of the patella classified?

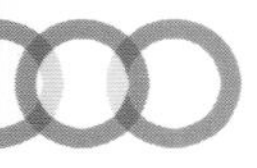

Answers

1. Patella fracture is the result of either direct trauma, such as a fall onto the knee, or an indirect trauma due to jumping or rapid flexion of knee against a fully contracted quadriceps muscle. Patella fractures are uncommon in the pediatric population. The low rate of injury is thought to be due to the thick cartilaginous layer that surrounds the patella during childhood and adolescence.

2. A transverse fracture is a fracture occurring in the medial-lateral plane. Vertical fractures occur in the superior-inferior direction and are very uncommon (see Case 20). Marginal fractures occur at the edge of the patella and do not disrupt the extensor mechanism. Fracture fragments separated by more than 3 mm are classified as displaced fractures and require operative intervention. A comminuted or stellate patella fracture has multiple fragments.

   Patella sleeve fractures account for approximately 50% of all patellar fractures and usually occur in patients between 8 and 12 years of age. The mechanism is an explosive acceleration with rapid quadriceps contraction while the knee is in flexion, resulting in avulsion of the periosteum, retinaculum, and cartilage from the patella. The lateral radiograph may show some swelling at the lower patellar pole and possibly a small bony fragment that has avulsed with the cartilage. Joint effusion is usually absent. MRI is critical for complete evaluation. Complications due to missed diagnosis or delay in presentation include avascular necrosis of inferior pole of the patella, patella alta, quadriceps wasting extensor lag, anterior knee pain, and ossification of the patellar tendon.

Keywords: orthopedics, extremity injury, blunt trauma

Bibliography

Carpenter JE, Kasman R, Matthews LS. Fractures of the patella. *J Bone Joint Surg Am* October 1993;75(10):1550–61.

Damrow DS, Van Valin SE. Patellar sleeve fracture with ossification of the patellar tendon. *Orthopedics* 2017;40(2):e357–9.

Ray JM, Hendrix J. Incidence, mechanism of injury and treatment of fractures of the patella in children. *J Trauma* April 1992;32(4):464–7.

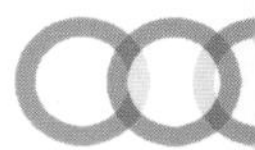

CASE 62

Lauren Allister

Question

A 6-year-old previously healthy male presents with persistent left-sided headache and neck pain. Three days ago, he had been hanging upside down on a door-mounted pull-up bar approximately 4–5 feet in the air when he fell straight down onto his head, landing on a hardwood floor. He had no loss of consciousness, upper extremity weakness, or paresthesias. He continued to complain of headache and neck pain, and was evaluated by his pediatrician the following day. At that time, his exam was notable for a left-sided torticollis, as well as a mild amount of lateral neck pain that was diagnosed as a muscle spasm. He was discharged home with acetaminophen and ibuprofen. The patient continued to complain of neck pain with worsening torticollis and decreasing activity, which prompted his emergency department visit.

On arrival to the emergency department, he was awake and interactive with stable vital signs. His exam was notable for left-sided torticollis, tenderness along the upper cervical spine, and paraspinal muscles bilaterally. His neurologic exam was completely intact.

Given his history of axial-load mechanism trauma and his findings on physical exam, a CT of the neck is ordered and is shown next.

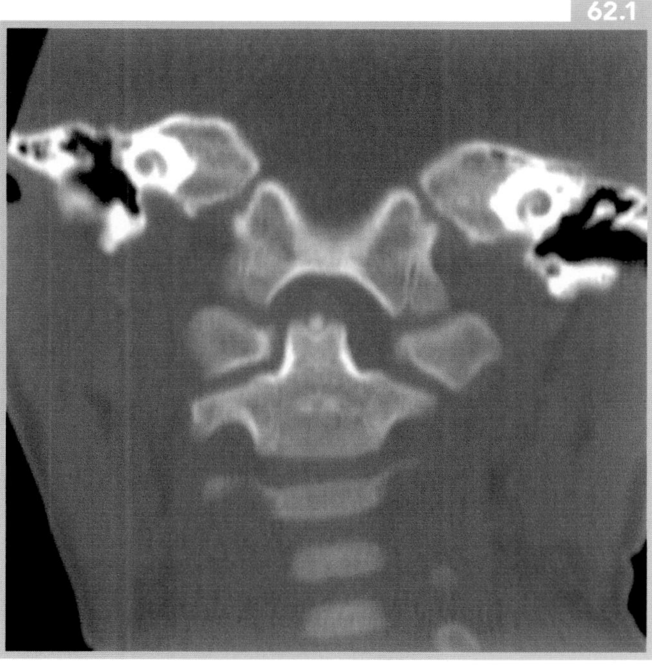

62.1

How common are these types of injuries in pediatric patients? How should this injury be managed at this time?

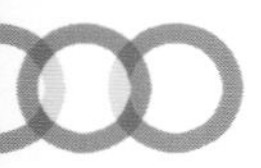

Answer

This CT demonstrates a mildly displaced, approximately 2–3 mm, fracture of the anterior C1 mass with associated left hinging/displacement.

Cervical spine injuries are rare in pediatric patients, with an incidence of 1%–1.5%. Some of the most common mechanisms of injury in pediatric patients are sports, motor vehicle collisions, falls from significant heights, and diving. In children under the age of 8, the upper cervical spine is more susceptible to injury, given certain anatomic features (a higher fulcrum) and more direct blunt mechanisms involving the head/upper cervical spine (Tilt et al., 2012). Upper cervical spine injuries carry a higher morbidity, including neurologic sequelae, and mortality, making prompt diagnosis imperative in a trauma evaluation.

This patient did not present with any neurologic symptoms. He was placed in cervical spine immobilization and followed closely as an outpatient. He did not require surgical intervention and recovered without sequelae.

Keywords: trauma, neurosurgery, neck injury, CT

Reference

Tilt L, Babineau J, Fenster D, Ahmad F, Roskind CG. Blunt cervical spine injury in children. *Curr Opin Pediatr* June 2012;24(3):301–6.

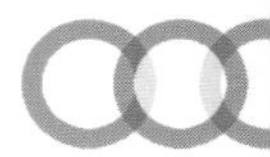

CASE 63

Lauren Allister

Question

An 18-year-old female with no past medical history presents with one day of mid- to lower-chest and left shoulder pain. She reports feeling mild pain early in the morning with worsening discomfort and associated left shoulder pain while taking an exam in school. There is some mild associated pain on inspiration without any other associated symptoms. She denies fever, cough, or trauma.

On examination, the patient is awake, alert, and conversant. Her vitals on arrival are T 98.7°F, HR 80, BP 118/60, RR 18, O_2 100% RA. Her physical exam is notable only for some mild mid-chest wall and upper abdominal discomfort with a soft abdomen; she has no lower abdominal pain, rebound, guarding, or organomegaly. She has a negative Murphy's sign. Her respiratory exam is clear with good aeration and no significant pleurisy. She has no reproducible left shoulder pain or limitation in range of motion.

Although her exam is reassuring, given her chest pain, an EKG and chest x-ray are ordered to evaluate for acute cardiopulmonary etiologies. Her EKG is normal for age. Her chest x-ray is shown.

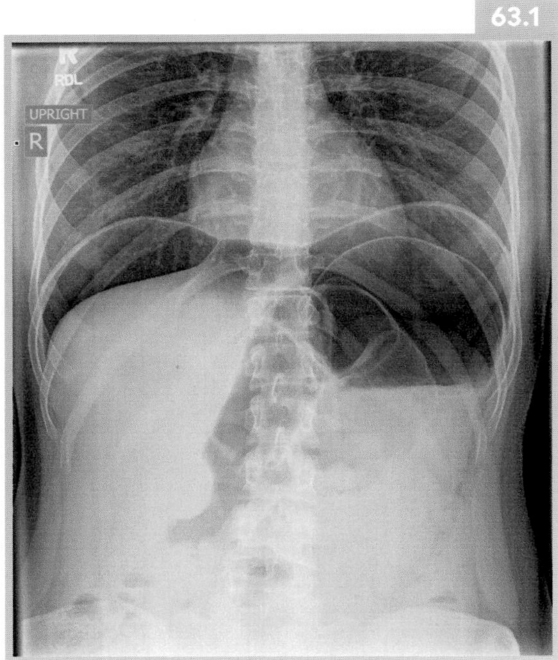

What is most notable about this chest x-ray? In hindsight, what clues in the patient's history could have led to this diagnosis? What are the immediate next steps in her emergency department evaluation?

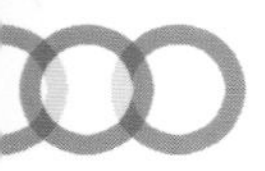

Answer

This patient's chest x-ray shows significant pneumoperitoneum consistent with bowel perforation. Given the emergent nature of this finding, pediatric surgery was consulted and the patient was taken immediately to the operating room (OR) for an exploratory laparotomy. There, she was found to have a 1 cm perforated gastric ulcer on the anterior wall of the stomach with leakage of gastric contents in the peritoneum.

Peptic ulcer disease is not common in children (Drumm et al., 1988) and perforation is an uncommon presenting symptom (Hua et al., 2007). Although acute abdominal pain may be a clinical manifestation of a perforated ulcer, symptoms of perforation may also include extra-abdominal symptoms, including chest pain and referred shoulder pain, from irritation of the diaphragm as in the case of this patient. For patients with a possible gastrointestinal complaint with any associated chest pain, perforation should always be suspected. Acute management includes making the patient NPO (nothing by mouth), initiating intravenous fluid resuscitation, starting broad-spectrum antibiotics, and surgical consultation.

Keywords: abdominal pain, acute abdomen, surgery

References

Drumm B, Rhoads JM, Stringer DA, Sherman PM, Ellis LE, Durie PR. Peptic ulcer disease in children: Etiology, clinical findings, and clinical course. *Pediatrics* September 1988;82(3 Pt 2):410–4.

Hua MC, Kong MS, Lai MW, Luo CC. Perforated peptic ulcer in children: A 20-year experience. *J Pediatr Gastroenterol Nutr* July 2007;45(1):71–4.

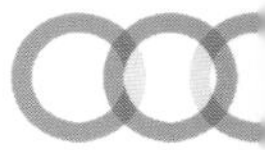

CASE 64

Lauren Allister

Questions

A 9-year-old female presents with one day of worsening abdominal pain, inability to ambulate secondary to pain, vomiting, and poor oral intake. Earlier in the week, she developed vomiting and diarrhea and was treated briefly with intravenous hydration, after which time she had improvement in her symptoms. Over the past 24 hours, she became more ill-appearing with worsening of her clinical status.

On examination, she is ill-appearing, actively vomiting with an abdominal examination made difficult by pain, and voluntary guarding. She is febrile to 39°C, tachycardic with a heart rate of 130, and a blood pressure of 100/60. Given her concerning examination and vital signs, her immediate workup includes IV placement for fluid resuscitation, laboratory studies, and an abdominal x-ray to assess for free air.

After the results of her abdominal x-ray, coupled with her clinical picture, a surgeon is consulted and an ultrasound is obtained.

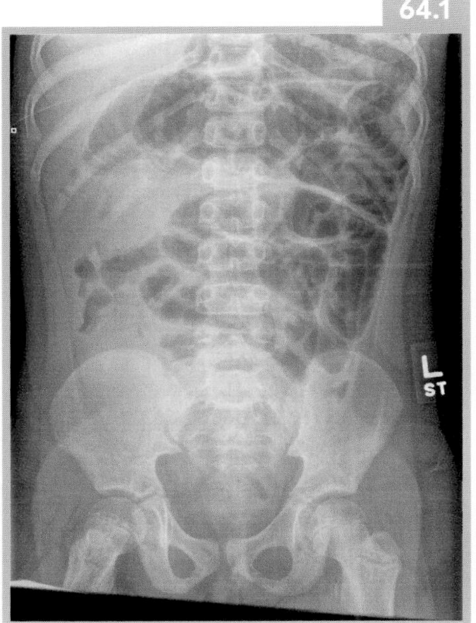

64.1

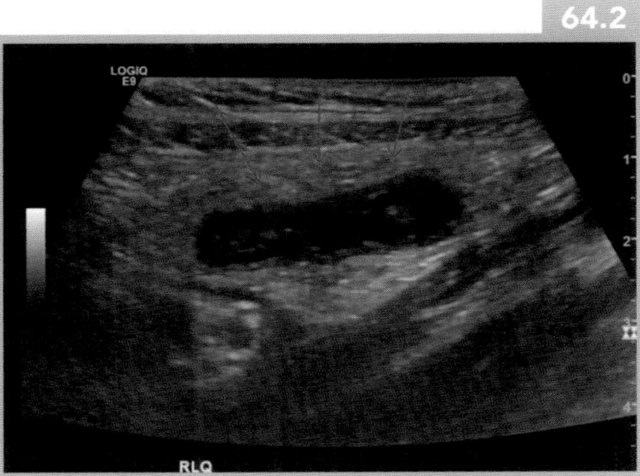

64.2

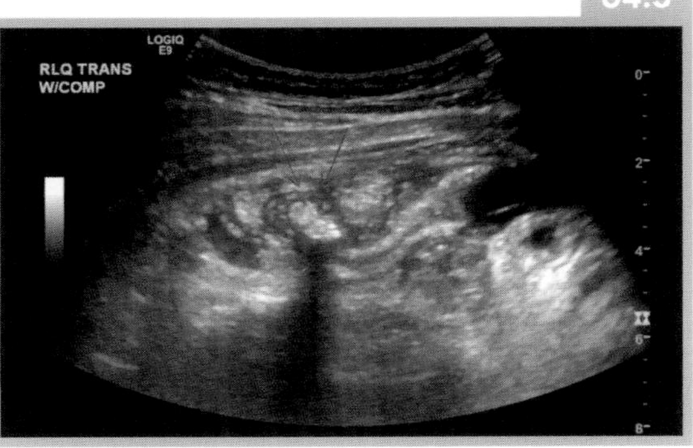

64.3

1. What is the notable finding on this patient's x-ray?
2. What is the classic diagnostic finding on this patient's ultrasound?

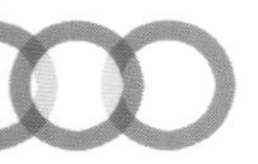

Answers

1. The abdominal film of this patient shows gas-distended loops of small bowel and multiple air-fluid levels consistent with small bowel obstruction. There is no free air to suggest a perforate viscous, but there is an unusual finding: an appendicolith or fecalith.

   Plain radiographs are typically not recommended in the evaluation of the acute abdomen, given the superiority of other diagnostic imaging modalities; however, they can be useful if there is clinical concern for obstruction or perforation, as in the case of this patient. A fecalith is not a common finding on plain films in cases of suspected appendicitis, but when present it is highly suggestive (Yamamoto, 2017).

2. Ultrasound is an ideal imaging modality in the initial evaluation of children with suspected appendicitis, given its ease of use and lack of radiation exposure. A non-compressible appendix with an outer diameter ≥6 mm, fecalith, hyperechoic periappendiceal fat, loss of echogenic submucosal layer, and increased flow of the appendix on the color Doppler scan are findings seen in appendicitis (Schuh et al., 2011). Periappendiceal fluid collections in the absences of a visualized abnormal appendix is also consistent with appendicitis. Screening ultrasound scans in obese children is less accurate.

   The ultrasound images demonstrate a dilated, inflamed appendix and a fecalith.

Keywords: abdominal pain, acute abdomen, surgery, ultrasound, fever

References

Schuh S, Man C, Cheng A, Murphy A, Mohanta A, Moineddin R, Tomlinson G, Langer JC, Doria AS. Predictors on non-diagnostic ultrasound scanning in children with suspected appendicitis. *J Pediatr* 2011;158:112–8.

Yamamoto L. Plain film radiographs of the pediatric abdomen. In *Clinical Emergency Radiology*, 2nd ed., Fox JC, ed. Cambridge, UK: Cambridge University Press, 2017:115.

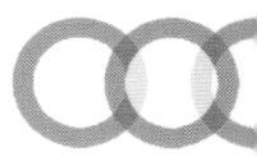

CASE 65

Lauren Allister

Question

A 9-year-old female presents with a few days of worsening right-sided abdominal pain, vomiting, fever, and inability to tolerate oral intake. On examination she is ill-appearing, with focal right-sided tenderness to palpation and some voluntary guarding. She has one episode of emesis in the emergency department. Her history and exam are concerning for a possible appendicitis so an IV is placed, labs are drawn, and an ultrasound is ordered as a first diagnostic imaging study. Her labs return unremarkable, with a normal white blood cell count and normal inflammatory markers. While the patient is in radiology getting her ultrasound, you receive a call from the radiologist alerting you to an abnormal and emergent finding (see Image 65.1).

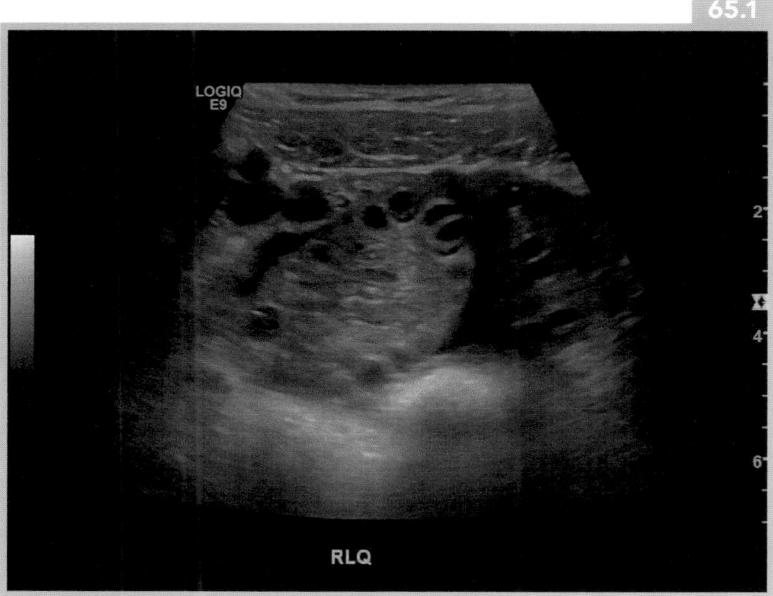

What is the finding on the ultrasound? How common is this clinical condition in this age group?

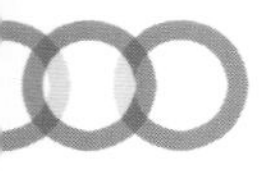

Answer

This patient's ultrasound shows diminished vascular flow and ovarian changes consistent with acute right-sided ovarian torsion.

Adnexal torsion is reported to be the fifth most common gynecologic emergency with a prevalence of 2.7% and incidence of 4.9 per 100,000 in women younger than 20 years (Childress and Dietrich, 2017). In pediatric patients, ovarian or adnexal torsion can be associated with a normal ovary, which is more prone to torsion secondary to small uterine size and a relatively long utero-ovarian ligament, making the adnexa more mobile (Childress and Dietrich, 2017). In up to 75% of cases, however, torsion is associated with ovarian or adnexal pathology (e.g. cysts, teratomas) (Childress and Dietrich, 2017).

Abdominal pain is the most common presenting symptom (Rey-Bellet Gasser et al., 2016) but other commonly associated symptoms include nausea and vomiting due to peritoneal reflexes, flank pain, and anorexia (Childress and Dietrich, 2017).

Ultrasound remains the mainstay for radiographic diagnosis, followed by CT scan (Rey-Bellet Gasser et al., 2016).

This is a true surgical emergency requiring immediate operative detorsion of the affected ovary. This patient was taken immediately to the operating room, but unfortunately her ovary was found to be necrotic and was removed. No associated ovarian or adnexal pathology was discovered. This case highlights both the difficulty in diagnosing this uncommon clinical entity in the pediatric population and how important prompt recognition and diagnosis must be to salvage an affected ovary.

Keywords: gynecology, acute abdomen, do not miss, ultrasound

References

Childress KJ, Dietrich JE. Pediatric ovarian torsion. *Surg Clin North Am* February 2017;97(1):209–21.

Rey-Bellet Gasser C, Gehri M, Joseph JM, Pauchard JY. Is it ovarian torsion? A systematic literature review and evaluation of prediction signs. *Pediatr Emerg Care* April 2016;32(4):256–61.

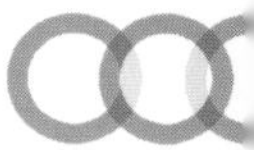

CASE 66

Lauren Allister

Question

A 19-year-female with no past history presents to the emergency department with confusion and altered speech. The patient was with two friends at school approximately 1 hour prior to arrival when she became confused, was unable to write or verbalize complaints, and was unable to speak clearly.

In the emergency department she is afebrile with stable vital signs. She is awake and alert but confused, has difficulty answering questions, and can only repeat short phrases. She has a non-focal examination with the exception of her neurologic exam, where she has receptive aphasia, decreased speech fluency, and frequent paraphasic errors which were more pronounced when responding to questions than with spontaneous speech. Her cranial nerve exam, strength, sensation, and gait testing are all intact.

Given the acuity of her change in mental status, a stat CT was ordered and showed a well-circumscribed lesion in the left parietal area concerning for a possible vascular event. An MRI with contrast is ordered for further clarification and is shown next.

66.1

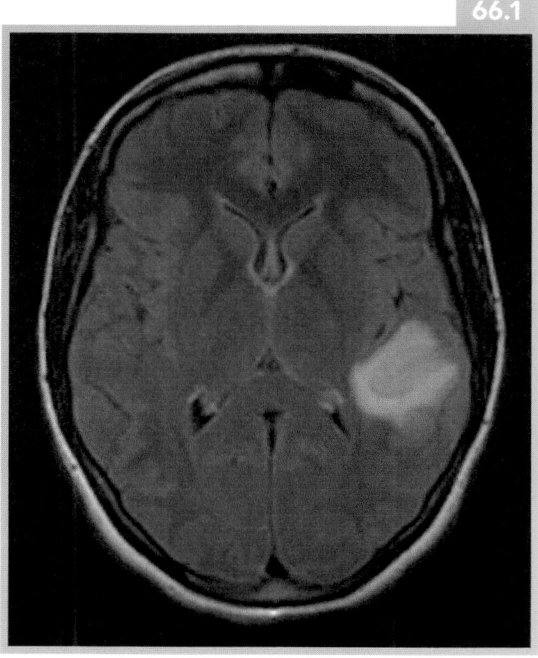

What are the defining features of this MRI? Is a cerebrovascular event the explanation for this patient's sudden-onset symptoms?

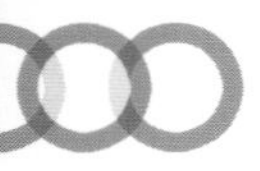

Answer

The patient's MRI demonstrates numerous T2 hyperintense lesions scattered throughout the supratentorial juxtacortical white matter, predominantly involving the frontal and parietal lobes bilaterally with a dominant expansile T2 hyperintense lesion in the left temporoparietal region, in the expected location of Wernicke's area. Many of the lesions demonstrate patchy or incomplete ring-like enhancement. The findings are highly suspicious for a demyelinating process, such as multiple sclerosis (MS). No acute infarction or intracranial hemorrhage is identified.

The patient's exam and MRI are most consistent with a new diagnosis of MS. The scattered lesions on MRI, as well as their patchy and incomplete ring enhancement, are consistent with a demyelinating process. Acute aphasia is not a common initial presentation of MS. MS primarily affects the white matter of the brain and spinal cord, whereas aphasia is typically seen with diseases involving the gray matter. In a multicenter trial of patients with MS, only 0.81% had aphasia as part of their symptom constellation (Lacour et al., 2004). In another small case series of MS patients who presented with acute aphasia, all patients were found to have left-sided lesions in areas of expressive and receptive language (Devere et al., 2000), similar to this patient's MRI findings.

While a cerebrovascular accident was appropriate to consider in this patient given her acute aphasia, the acute onset of any neurologic symptoms in a pediatric patient should always raise concern for a possible demyelinating process, such as acute disseminated encephalomyelitis (ADEM) or MS.

Keywords: neurology, MRI, CT, mimickers

References

Devere TR, Trotter JL, Cross AH. Acute aphasia in multiple sclerosis. *Arch Neurol* August 2000;57(8):1207–9.

Lacour A, De Seze J, Revenco E, Lebrun C, Masmoudi K, Vidry E, Rumbach L, Chatel M, Verier A, Vermersch P. Acute aphasia in multiple sclerosis: A multicenter study of 22 patients. *Neurology* March 23, 2004;62(6):974–7.

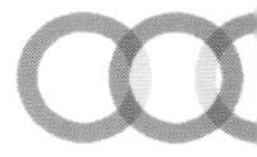

CASE 67

Lauren Allister

Question

A 6-year-old male presents with abdominal pain. His mother reports that he has had diffuse abdominal pain for 1–2 days with infrequent, hard stools. She denies a history of constipation, fever, localizing pain, vomiting, trauma, or urinary symptoms. She reports she has been giving him a few over-the-counter medications for his pain without effect.

On exam the patient is uncomfortable but without signs of an acute abdomen. His exam is notable only for some mild diffuse discomfort to deep palpation. Although you suspect constipation, given the patient's pain and lack of true constipation history, you order an abdominal x-ray, which is shown next.

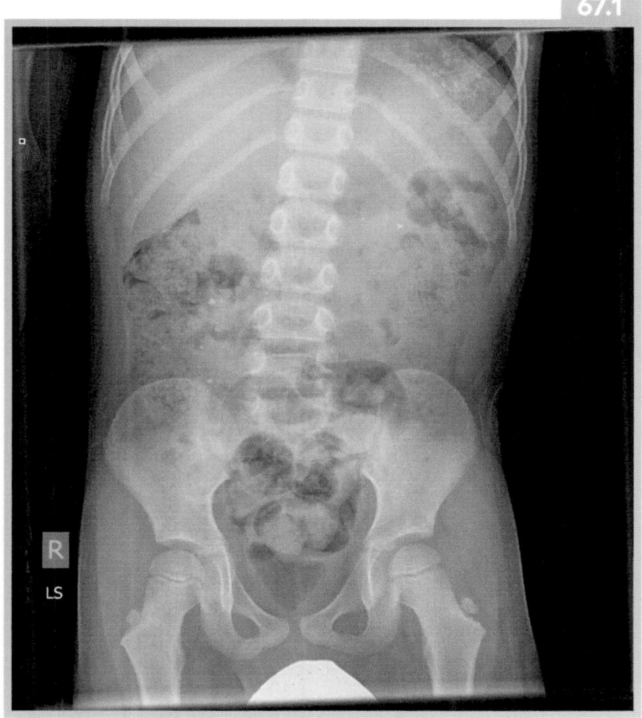

67.1

Is constipation the right diagnosis for this patient? What in the patient's history can explain the radiographic abnormality shown here?

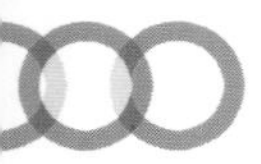

Answer

This patient's x-ray demonstrates a large stool burden with a non-obstructive bowel gas pattern, supporting a diagnosis of constipation. Of note, there are diffuse, granular radiopaque foreign bodies scattered throughout the large bowel. When further questioned about the patient's intake over the past week, the patient's mother reports having given the patient Pepto-Bismol for his constipation.

The active ingredient of Pepto-Bismol is bismuth salicylate. Bismuth is a heavy, white, crystalline metal in the same row of the periodic table as barium and lead, hence its radiopaque properties.

While this patient's x-ray was consistent with his mother's report of Pepto-Bismol administration, it is important to consider toxic ingestions with this x-ray pattern as well, including chloral hydrate/calcium, heavy metals (lead, arsenic, mercury), iodides/iron (vitamin pills), phenothiazines and psychotropics, enteric-coated tablets, and some slow-release capsules.

Keywords: abdominal pain, medications, benign

Bibliography

Haferbecker D, Phllipi C. Case 2: What is that in your bowel? *Paediatr Child Health* March 2008;13(3):197–200.

Yamamoto L. Abdominal pain with faint intra-abdominal calcifications. *Radiol Cases Pediatr Emerg Med* 3, Case 10.

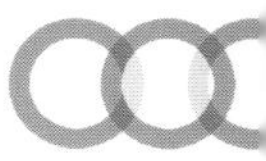

CASE 68

Kevin R. Schwartz

Question

A 2-year-old boy fell while running with a clothes hanger in his mouth. On exam, there is a clothes hanger hanging from his lower mouth. He appears anxious but is maintaining his airway. He is drooling but has no stridor, no active bleeding, no work of breathing, and his lungs are clear. Plain film x-rays were obtained and are shown here.

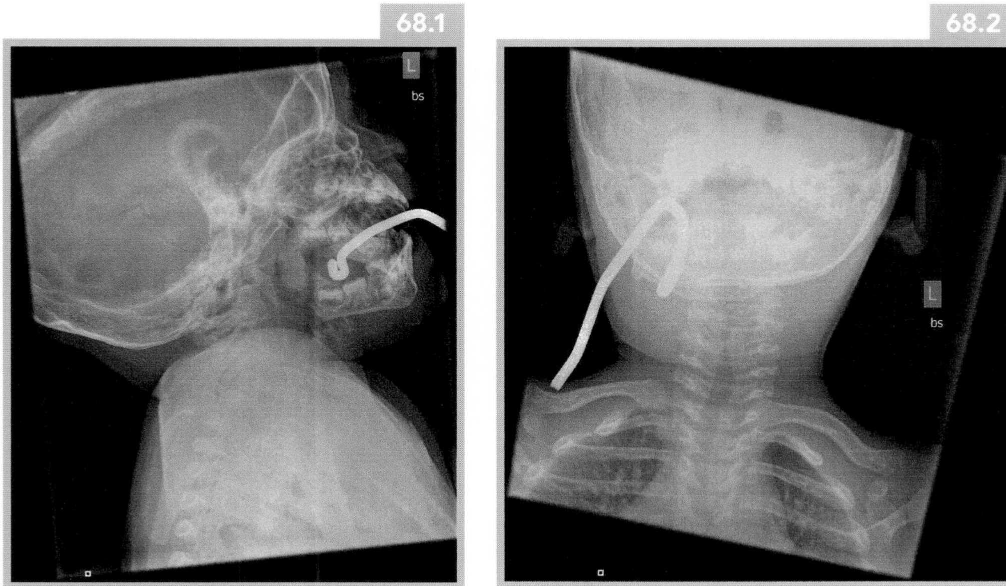

How should this patient be managed and what complications should he be monitored for?

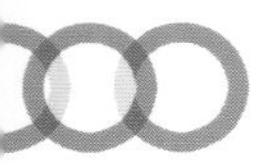

Answer

The patient has penetrating trauma to the floor of the mouth. A number of cases have been reported in the literature of similar injuries. In the majority of cases, surgical removal in the operating room is recommended rather than removal at bedside. The primary immediate complication is bleeding. After removal, the patient should be observed for airway edema. Dexamethasone has been used in an effort to prevent airway swelling though evidence for this application is lacking. Infection has been reported as a later complication in a number of case reports, though there are limited data to support routine antibiotic prophylaxis.

Keywords: airway, head and neck/ENT, penetrating trauma, foreign body

Bibliography

Chauhan N, Guillemaud J, El-Hakim H. Two patterns of impalement injury to the oral cavity: Report of four cases and review of the literature. *Int J Pediatr Otorhinolaryngol* August 2006;70(8):1479–83.

Cheng J, Kleinberger A, Dunham B. Don't hang your coat here. *Int J Pediatr Otorhinolaryngol* 2012;76:750–1.

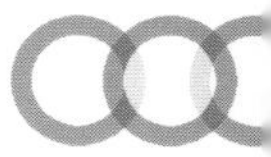

CASE 69

Kevin R. Schwartz

Question

A 12-year-old, previously healthy male presents to the emergency department with 5 days of worsening eye pain, tearing, redness, and a spreading rash around the eyelid over the past 3 days. He was seen in another emergency department prior to the onset of the rash and was prescribed erythromycin ophthalmic ointment without improvement.

On exam, vital signs are normal and visual acuity is 20/20 in both eyes. The sclera appears red in the right eye and you note the findings shown here.

69.1

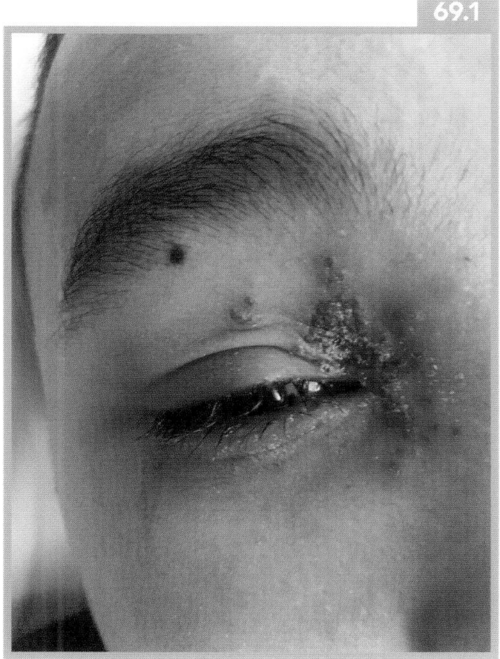

What infection is likely responsible for these findings and what sequelae should you be concerned for?

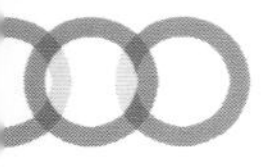

Answer

This patient has herpes simplex virus (HSV) blepharoconjunctivitis. HSV-1 is the leading cause of blindness worldwide. Primary or secondary herpes infection can lead to keratitis affecting the epithelium and/or stroma of the cornea and ultimately result in corneal scarring. Children have poorer visual outcomes compared with adults because difficulties in examination delay the diagnosis and cooperation with topical ophthalmic medications is challenging. HSV eye disease may present with pain, visual blurring, eye discharge, and/or eye redness. Vesicular lesions on the lids (as seen in HSV blepharoconjunctivitis) are often not present. Unilateral presentations of HSV eye disease are more common, however, bilateral disease can occur. Up to 80% of children with HSV keratitis may develop corneal scarring, though this is far less common with isolated blepharoconjunctivitis without concurrent keratitis. Recurrence is common with over 80% of children with HSV eye disease experiencing recurrent disease with a mean time to recurrence of 13 months.

When HSV eye disease is suspected, urgent ophthalmology referral is indicated. Treatment consists of oral acyclovir or valacyclovir and a close ophthalmology repeat examination. Given the high rates of HSV recurrence, there is some evidence to support long-term acyclovir prophylaxis, particularly for those patients with stromal keratitis on presentation. Ophthalmic steroid drops are contraindicated in all cases where there is any suspicion for HSV keratitis, as they can exacerbate disease and significantly worsen visual prognosis.

Keywords: ophthalmology, dermatology, do not miss, infectious diseases

Bibliography

Liu S, Pavan-Langston D, Colby KA. Pediatric herpes simplex of the anterior segment. *Ophthalmology* 2012;119(10):2003–8.

Revere K, Davidson SL. Update on management of herpes keratitis in children. *Curr Opin Ophthalmol* 2013;24:343–7.

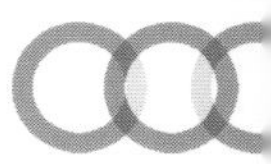

CASE 70

Kevin R. Schwartz

Question

A 16-year-old female with no significant past medical history presents to the emergency department (ED) after being struck by a car. The patient was struck on her right side and knocked to the ground, striking her left parietal scalp. She had no loss of consciousness. A cervical collar and backboard were applied by emergency personnel on scene. On arrival to the ED, she is awake, alert, and in no significant discomfort.

On exam: HR 105, BP 130/86, RR 16, SaO_2 100% on RA.

Her primary survey is intact; a secondary survey reveals no signs of head or torso trauma. Her abdominal exam is significant for moderate right upper quadrant and epigastric tenderness without guarding, but is otherwise normal.

Laboratory studies are notable for elevation in her transaminases with AST 320 U/L, ALT 280 U/L. A CT scan of her abdomen and pelvis with IV contrast was obtained and is shown here.

70.1

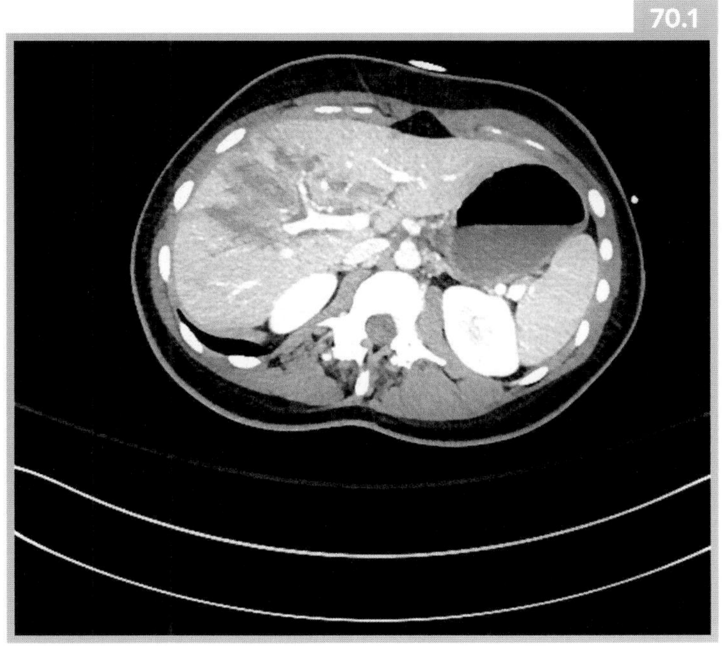

What are the indications for abdominal imaging in blunt abdominal trauma and how is this type of injury typically managed?

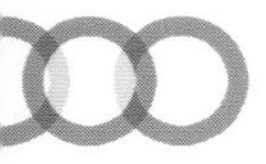

Answer

This patient has sustained a grade IV liver laceration secondary to blunt abdominal trauma. Blunt abdominal trauma may cause solid organ or hollow viscous organ injury. The solid organs most frequently injured are the spleen followed by the liver. Patients with unstable vital signs after blunt abdominal trauma should be resuscitated according to Advanced Trauma Life Support guidelines. Operative exploration by a trauma surgeon may be indicated in the setting of persistent hemodynamic instability. For stable patients, indications for imaging after blunt abdominal trauma include

- A physical exam suggestive of injury (tenderness to palpation, bruising, a "seatbelt sign")
- Elevation of transaminases (AST > 200 U/L or ALT > 125 U/L)
- Gross hematuria or microscopic hematuria >50–100 RBCs/hpf
- Declining hematocrit or hematocrit <30%
- Inability to perform an adequate examination in a patient with history or mechanism suggestive of intra-abdominal injury

Abdominal CT with IV contrast is the preferred diagnostic modality for pediatric patients with blunt abdominal trauma. Ultrasound imaging and the focused assessment with sonography for trauma (FAST) have not been demonstrated to have adequate sensitivity to identify solid and hollow organ injuries in pediatric patients. The utility of ultrasound for evaluating injury can be increased when combined with lab findings and physical exam findings, but contrast-enhanced CT remains the gold standard for evaluating intra-abdominal injuries after blunt trauma.

The vast majority of patients with liver and spleen injuries are managed non-operatively and less than 10% require blood transfusion. The American Pediatric Surgical Association has developed evidence-based guidelines regarding management of clinically stable patients with isolated liver and/or spleen injuries which recommend clinical observation on either the general pediatric ward or the pediatric ICU depending on the severity of injury. Operative intervention is indicated only for those with hemodynamic instability or ongoing blood loss requiring >20 cc/kg of RBC transfusions, which occurs in less than 10% of cases.

Keywords: blunt trauma, acute abdomen, CT

Bibliography

Notrica DM, Eubanks JW 3rd, Tuggle DW, Maxson RT et al. Nonoperative management of blunt liver and spleen injury in children: Evaluation of the ATOMAC guideline using GRADE. *J Trauma Acute Care Surg* 2015;79:683.

Pediatric Trauma Society Clinical Resources Website. The evaluation of pediatric blunt abdominal trauma, 2016. http://pediatrictraumasociety.org/benchmark/clinical-resources.cgi.

Schonfeld D, Lee LK. Blunt abdominal trauma in children. *Curr Opin Pediatr* 2012;24:314–8.

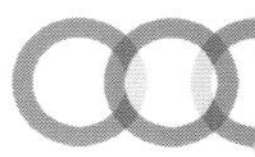

CASE 71

Kevin R. Schwartz

Question

A 13-year-old female with no significant past medical history presents to the emergency department complaining of 2 weeks of hoarse voice, periorbital edema, and morning headaches.

On exam, the patient is afebrile with normal vital signs. She has periorbital edema and her neck feels full to palpation particularly on the right. The remainder of exam is normal. As part of her evaluation, chest x-rays are obtained and shown here.

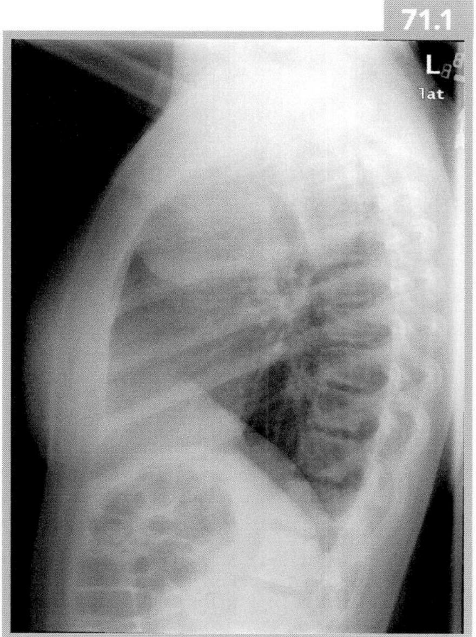

71.1

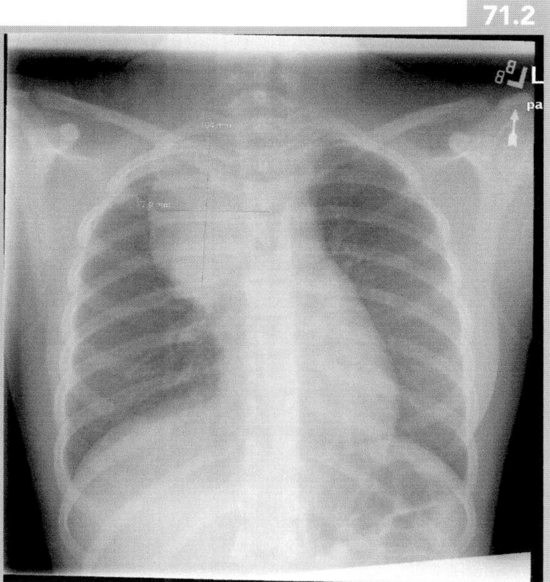

71.2

What are the most common etiologies for this finding and what are the considerations for its initial management?

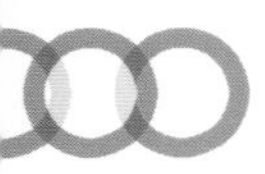

Answer

This patient has an anterior mediastinal mass and has developed superior vena cava (SVC) syndrome. About 90% of mediastinal masses in children are related to malignancy. The most common malignant causes of pediatric mediastinal masses include acute lymphoblastic leukemia (see Case 109) (especially T-cell immunophenotype) and lymphoma, followed by sarcomas, neuroblastoma, and germ cell tumors. Non-malignant causes including teratomas and cysts comprise the remaining 10% of mediastinal masses.

Airway compression is of paramount concern in children with a mediastinal mass, and symptoms such as cough, dyspnea, and orthopnea are common. It is critical to avoid sedation and anesthesia in the emergency department in these patients, as loss of airway tone is associated with tracheal collapse and cardiorespiratory arrest. Care should be taken to minimize patient agitation.

CT chest with contrast may be utilized to better characterize the mass and should be performed in a position that is comfortable for the patient.

Initial management consists of elevating the head of the bed, supplemental O_2 as needed, and admission to an intensive care unit for close monitoring. Consultation with a pediatric oncologist to determine when to potentially administer systemic steroids and/or radiation therapy is recommended. Ideally these therapies are initiated after diagnostic tissue sampling has occurred, but, in some instances, the clinical situation merits more urgent administration.

SVC syndrome refers to the increased venous pressure which results from compression of the superior vena cava by a mass of the middle or anterior mediastinum. It can present with edema of the head, neck and arms, plethora, distended subcutaneous vessels as well as cough, hoarseness, dyspnea, and stridor, all of which result from edema of the larynx and/or pharynx. Symptoms usually develop over weeks. Treatment of SVC syndrome is as described for treatment of mediastinal mass with the addition that when a thrombus is present in the SVC, anticoagulation and/or thrombolysis may be indicated.

Keywords: oncology, airway, do not miss, life-threatening

Bibliography

Ingram L, Rivera GK, Shapiro DN. Superior vena cava syndrome associated with childhood malignancy: Analysis of 24 cases. *Med Pediatr Oncol* 1990;18:476.

Perger L, Lee EY, Shamberger RC. Management of children and adolescents with a critical airway due to compression by an anterior mediastinal mass. *J Pediatr Surg* 2008;43(11):1990–7.

Wilson LD, Detterbeck FC, Yahalom J. Superior vena cava syndrome with malignant causes. *N Engl J Med* 2007;356(18):1862–9.

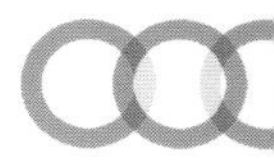

CASE 72

Kevin R. Schwartz

Question

A 13-year-old female with no significant past medical history presents to the emergency department complaining of one week of abdominal pain and a sense of abdominal fullness. She is otherwise well. She has not yet begun to menstruate.

On exam, the patient is well-appearing with a distended firm abdomen which is mildly tender throughout.

An abdominal ultrasound is obtained prompting a follow-up abdominal MRI with the images shown.

72.1

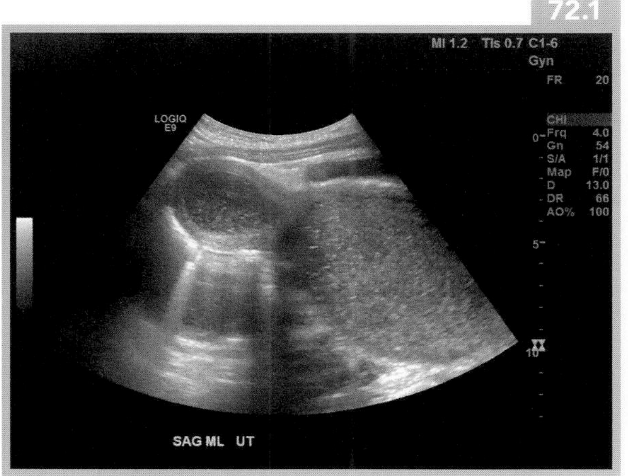

72.2

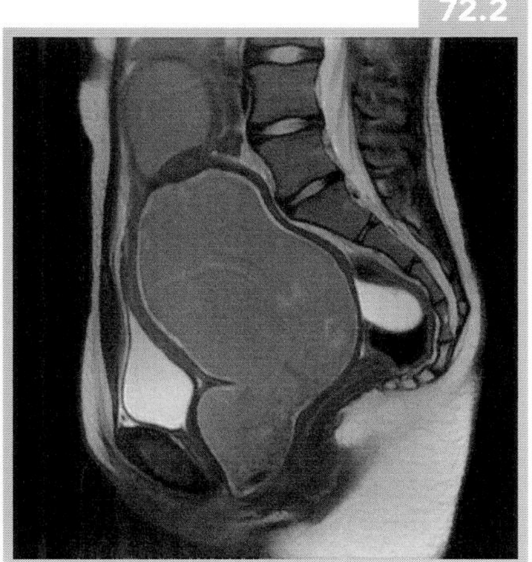

What is the typical presentation of this disorder and how is it managed?

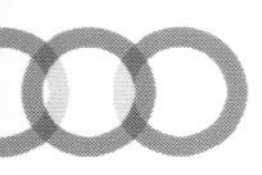

Answer

This patient has hematometrocolpos, the collection of menstrual blood in the vagina and uterus, secondary to onset of menses with an imperforate hymen. An imperforate hymen occurs in 1:1000 to 1:30,000 girls and is generally an isolated condition but may be associated with other congenital malformations including multicystic kidney dysplasia and bifid clitoris. Although many cases are detected prior to puberty on routine physical exam, if undiagnosed, patients may present with hematometrocolpos soon after menarche.

Variably present symptoms of hematometrocolpos include abdominal pain, urinary retention, lower back pain, buttock pain, and sciatica.

The condition can be visualized on abdominal ultrasound, whereas an abdominopelvic MRI is frequently used to search for other abnormalities pre-operatively. Surgical hymenectomy is curative and the majority of patients have complete resolution of symptoms once blood is released. Clues to this diagnosis include worsening abdominal or back pain in a Tanner V stage female who reports not having yet had menses. The classic physical exam feature on genitourinary exam is a bulging, bluish hymen.

Keywords: abdominal pain, gynecology, congenital anomaly, ultrasound, MRI

Bibliography

Bapat R, Bergsman C. Hematometrocolpos presenting as sciatica, constipation, and urinary retention. *Clin Pediatr* 2008;47(1):71–3.

Domany E, Gilad O, Shwarz M, Vulfsons S, Garty BZ. Imperforate hymen presenting as chronic low back pain. *Pediatrics* 2013;132(3):e768–70.

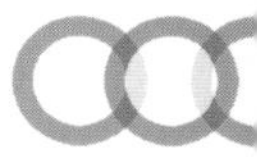

CASE 73

Kevin R. Schwartz

Question

A previously healthy 3-year-old with a reported history of rolling off a 3-foot-high bed was found to be apneic and unresponsive on the scene by EMS (emergency medical services). He was intubated and brought to the emergency department, where it is found to be obtunded with no spontaneous movement on no sedation. Pupils are 6 mm on the right and fixed, 4 mm on the left and fixed. Mannitol and hypertonic saline are given and a CT scan of the head was obtained with images shown.

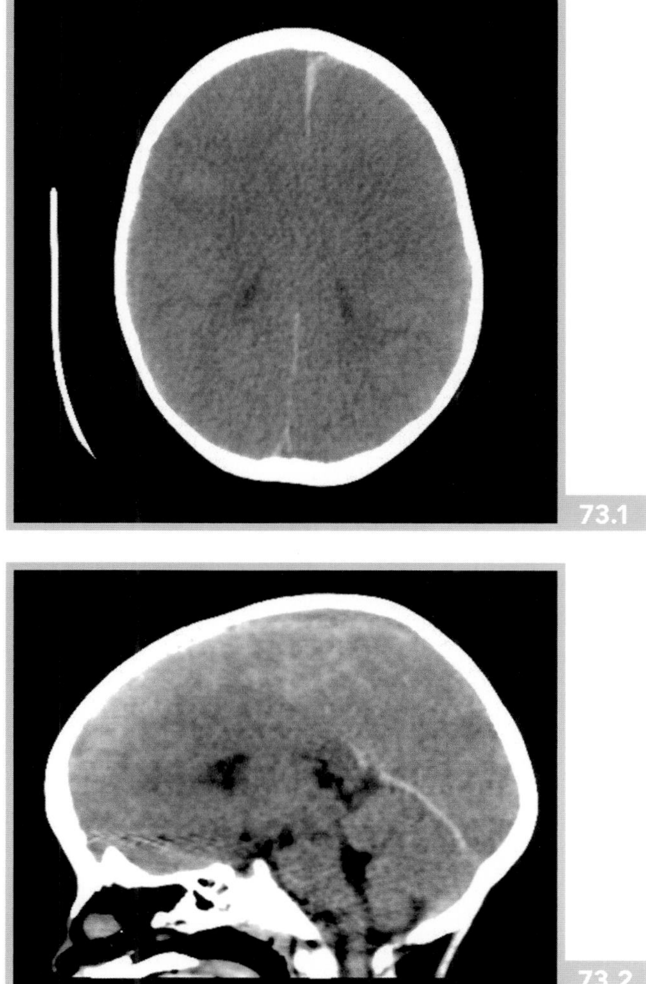

73.1

73.2

What is the most likely mechanism for these findings?

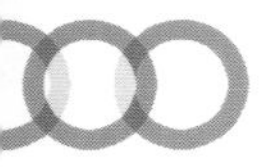

Answer

The patient has subdural hematomas (SDH) within the anterior and posterior falx. The majority of cases of subdural hemorrhage in children less than 2 years of age are caused by inflicted, non-accidental trauma. Subdural hemorrhage occurs when rotational or coup–countrecoup forces cause injury to veins, arteries, and brain parenchyma leading to bleeding into the potential space between the dura and arachnoid membranes. Whereas epidural hemorrhages do not cross cranial sutures and appear convex on CT, subdural hemorrhages can cross suture lines and appear concave on CT. Subdural hemorrhage may occur with significant falls, car crashes, and other high-impact mechanisms. Rarely, inherited conditions including bleeding disorders, osteogenesis imperfecta, glutaric aciduria, and cerebral atrophy can cause SDH with milder trauma.

Management of SDH consists of C-spine immobilization, airway, breathing, and circulatory support including intubation for patients with a Glasgow Coma Scale (see Case 40) score <8 and measures to reduce intracranial hypertension with immediate consultation with a neurosurgeon. Surgical decompression is generally indicated for patients with epidural hematoma. In contrast, patients with subdural hematomas and significantly depressed mental status are sometimes managed non-operatively, as surgical decompression may not improve the ultimate prognosis in the setting of significant neurologic symptoms.

Once clinically stable, a skeletal survey and fundoscopic exam looking for retinal hemorrhages should be undertaken for all children <2 years of age and any child without a clear significant mechanism for their injury. Child protection services should be consulted.

Keywords: child abuse, head injury, blunt trauma, neurosurgery, CT

Bibliography

Hoskote A, McShane T. Subdural haematoma and non-accidental head injury in children. *Child Nerv Syst* 2002;18:311–7.

Ortega HW, Vander Velden H, Kreykes KS, Redi S. Childhood death attributable to trauma: Is there a difference between accidental and abusive fatal injuries? *J Emerg Med* 2012;45(3):332–7.

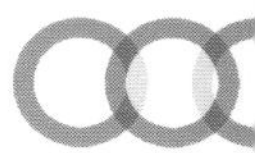

CASE 74

Lauren Allister

Question

An 18-year-old male with no past medical history presents with the acute onset of left-sided chest pain while watching a hockey game with his parents. He describes it as a sudden, sharp pain which worsens with inspiration. He denies any trauma, palpitations, right-sided chest pain, dizziness, nausea, or vomiting. He has no fever and has not had any recent illnesses.

On examination, he is calm and in no respiratory distress. He is afebrile with a respiratory rate of 18 and his O_2 saturation is 100% on room air. His exam is notable for no reproducible chest wall tenderness, a normal cardiac exam, and diminished breath sounds on the left. A chest x-ray is ordered and shown next.

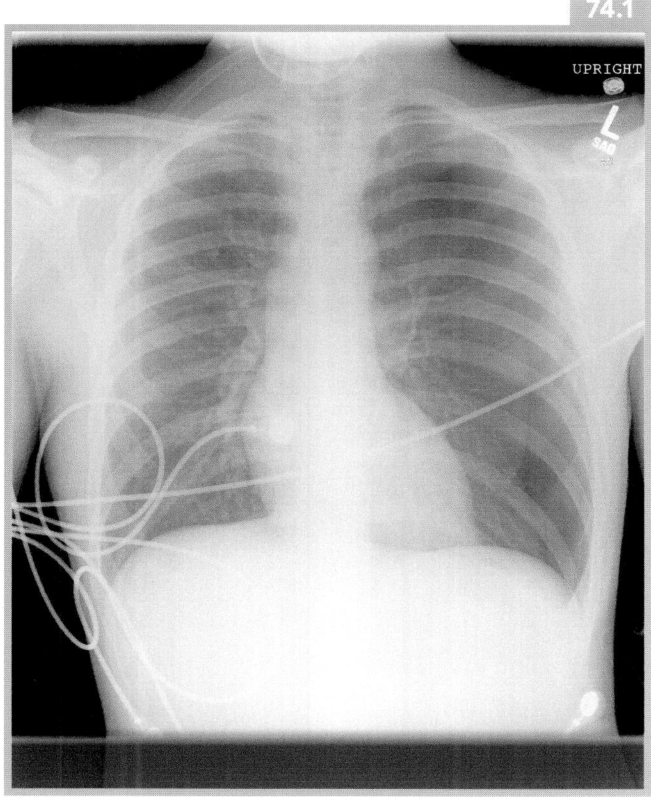

What is the finding on this chest x-ray? What is the next intervention for this patient?

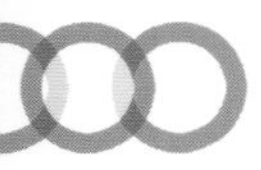

Answer

This patient's x-ray shows a left-sided pneumothorax without tracheal or midline shift.

This case is an example of a spontaneous primary pneumothorax: one that occurs without trauma, antecedent illness, or infection and without a predisposing underlying medical condition. The pathophysiologic mechanisms responsible for a spontaneous pneumothorax seem to be a combination of connective tissue leakage of air out of the pleural space often associated with blebs or bullae.

Symptoms of a pneumothorax include acute onset of chest pain and shortness of breath. Diagnosis of spontaneous pneumothorax is often clinically suspected based on history and physical examination, and confirmed by an erect posterior–anterior (PA) chest radiograph. The treatment options for spontaneous pneumothorax in a clinically stable patient include observation alone, observation with 100% high-flow oxygen delivery via mask, simple aspiration, large or small bore pleural catheter, and placement of a thoracostomy tube. Multiple formulas and guidelines exist as to which intervention is necessary based on the size of the pneumothorax. The existing adult guidelines call for those patients who are clinically stable with a large primary spontaneous pneumothorax (>20%) to have placement of a pleural catheter or appropriately sized chest tube; those who continue to have symptoms or are clinically unstable must be admitted to the hospital with high-flow oxygen administration.

As this patient's pneumothorax was felt to occupy >25% of his right lung field, he was placed on 100% oxygen, a chest tube was inserted, and he was hospitalized for pain control and serial x-rays with eventual resolution of his symptoms.

Keywords: pulmonary, chest pain, respiratory distress

Bibliography

Dotson K, Johnson LH. Pediatric spontaneous pneumothorax. *Pediatr Emerg Care* July 2012;28(7):715–20.

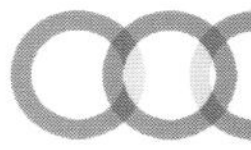

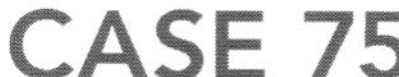

CASE 75

Michael Gottlieb

Questions

A 10-month-old girl presents to the pediatric emergency department with abdominal pain and swelling. Her parents had noticed an outpouching of the umbilicus since birth, but it is now larger and they are unable to reduce it. Examination of the abdomen reveals this finding.

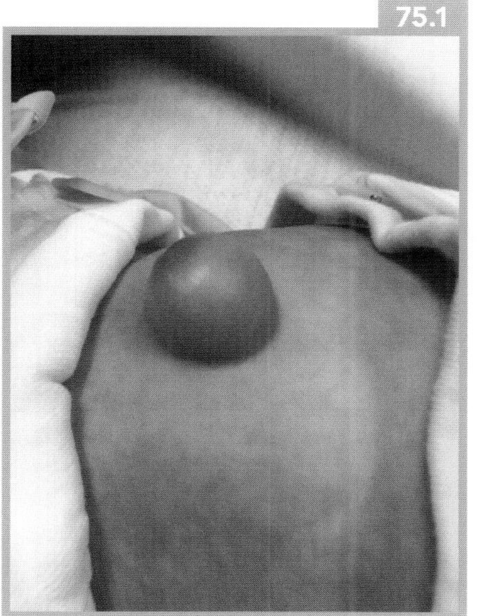

75.1

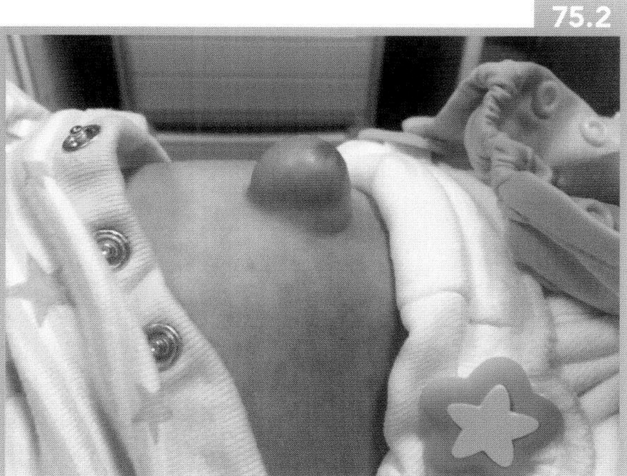

75.2

1. What is the difference between an incarcerated and a strangulated hernia?
2. What is the treatment of an incarcerated umbilical hernia?

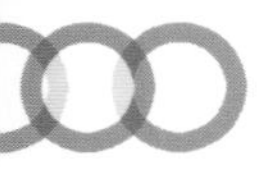

Answers

1. Umbilical hernias are usually benign and resolve as the child grows older and begins to use abdominal muscles for trunk support. However, some cases may not resolve. Rarely, loops of bowel may become stuck in the hernia. Incarcerated hernias refer to hernias that are unable to be reduced. Strangulated hernias are a subset of incarcerated hernias where the bowel has insufficient blood supply and may become necrotic. Strangulated hernias are more painful and associated with skin color changes, increased warmth, systematic symptoms, and ill appearance.

2. Providers should attempt an initial reduction of suspected incarcerated hernias. This may be facilitated by providing pain control and using an ice pack to reduce the edema. Cases that are not reducible at the bedside may require operative reduction. Any signs of strangulation should prompt immediate surgical consultation as closed reduction is contraindicated in these cases.

Keywords: surgery, vomiting, mass, acute abdomen

Bibliography

Blay E Jr, Stulberg JJ. Umbilical hernia. *JAMA* June 6, 2017;317(21):2248.

Earle DB, McLellan JA. Repair of umbilical and epigastric hernias. *Surg Clin North Am* October 2013;93(5):1057–89.

Summers A. Congenital and acquired umbilical hernias: Examination and treatment. *Emerg Nurse* March 2014;21(10):26–8.

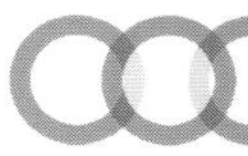

CASE 76

Barbara Pawel

Question

A 10-year-old child presents with a left arm injury after falling on his outstretched hand with the arm in pronation while skateboarding.

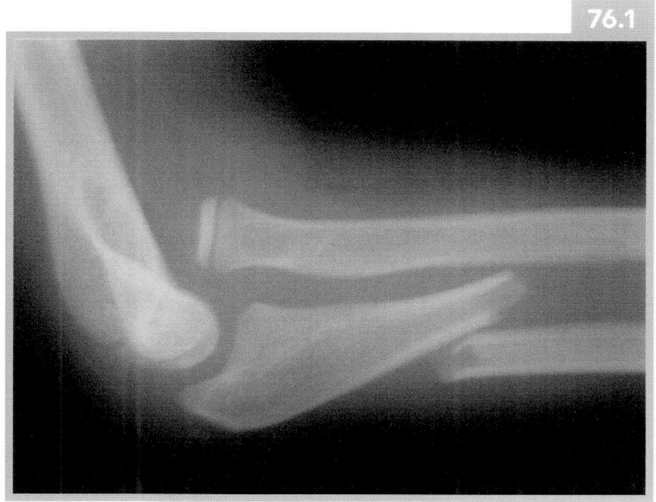
76.1

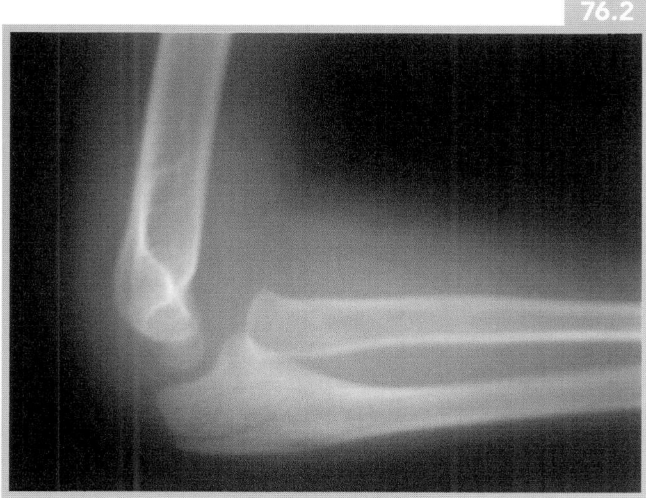
76.2

On the true lateral radiograph of the elbow, which line should be assessed to make the diagnosis of a Monteggia fracture?

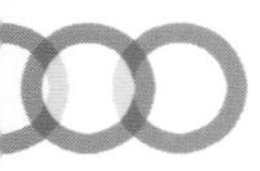

Answer

The radiocapitellar line is drawn through the center of and parallel to the long axis of the radius and should always pass through the center of the capitellum unless there is a radial head dislocation as seen in Image 76.1. A subtle dislocation is shown in Image 76.2.

A Monteggia fracture is a radial head dislocation plus a proximal ulna fracture. In children, the ulna fracture forms include plastic deformation, metaphyseal buckle fracture, greenstick fracture, or a complete displaced fracture. It is unusual to have an isolated radial head dislocation in children; the ulna must be carefully examined for the presence of an incomplete fracture. It is also important to carefully examine the radial head for tenderness in all ulna fractures since it is common for the head to spontaneously relocate. Treatment is often non-operative in children: closed reduction of both the ulnar fracture and the radial head dislocation followed by long arm cast application. Children with closed physes or those with an unstable closed reduction may require ORIF (open reduction and internal fixation). Increased complication rates from delayed diagnosis can be avoided by obtaining elbow radiographs with every suspected forearm fracture to assess for radial head dislocation.

Keywords: orthopedics, extremity injury, pitfalls

Bibliography

Ring D. Monteggia fractures. *Orthop Clin N Am* 2013;44:59–66.

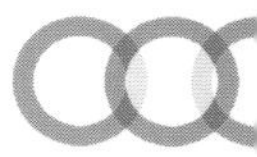

CASE 77

Lauren Allister

Question

A 12-year-old boy presents with one day of left hemiscrotal pain and swelling. He denies trauma, dysuria, hematuria, abdominal pain, or back pain. He has no right-sided symptoms.

On exam, he is afebrile with normal vital signs. His genitourinary exam is notable for tenderness of the left testicle with some associated edema, erythema, and a difficult to elicit cremasteric reflex on the left side. His testicle had a normal lie, and he had neither right testicular pain nor overlying signs of trauma or discoloration.

Given the etiologies for hemiscrotal pain, including testicular torsion, a scrotal ultrasound is ordered.

77.1

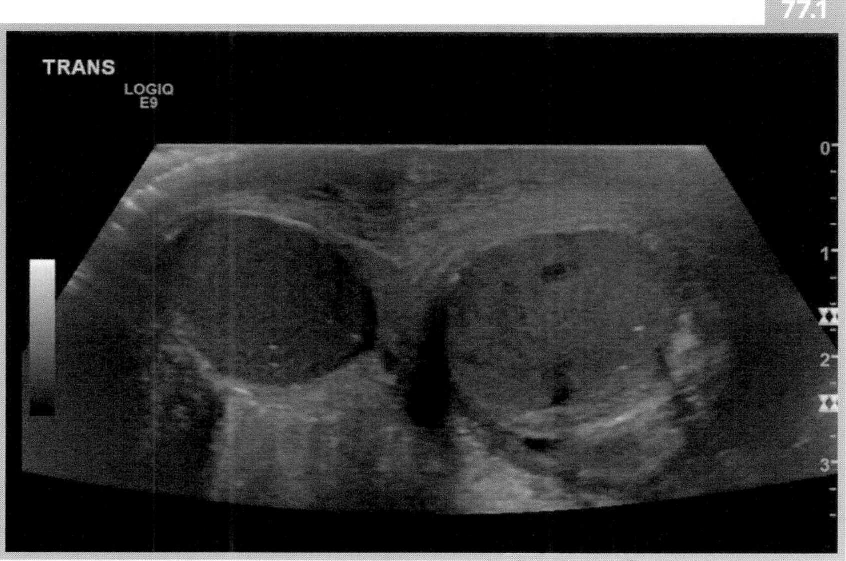

What does this ultrasound show? What are the next steps for this patient?

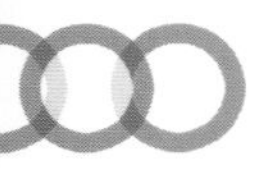

Answer

This patient's ultrasound shows a lack of Doppler blood flow to an enlarged testicle consistent with acute testicular torsion.

Although other diagnoses can present with acute testicular pain, it is important to recognize the possibility of testicular torsion because the best chance of testicular preservation occurs with expeditious management.

Diagnosis can often be made on history and physical exam alone, with the most predictive features being acute onset of unrelenting pain accompanied by unilateral testicular tenderness, elevation (high-riding) of the testicle, transverse testicular orientation, palpation of the epididymis anteriorly, and an absent cremasteric reflex.

If torsion is suspected, management should include manual detorsion and prompt surgical consultation. While an ultrasound is sensitive for the detection of torsion, and useful in identifying other etiologies of hemiscrotal pain, imaging should be deferred for the aforementioned practices if torsion is highly suspected. Testicular salvage rates are associated with the duration of ischemia with a "golden" window of 4–8 hours from the time of torsion to time of detorsion, so expeditious recognition and definitive management are the cornerstones of optimal emergency department care.

Keywords: genitourinary, ultrasound, do not miss

Bibliography

Bowlin PR, Gatti JM, Murphy JP. Pediatric testicular torsion. *Surg Clin North Am* February 2017;97(1):161–72.

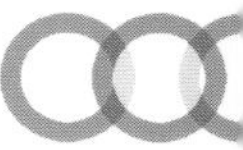

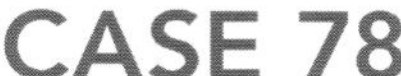

CASE 78

Lauren Allister

Question

A 16-year-old male arrives in the emergency department reporting that he swallowed a nail on a whim. He denies any pain, vomiting, or difficulty breathing, but once he disclosed to his family, they brought him into the emergency department. He denies any co-ingestions.

On examination, he is afebrile with stable vital signs. He has a benign abdominal exam.

Given his history, x-rays are ordered to evaluate for the foreign body and to localize the object.

78.1

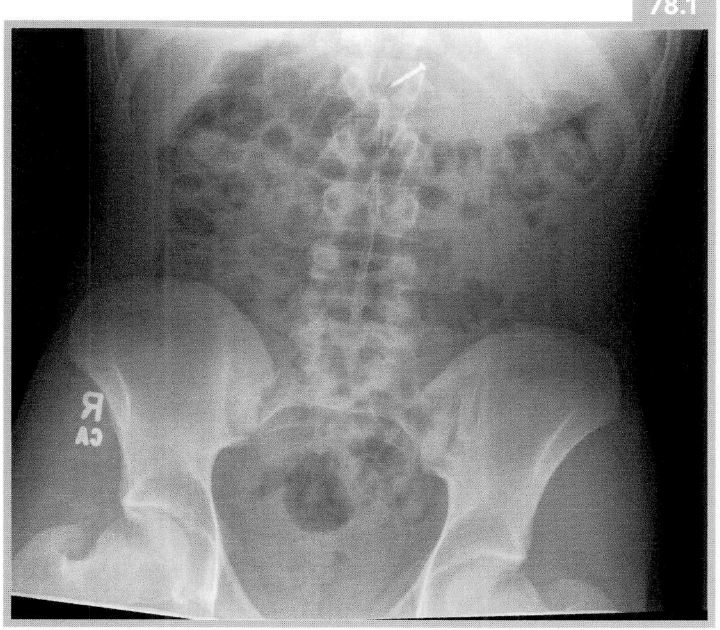

What is the next step for this patient, based on the location and nature of this foreign body? Are there special considerations for a nail or other ingested sharp object?

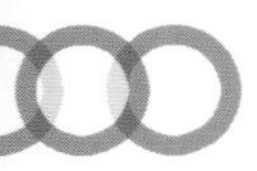

Answer

Foreign body ingestion is a common pediatric complaint in the emergency department.

Sharp objects warrant special consideration given their higher associated morbidity following ingestion. There is a higher risk of complications after ingestions with sharp objects than with other foreign bodies, including risk of perforation either in the esophagus or at angulated areas of the gastrointestinal (GI) tract, such as the C loop of the duodenum and ileocecal valve. Other potential sequelae include aortoesophageal fistula, retropharyngeal abscess, and mediastinitis.

For all suspected foreign body ingestions, plain x-rays are the mainstay both of confirmation of a reported ingestion and localization of the foreign body.

Many objects are not visible on x-ray, so endoscopy should still be considered if an x-ray is negative. Sharp objects in the esophagus should be removed immediately. Most sharp objects in the stomach or duodenum pass through the GI tract uneventfully; because these objects still carry a high risk of complications, they should be removed endoscopically if possible. If the object has passed beyond the duodenum, it should be followed with serial x-rays. If the object does not move distally for 3 days, surgical intervention should be considered. In addition, patients should be instructed to watch for signs and symptoms of GI obstruction or bleeding such as abdominal pain, vomiting, fever, hematemesis, or melena.

For this patient, the x-ray shows the ingested nail in the stomach/early small intestine. Given his lack of symptoms and the potential difficulty in retrieving the nail, the decision was made in collaboration with pediatric gastroenterology and surgery consultants to discharge the patient home with close symptom observation and follow-up x-rays in 3 days if the nail had not passed spontaneously in his stool.

Keywords: foreign body, gastrointestinal

Bibliography

Wright CC, Closson FT. Updates in pediatric gastrointestinal foreign bodies. *Pediatr Clin N Am* 2013;60(5):1221–39.

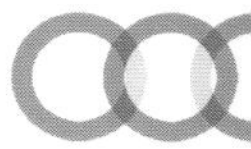

CASE 79

Emily Obringer

Questions

An 11-year-old girl returns with this rash a week after camping in the woods. She is otherwise feeling well. You learn that the campsite was in a Lyme-endemic area.

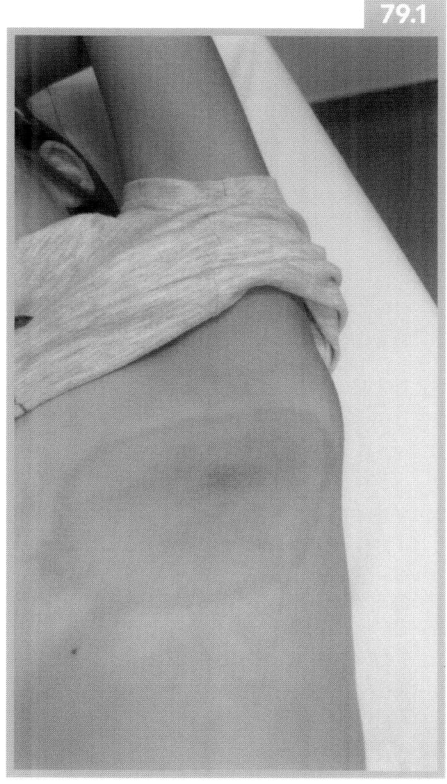
79.1

1. What diagnostic tests should be performed in early Lyme disease?
2. Early localized Lyme disease is best treated with doxycycline for 14–21 days. What alternative therapy should be prescribed for children under 8 years of age? Why?

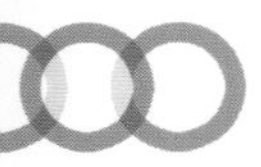

Answers

1. In the early stages of Lyme disease, the diagnosis is best made based on clinical presentation with the characteristic rash—a single erythema migrans lesion in localized disease or multiple erythema migrans lesions in early disseminated disease. Antibody testing for *Borrelia burgdoferi* in the first several weeks of disease is insensitive and not recommended (American Academy of Pediatrics, 2018). Early disseminated disease without rash and late Lyme disease should be diagnosed based on clinical presentation and serologic testing.

2. Doxycycline is the treatment of choice for early localized Lyme disease. However, prolonged administration (>10 days) of doxycycline is associated with permanent dental discoloration in children younger than 8 years of age and is therefore not recommended in this age group, with the exception of treatment of neurologic symptoms. Alternative therapy includes amoxicillin or cefuroxime.

Keywords: infectious diseases, dermatology, environmental

Reference

American Academy of Pediatrics. Lyme disease. In *Red Book: 2018–2021 Report of the Committee on Infectious Diseases*, Kimberlin DW, Brady MT, Jackson MA, and Long SS eds. Itasca, IL: American Academy of Pediatrics, 2018:515–23.

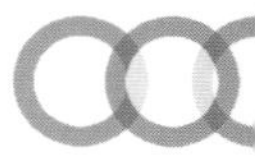

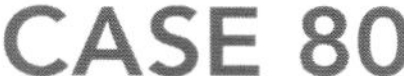

CASE 80

Michael Gottlieb

Questions

A 14-year-old boy presents to the emergency department with right shoulder pain after being tackled while playing football. He denies any other injuries. He has good sensation and strength distally, but is unable to elevate his right arm or touch his opposite shoulder. He has good pulses, strength, and sensation distally.

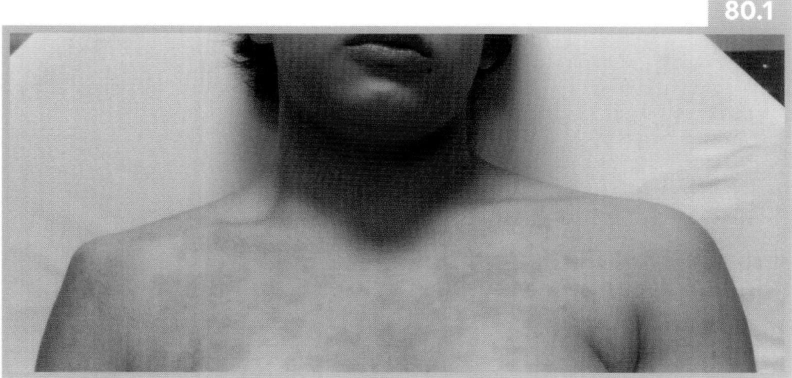

80.1

1. What is the diagnosis?
2. What are the most common complications associated with this?

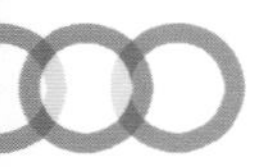

Answers

1. This patient is presenting with a shoulder (glenohumeral) dislocation. This is one of the most common joint dislocations seen in the emergency department. Classically, patients will demonstrate a squared-off shoulder (demonstrated in Image 80.1) with an inability to touch the opposite shoulder. In repeat dislocations without acute trauma and a supporting physical exam, radiographs may be unnecessary. However, if there was significant trauma or the diagnosis is in question, one should obtain anteroposterior, lateral, and scapular Y-view shoulder radiographs.
2. The four most common complications are Bankart lesions (up to 87%), Hill-Sachs lesions (54%–76%), rotator cuff tears (14%), and axillary nerve injuries (3%). A Bankart lesion is a deformity of the glenoid rim which can lead to joint instability. A Hill-Sachs deformity is a cortical depression in the posterolateral head of the humerus that occurs as a result of the force of the humeral head against the glenoid rim during the dislocation. Rotator cuff tears can also occur due to the force of the dislocation and can cause shoulder instability. The axillary nerve, which travels in close proximity to the humeral head, can be damaged during the dislocation, resulting in loss of sensation over the deltoid and difficulty with arm abduction.

Keywords: orthopedics, extremity injury, blunt trauma

Bibliography

Bonz J, Tinloy B. Emergency department evaluation and treatment of the shoulder and humerus. *Emerg Med Clin North Am* May 2015;33(2):297–310.

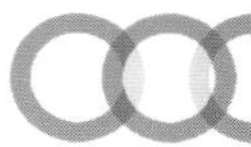

CASE 81

Michael Gottlieb

Questions

A 6-year-old boy presents to the emergency department with left arm pain after a tripping and falling onto his outstretched left arm. He is holding his arm with his other hand. He has significant swelling and tenderness near the elbow joint. Elbow radiographs are obtained.

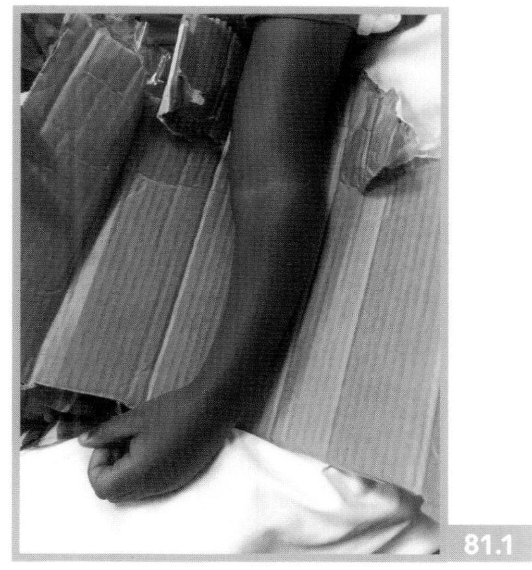

81.1

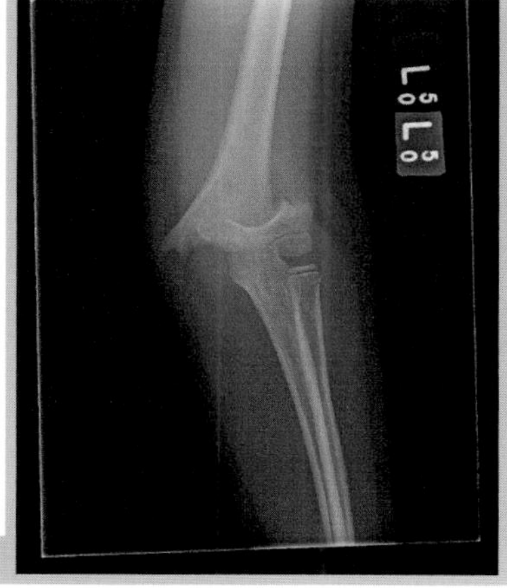

81.2

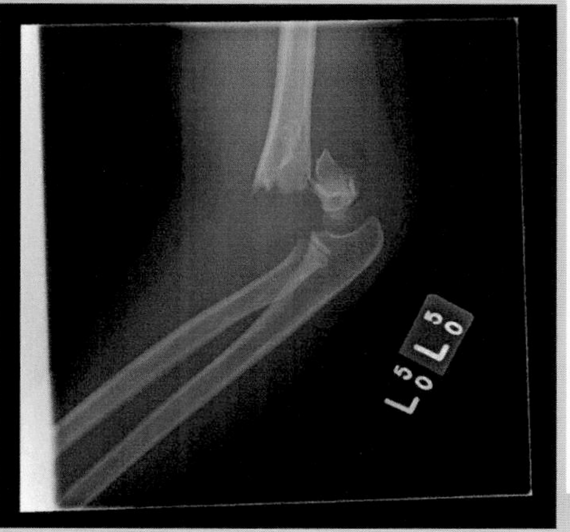

81.3

1. What type of fracture is displayed?
2. What are the most common complications from this type of injury?

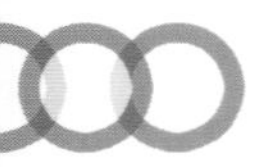

Answers

1. This patient is presenting with a type III supracondylar fracture. Supracondylar fractures are the most common elbow fractures in childhood with a peak incidence between 5 and 7 years of age. The most common etiology is a fall on an outstretched hand. Type I (non-displaced) fractures may or may not demonstrate a fracture line. Indirect findings supporting a type I fracture include a posterior fat pad, a large anterior fat pad (referred to as the sail sign), an abnormal anterior humeral line (see Case 116), or an abnormal radiocapitellar line (see Case 76). Type II fractures involve partial displacement, whereas type III fractures involve complete displacement and are at highest risk for complications.

2. The three most common complications include neurologic injury, vascular injury, and compartment syndrome. The anterior interosseous nerve is the most commonly injured nerve (80%) and should be tested by having the patient make an "OK" sign with their thumb and first finger. The next most commonly injured nerves include the median nerve (28%–60%), radial nerve (26%–61%), and ulnar nerve (11%–15%). The most common vascular injury is the brachial artery (5%–20%) and should be assessed with pulse, color, temperature, and capillary refill. Finally, all patients require hospital admission for urgent or emergent operative fixation to reduce swelling, as well as for monitoring for evidence of compartment syndrome.

Keywords: orthopedics, extremity trauma, blunt trauma

Bibliography

Sherman SC. Pediatric supracondylar fracture. *J Emerg Med* February 2011;40(2):e35–7.

Wu J, Perron AD, Miller MD, Powell SM, Brady WJ. Orthopedic pitfalls in the ED: Pediatric supracondylar humerus fractures. *Am J Emerg Med* October 2002;20(6):544–50.

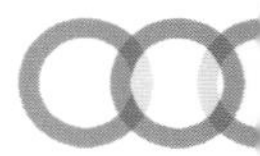

CASE 82

Timothy Ketterhagen

Question

The mother of a 4-year-old boy brings him to the emergency department because he has "a ring stuck on his finger." The patient was reportedly playing in the family's garage when he put a metal nut on his middle finger but was unable to remove it. The patient's mother attempted to pull the object off, but this only caused more swelling of the finger. The patient is complaining of pain of the middle finger. No other injuries are reported.

Physical exam shows a large metal nut on the middle finger of the left hand. The distal third digit is swollen. Cap refill <2 seconds. The patient is able to move his finger but range of motion is limited by pain. The rest of the physical exam is unremarkable. The affected hand is shown here.

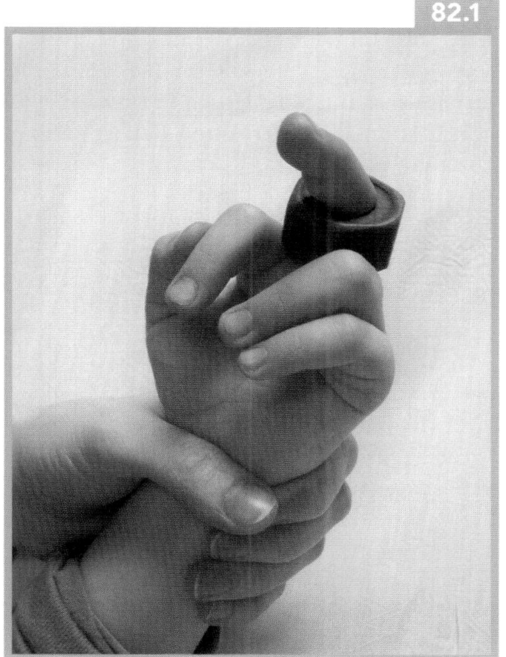

82.1

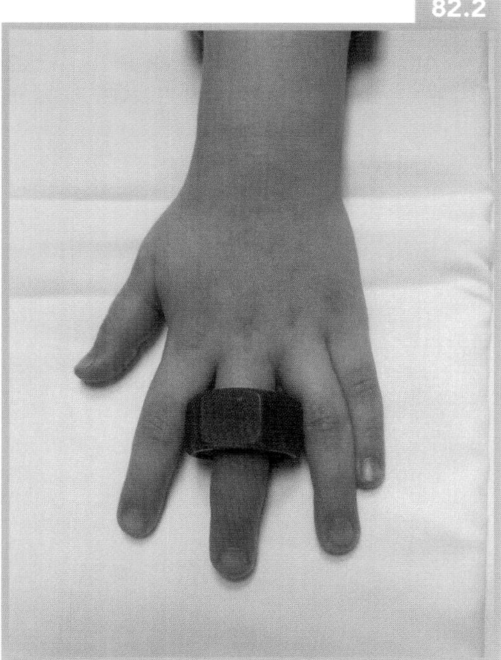

82.2

What techniques might be used to remove an incarcerated ring from a digit?

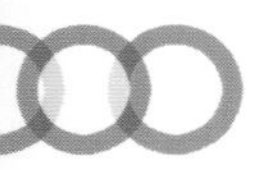

Answer

Rings can be difficult to remove from a swollen digit. The degree of vascular compromise of the digit depends on the magnitude and duration of swelling. Imaging may be indicated if a fracture or dislocation is suspected as the deformity itself may prevent ring removal. Tetanus status should be addressed.

There are several techniques that can be utilized to remove an incarcerated ring. Wound cleansing and local anesthesia should be implemented in all cases. The digital block technique should be used judiciously depending on the patient's cooperation and severity of discomfort. The hand should be kept elevated as much as possible. Ice may be applied to decrease swelling.

- *Lubrication*: Apply soap or petroleum jelly to the finger and attempt to slide the ring off the finger.
- *String pull method*: To a lubricated finger, pass one end of string/suture/rubber band under the ring. Grasp both ends of the string and pull in a circular motion around the finger to gradually advance the ring off distally.
- *String wrap method*: Pass one end of string or suture under the ring. Wrap the suture on the distal end of the ring around the finger. Continue wrapping past the PIP (proximal interphalangeal) joint to compress the soft tissue swelling. Grasp the ring and exert back-and-forth pressure while pulling the ring over the string/suture. The proximal end of the string may also be pulled to gradually advance the ring off the finger distally.
- *Ring cutter*: Insert the guard between the ring and finger. Apply pressure while rotating the blade of the ring cutter. Electric cutting devices are also available. Care must be taken to avoid skin burns as the metal may heat up from friction alone. Irrigation during cutting may help dissipate heat. After the ring is cut through, pull the ring apart with a hemostat and remove from the finger.

Keywords: foreign body, hand injury, procedures

Bibliography

Bothner J. Ring entrapment and removal. http://www.uptodate.com/contents/ring-removal-techniques. Last updated June 6, 2018.

Fleisher GR, Ludwig S, eds. *Textbook of Pediatric Emergency Medicine*. 6th ed. Philadelphia: Lippincott Williams & Wilkins, 2010.

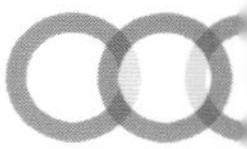

CASE 83

Emily Obringer

Questions

A 10-year-old girl presents with a limp. On exam she is noted to have cellulitis of the plantar aspect of her foot. Upon further questioning, the girl admits to playing in a construction site near her home a few days ago and recalls stepping on something sharp. She was able to remove the object that punctured her tennis shoe but cannot describe what it was. Since then she has had increasing pain in the area.

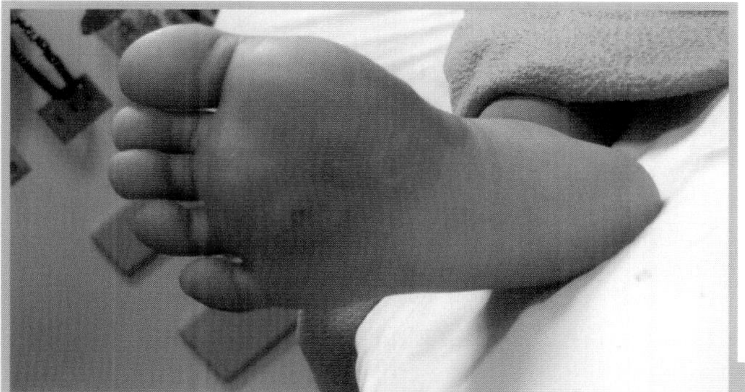

83.1

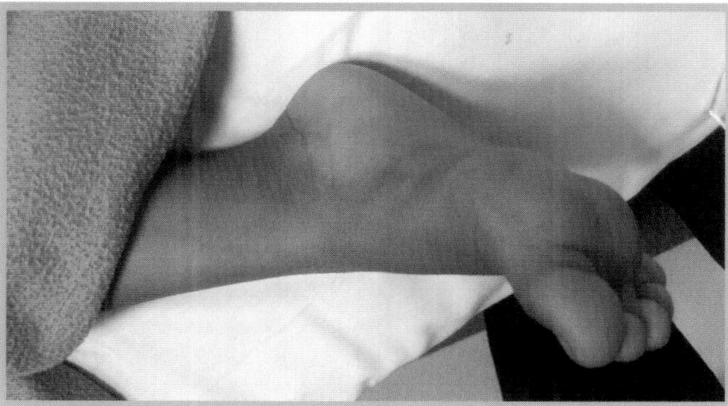

83.2

1. Cellulitis of the foot after a puncture wound is most likely caused by what organism(s)?
2. Should antibiotic prophylaxis be given at the time of injury to prevent cellulitis and other complications, such as osteomyelitis?
3. What imaging studies are indicated?

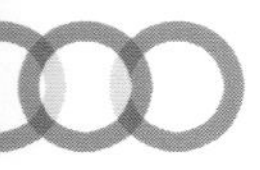

Answers

1. Cellulitis is most frequently caused by normal skin flora, such as staphylococcal and streptococcal species. In the case of cellulitis of the foot related to puncture wound, *Pseudomonas aeruginosa* is also common (Fisher et al., 1985). Additionally, special consideration should be given to the environment when the puncture wound injury occurred. Infection related to waterborne organisms, fungi, and other mycobacteria should be suspected in the appropriate clinical setting. Whenever possible, culture of the infected wound should be obtained.

2. Antibiotic prophylaxis for puncture wounds is not well studied and therefore recommendations are controversial. Generally, if a patient presents within 24 hours of an uncomplicated puncture injury, thoroughly cleaning the area and investigating for a potential retained foreign body is sufficient (Chisholm and Schlesser, 1989; Chachad and Kamat, 2004). A patient who presents after 24 hours frequently has local signs of infection and therefore antibiotic treatment, rather than prophylaxis, is indicated. If a patient presents between 24 and 72 hours after the injury and does not have signs of infection, antibiotic prophylaxis may be given (Chachad and Kamat, 2004).

3. Unless the puncture wound is superficial or the patient is certain that the foreign body was removed intact, plain radiographs should be obtained to evaluate for a retained foreign body (Chisholm and Schlesser, 1989; Chachad and Kamat, 2004). Metal, glass, and plastic are generally well visualized with this technique. If a radiolucent object, such as wood, is suspected, an ultrasound should be considered (Chisholm and Schlesser, 1989). Concern for osteomyelitis should lead the clinician to perform additional imaging studies, such as an MRI with and without contrast.

Keywords: infectious diseases, pitfalls, penetrating trauma

References

Chachad S, Kamat D. Management of plantar puncture wounds in children. *Clin Pediatr (Phila)* 2004;43(3):213–6.

Chisholm CD, Schlesser JF. Plantar puncture wounds: Controversies and treatment recommendations. *Ann Emerg Med* 1989;18:1352–57.

Fisher MC, Goldsmith JF, Gilligan PH. Sneakers as a source of Pseudomonas aeruginosa in children with osteomyelitis following puncture wounds. *J Pediatr* 1985;106(4):607–9.

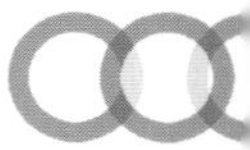

CASE 84

Timothy Ketterhagen

Question

A mother brings her 13-year-old son to the emergency department with a right eye injury. The patient states that he was running through the forest behind his house when he ran into the end of a small branch approximately 20 minutes prior to arrival. The branch made direct contact with the right eye and he felt immediate pain. The mother reports that the patient does not wear glasses and he had "perfect vision" prior to the incident. The patient denies any loss of consciousness and no other injuries were reported.

On physical exam he is awake and alert. There is a 1.5 cm vertical laceration to the sclera medial to the iris. There is surrounding subconjunctival hemorrhage. Extraocular movements are intact. The pupil is central and round. No hyphema is appreciated. Visual acuity is normal. No foreign body is visualized. No other injuries are appreciated. The injury is shown here.

84.1

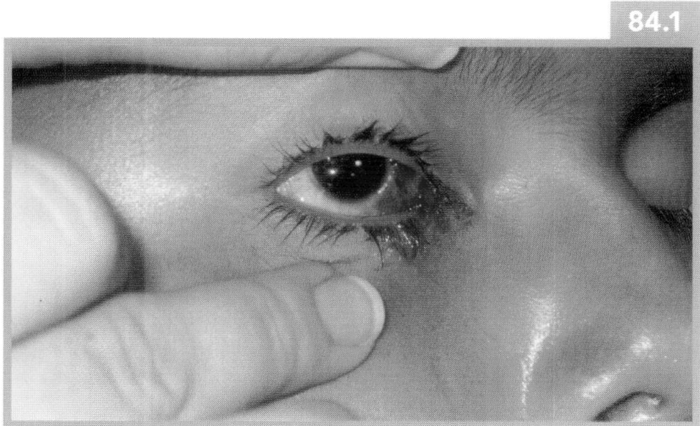

How should this injury be evaluated and managed?

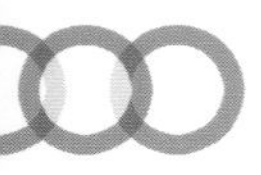

Answer

Lacerations to the cornea or sclera can occur following trauma by a sharp object, projectile, or by blunt trauma. The clinician should consider the possibility of a retained foreign body. Delayed presentation increases the risk of infection. Previous visual acuity should be considered. The presence of 360° subconjunctival hemorrhage, impaired extraocular movements, volume loss to the eye, decreased visual acuity, or hyphema may indicate globe rupture.

All corneal and scleral lacerations should be discussed with an ophthalmologist. If the laceration is deemed to be superficial (<1 cm) and not associated with intraorbital injury, antibiotic ointment may be prescribed and the patient may follow up with an ophthalmologist as an outpatient. For larger lacerations or if globe rupture is suspected, immediate evaluation by an ophthalmologist is warranted. A loose fitting eye shield should be applied. A slit lamp should be used to evaluate the injury. All eye drops should be avoided. Foreign bodies should be left in place. A CT scan is the imaging study of choice in the emergency department, although MRI may provide superior images if a metal foreign body is not suspected. Provide appropriate analgesia, antiemetic agents, and sedation (if indicated). IV antibiotics should be started. Tetanus status should be addressed. An ophthalmologist should determine definitive management.

A corneal abrasion is a violation of the most superficial layer of the cornea. Corneal abrasions can be evaluated with a fluorescein exam. If symptoms persist or a large defect is seen, consult an ophthalmologist. The patient may be discharged with supportive care, topical antibiotics, and instructions to follow up in 24–48 hours with a primary care provider or, in the case of large abrasions or those involving the visual axis, with an ophthalmologist. Healing is expected within 24–48 hours. Topical anesthetics should not be prescribed, as wound healing and the normal corneal reflex can be disrupted.

Keywords: ophthalmology, penetrating trauma, do not miss

Bibliography

Gardiner MF, Kloeck CE. Conjunctival injury. http://www.uptodate.com/contents/conjunctival-injury. Last updated July 28, 2017.

Hoffman RJ, Wang VJ, Scarfone R. *Fleisher & Ludwig's 5-Minute Pediatric Emergency Medicine Consult.* Philadelphia: Wolters Kluwer Health/Lippincott Williams & Wilkins, 2012.

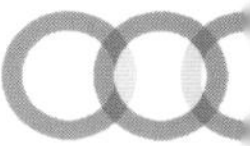

CASE 85

Emily Obringer

Questions

A 9-year-old boy presents to the emergency department in the summer with worsening bilateral ear discharge. He is active on his neighborhood swim team. He describes intense pruritis and there is tenderness on exam when the pinnae are manipulated. You suspect a diagnosis of acute otitis externa.

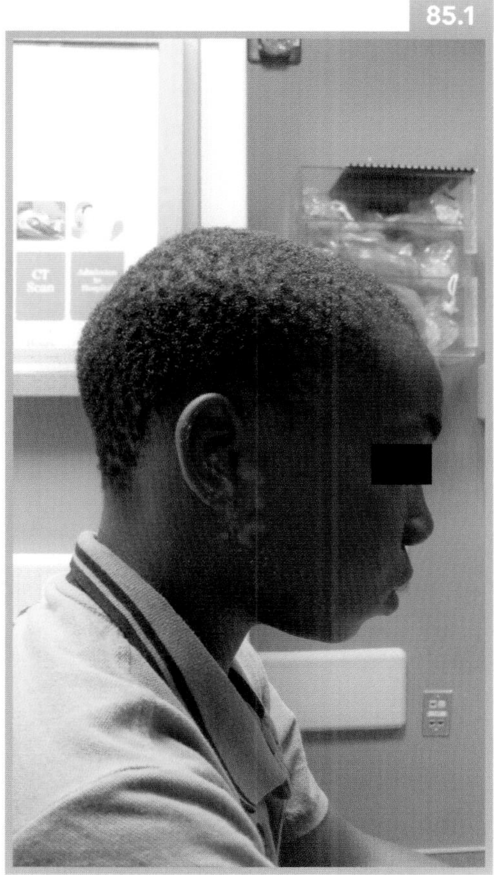

85.1

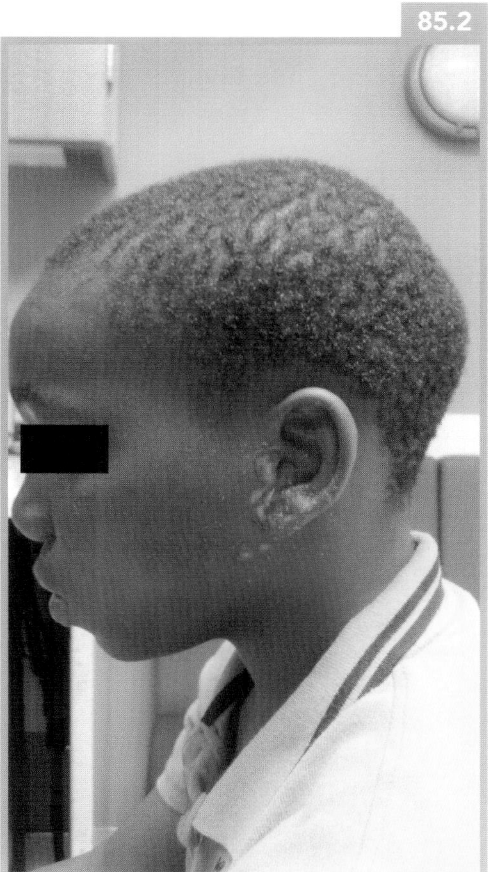

85.2

1. What is the most common etiologic agent for this disease?
2. How is acute otitis externa best treated?

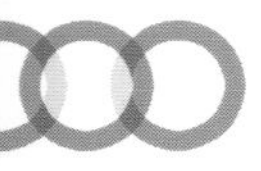

Answers

1. *Pseudomonas aeruginosa* is the most common etiologic agent of acute otitis externa, especially in those cases associated with prolonged exposure to water (such as swimming pools) (Boyce, 2012). Other otic syndromes that may be caused by *Pseudomonas aeruginosa* include chronic suppurative otitis media, necrotizing otitis externa, and otorrhea in the presence of tympanostomy tubes.

2. Uncomplicated acute otitis externa should be managed without the use of systemic antibiotics. The American Academy of Otolaryngology–Head and Neck Surgery recommends that topical therapy alone be prescribed initially, along with adequate analgesia (Rosenfeld et al., 2014). Topical otic preparations are available in a variety of formulations, including antibiotic alone or in combination with a steroid, and antiseptic alone or in combination with a steroid. Two meta-analyses have shown no difference in clinical outcomes among the various preparations; therefore, the clinician should consider patient preference, cost, and potential adherence to therapy when deciding (Rosenfeld et al., 2006; Kaushik et al., 2010). Additionally, if the tympanic membrane cannot be visualized and there is concern for possible tympanic membrane rupture, topical ototoxic agents, such as neomycin, should not be used. A 7- to 10-day course of topical therapy is usually sufficient.

Keywords: infectious diseases, head and neck/ENT

References

Boyce TG. Otitis externa and necrotizing otitis externa. In *Principles and Practice of Pediatric Infectious Diseases*, 4th ed., Long SS, Pickering LK, Prober CG, eds. Edinburgh: Elsevier-Saunders, 2012:220–2.

Kaushik V, Malik T, Saeed SR. Interventions for acute otitis externa. *Cochrane Database Syst Rev* 2010; Jan 20 (1):CD004740.

Rosenfeld RM, Schwartz RT, Cannon CR, Roland PS, Simon GR, Kumar KA, Huang WW, Haskell HW, Robertson PJ. Clinical practice guideline: Acute otitis externa. *Otolaryngol Head Neck Surg* 2014;150(1 Suppl.):S1–24.

Rosenfeld RM, Singer M, Wasserman JM, Stinnett SS. Systematic review of topical antimicrobial therapy for acute otitis externa. *Otolaryngol Head Neck Surg* 2006;134(4 Suppl.):S24–48.

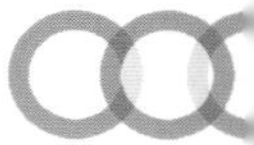

CASE 86

Emily Obringer

Questions

A toddler presents with a non-pruritic, diffuse, erythematous maculopapular rash with areas of coalescence over the face, trunk, and extremities. He is afebrile and otherwise has been acting appropriately. Five days prior, he was seen by his pediatrician for fever and fussiness. At that time, he was diagnosed with an ear infection and started on amoxicillin.

86.1

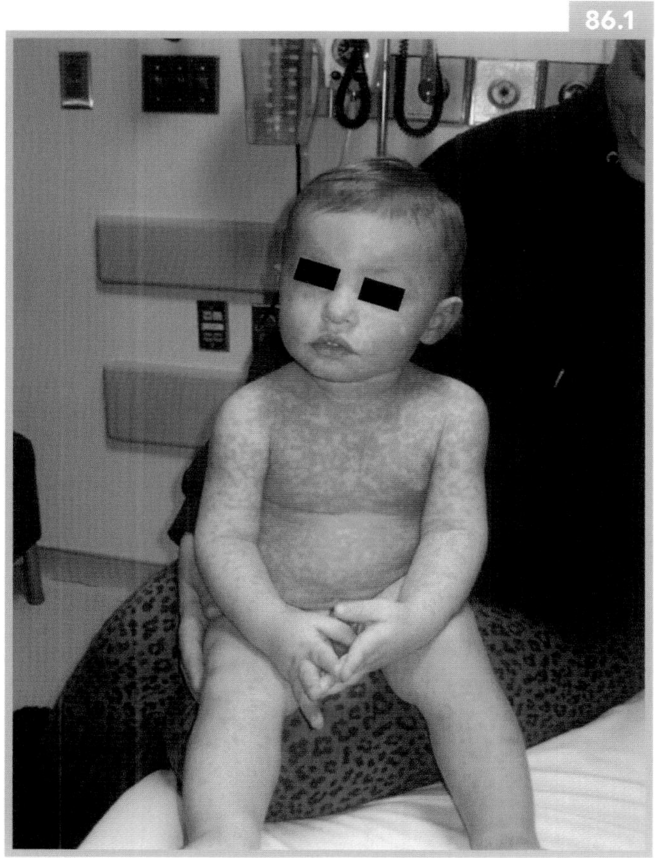

1. Can this child receive beta-lactam antibiotics in the future?
2. What viral infections are in the differential diagnosis for this patient?

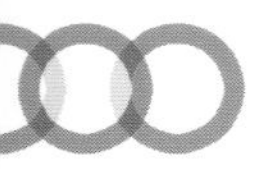

Answers

1. Non-pruritic maculopapular rashes are a common adverse effect associated with amoxicillin. About 3%–7% of patients may develop this type of reaction during treatment with an aminopenicillin (Bass et al., 1973). Frequently, the non-pruritic rash develops 3 to 10 days after initiating the antibiotic. The rash is thought to be idiopathic and is unlikely to be IgE-mediated (Pichichero 2005). In most cases, a child such as the one in the description can receive beta-lactam antibiotics in the future (Bierman et al., 1972). Careful documentation of the rash in the patient's allergies is important to ensure appropriate future antibiotic treatment options.

   IgE-mediated (type I) reactions, also known as immediate hypersensitivity reactions, range in severity from urticaria to anaphylaxis. Patients who experience this type of reaction to amoxicillin (or other penicillins) should consult an allergist prior to exposure to other penicillins.

2. Acute Epstein-Barr virus (EBV) infection could be considered. It has long been described that amoxicillin use during acute EBV infection produces a maculopapular rash (Shapiro et al., 1969). The rash is not an allergic reaction to the antibiotic. Unlike the patient described here, the rash associated with amoxicillin use during acute EBV infection is typically pruritic. Roseola may also be considered in this patient depending on additional history. Classically, roseola presents in children 6–24 months of age with 3–5 days of high fevers, and as the fever subsides a maculopapular rash may develop.

Keywords: infectious diseases, drug reactions, mimickers

References

Bass JW, Crowley DM, Steele RW, Young FSH, Harden LB. Adverse effects of orally administered ampicillin. *J Pediatr* 1973;83:106–8.

Bierman CW, Pierson WE, Zeitz SJ, Hoffman LS, VanArsdel PP Jr. Reactions associated with ampicillin therapy. *JAMA* 1972;220:1098–100.

Pichichero M. A review of evidence supporting the American Academy of Pediatrics Recommendation for prescribing cephalosporin antibiotics for penicillin-allergic patients. *Pediatrics* 2005;115(4):1048–57.

Shapiro S, Siskind V, Slone D, Lewis GP, Jick H. Drug rash with ampicillin and other penicillins. *Lancet* 1969;2:969–72.

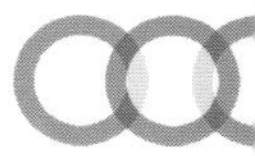

CASE 87

Veena Ramaiah

Question

A 21-month-old presents to the pediatric emergency department with a blistering rash to the buttocks. Her mother noticed the rash upon arrival home from work. The child was in his grandparents care today in their home as per routine childcare arrangement, and they report no vomiting, fevers, or history of sitting in or spilling hot liquid. He does have diarrhea and has pain when sitting on his buttocks.

His vital signs are normal and examination is normal except for blistering and erythema to medial buttocks in diamond-shaped pattern consistent with outline of diaper. The blistering and erythema extends up to the inferior scrotum, but the penis, peri-anal area, and inguinal folds spared. A 2 × 2 cm denuded area with erythematous, blanching base is present on the right buttock. Lesions are tender to palpation.

87.1

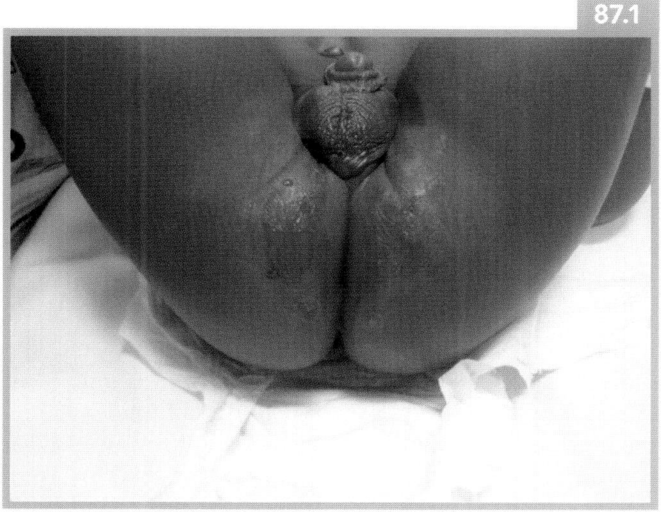

What does this look like, and what else would you like to know?

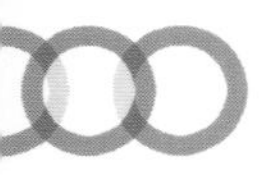

Answer

After a physical exam and on further questioning, Mom was unsure of medications in home. However, when asked directly about stool softeners, she thought maybe the grandfather takes a stool softener. We contacted the patient's grandfather by phone. Both grandparents deny any hot liquid spills or possible burns to the child. The grandfather does take Ex-Lax® (stimulant laxative) and keeps it in a drawer in the bedroom. The patient had been playing in there today. The grandfather was asked to look for the Ex-Lax and he could not find it in the drawer. He is unsure how many were in the drawer.

In light of the diarrhea and the distinctive pattern of the lesions, the conclusion was chemical burn/dermatitis due to Ex-Lax ingestion.

Discussion

Blistering lesions to the buttocks are often very concerning for burns. In addition, the absence of an explanation for the possible burn requires one to consider the possibility of inflicted injury. This case highlights the importance of considering a wider differential diagnosis, paying particular attention to the review of systems and taking the time to obtain a detailed history from the person at the bedside and caretakers who may not be present at the time.

There are case reports in the literature of laxative-induced dermatitis of the buttocks mimicking inflicted burns (Leventhal et al., 2001; Spiller et al., 2003), particularly in the setting of senna-containing laxatives.

Laxatives containing senna are not recommended for children under 2 years of age. However, the appearance, especially of Ex-Lax, makes it very attractive to toddlers who do not realize it is a medication. Ex-Lax is a chocolate-flavored medication with squares wrapped in foil that appears very similar to candy. Each square can contain 15–25 mg of sennosides. Senna is an herb from which the extracts are obtained. The active components in senna extracts are anthraquinone derivatives and their glucosides, referred to as senna glycosides or sennosides. Sennosides irritate the lining of the colon causing peristalsis and promoting evacuation of stool. Senna may also enhance intestinal fluid accumulation and increase the moisture content of stool by inhibiting electrolyte and water re-absorption from the colon.

The exact mechanism for the evolution of the dermatitis/burn is unknown. Possible theories include prolonged contact of senna-containing diarrheal stool against the buttocks due to the diaper or injury from increased concentrations of digestive enzymes in the diarrheal stool due to increased gut transit time (Leventhal et al., 2001; Durani et al., 2006). The sparing of the peri-anal area and the presence of blistering in only children in diapers is indicative of the prolonged contact playing a role in the evolution of the burn.

This patient's blistering was superficial partial thickness. No debridement was necessary, and the child was discharged with silver sulfadiazine cream applied topically twice a day for a week.

Keywords: child abuse mimickers, dermatology, medications

References

Durani P, Agarwal R, Wilson DI. Laxative induced burns in a child. *J Plast Reconstr Aesthet Surg* 2006;59(10):1129.

Leventhal JM, Griffin D, Duncan KO, Starling S, Christian CW, Kutz T. Laxative-induced dermatitis of the buttocks incorrectly suspected to be abusive burns. *Paediatrics* 2001;107(1):178–9.

Spiller HA, Winter ML, Weber JA, Krenzelok MP, Anderson DL, Ryan ML. Skin breakdown and blisters from senna-containing laxatives in young children. *Ann Pharmacother* 2003;37(5):636–9.

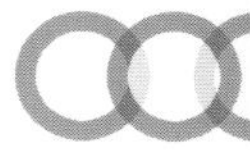

CASE 88

Justin Triemstra

Question

A 19-month-old male presents with an evanescent rash and swelling of his feet following a viral illness. He has no mucosal lesions and otherwise appears well.

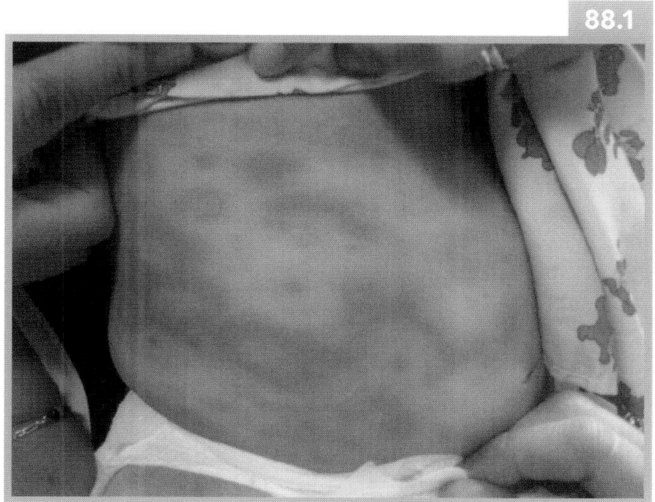

88.1

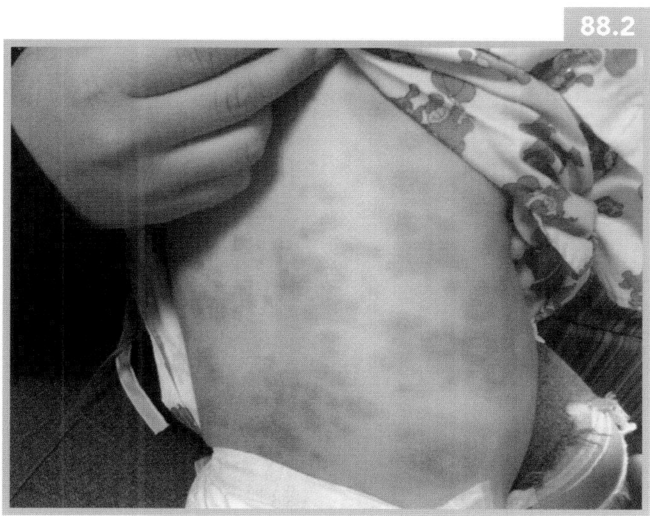

88.2

(Courtesy of Dr. Mara Beveridge.)

What is the condition? What is the common differential diagnosis for this type of rash? What is the treatment for this condition?

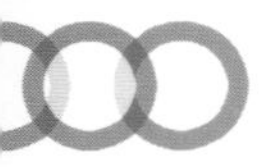

Answer

The diagnosis is consistent with acute annular urticarial hypersensitivity, also known as urticaria multiforme. Urticaria multiforme is an allergic hypersensitivity reaction that presents initially as small erythematous lesions that rapidly expand to form annular, arcuate wheals with central clearing or a dusky, ecchymotic appearance. The diagnosis is typically made clinically, and a skin biopsy is usually not warranted.

Urticaria multiforme is commonly confused with erythema multiforme or serum sickness–like reaction. The important distinction can be found in the duration of the lesions. In urticaria multiforme, the lesions usually last minutes to hours as opposed to days to weeks as in erythema multiforme and serum sickness–like reaction. Furthermore, dermatographism is common in urticaria multiforme, unlike in erythema multiforme or serum sickness–like reaction.

Most cases resolve following supportive care with antihistamines. Systemic corticosteroids should be reserved for only severe cases. Any new or unnecessary antibiotics should be discontinued. If symptoms persist or the rash is associated with other systemic findings such as arthralgias, fevers, or other abnormal laboratory values, other conditions should be considered.

Keywords: dermatology, drug reactions, mimickers

Bibliography

Shah K, Honig P, Yan A. "Urticaria multiforme": A case series and review of acute annular urticarial hypersensitivity syndromes in children. *Pediatrics* 2007;119:1177–83.

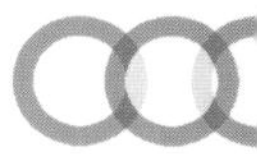

CASE 89

Timothy Ketterhagen

Question

A 7-year-old male is brought to the emergency department due to discoloration of his tongue. His mother noticed the darkening of the tongue one night previously, but it has not improved. The patient has had upset stomach and loose stools for the past 2 days. However, the mother states that the patient has not had vomiting and has been drinking a normal amount. Urine output has been normal. No fevers. Activity level is normal. He denies any recent ingestion of any dark-colored foods.

Physical exam reveals black discoloration of the tongue. No dental or lip discoloration is appreciated. The posterior pharynx is normal and his abdominal exam is reassuring. His physical exam is otherwise unremarkable.

89.1

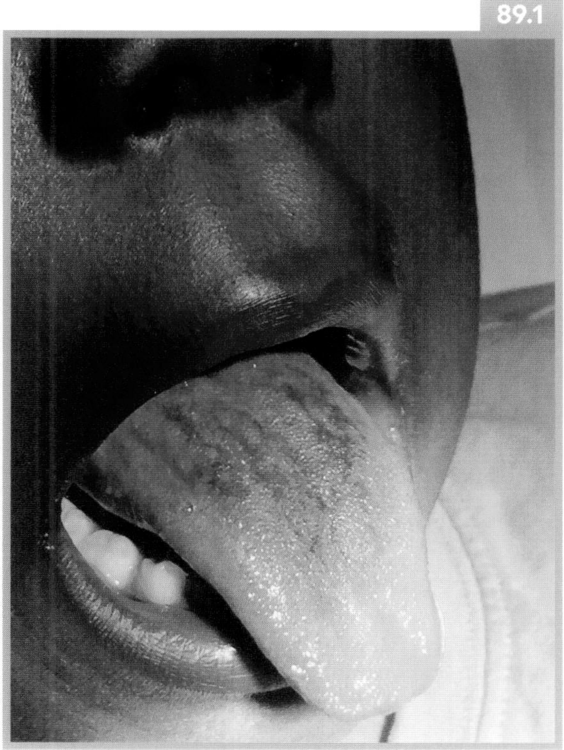

Additional historical information is elicited that suggests the etiology. What is the etiology of the tongue discoloration?

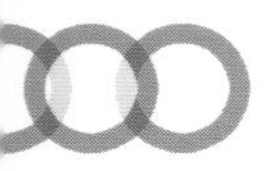

Answer

The mother has been giving the patient Pepto-Bismol (bismuth subsalicylate) intermittently for his stomach discomfort, which is the likely cause of this patient's tongue discoloration. Patients may also report darkening of the stools. According to the product website, "when a small amount of bismuth combines with trace amounts of sulfur in your saliva and gastrointestinal tract, a black-colored substance (bismuth sulfide) is formed." This is a temporary and benign side effect of Pepto-Bismol. Symptoms should resolve several days after stopping the medication. No workup is required unless an alternate cause is suspected.

Keywords: medications, head and neck/ENT, benign

Bibliography

Lexicomp Online®, Pediatric & Neonatal Lexi-Drugs®, Hudson, Ohio: Lexi-Comp, Inc.; February 23, 2017. https://www.wolterskluwercdi.com/lexicomp-online/

"Why can Pepto-Bismol sometimes darken the tongue or stool?" http://www.pepto-bismol.com/en-us/faq/black-stool-black-tongue.

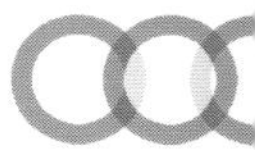

CASE 90

Michael Gottlieb

Questions

A 12-year-old girl was running down the stairs and jumped down the last five steps, landing on her right foot. She had immediate pain and was unable to ambulate. Her exam was significant for diffuse pain and swelling of the ankle joint. The following images were obtained:

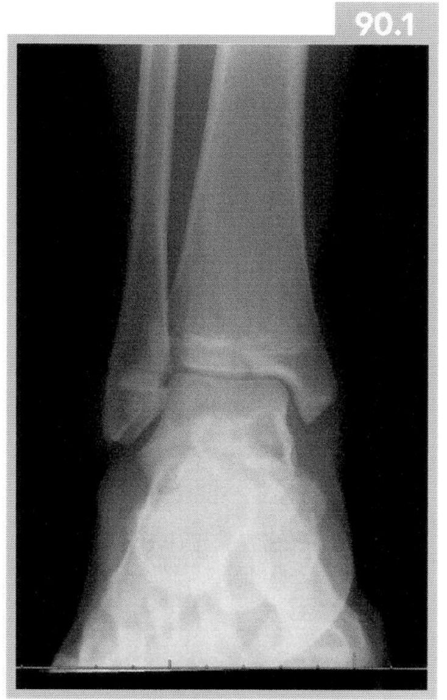

90.1

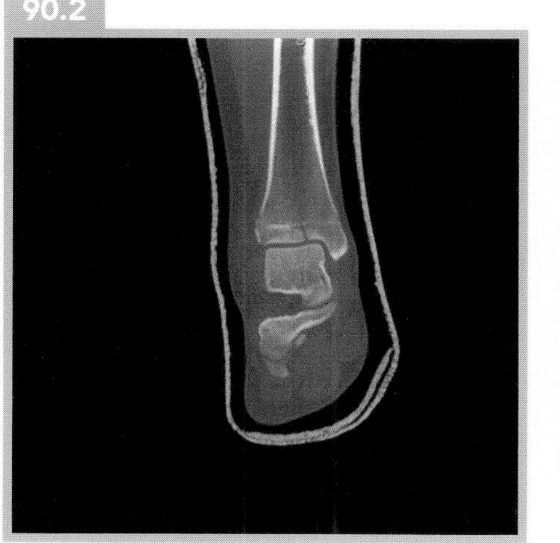

90.2

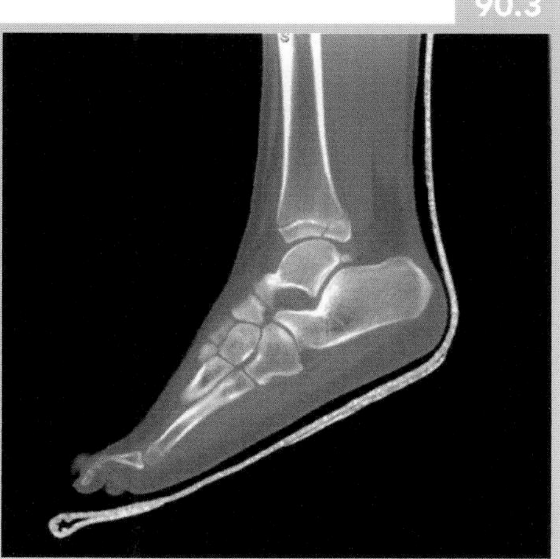

90.3

1. Using the Salter-Harris (S-H) classification, what type of fracture is this?
2. Which Salter-Harris fracture has the best prognosis? Which has the worst?

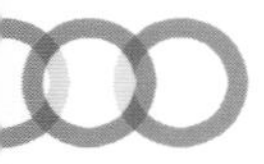

Answers

1. This patient is presenting with a Tillaux fracture, which is a special type of Salter-Harris III fracture that occurs in adolescents between the ages of 12 and 15 when the medial growth plate has closed, but the lateral aspect is still open.

   Salter-Harris classification is a commonly used criteria to describe fractures in children with respect to the growth plate. S-H I describes fractures through the growth plate. S-H II describes fractures above the growth plate (toward the metaphysis). S-H III describes fractures below the growth plate (toward the epiphysis). S-H IV describes fractures extending both above and below the growth plate. S-H V describes fractures that involve a compressive force directly on the growth plate. This may be easily recalled using the mnemonic:

   I—S: Straight across
   II—A: Above
   III—L: Lower
   IV—TE: Through everything
   V—R: Rammed

2. Salter-Harris I fractures typically have the best prognosis and are typically treated conservatively with immobilization until the fracture has healed. Salter-Harris V fractures are associated with the worst prognosis due to the significant damage to the growth plate. Unfortunately, these fractures are often diagnosed after the fact when subsequent radiographs demonstrate a bony bar across the physis or after a leg length discrepancy occurs.

Keywords: orthopedics, blunt trauma, extremity injury

Bibliography

Chasm RM, Swencki SA. Pediatric orthopedic emergencies. *Emerg Med Clin North Am*. November 2010;28(4):907–26.

Kennedy MA, Sama AE, Padavan S. The Tillaux fracture: A case report. *J Emerg Med* July–August 1998;16(4):603–6.

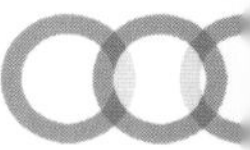

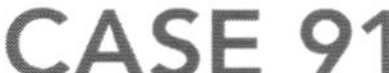

CASE 91

Leah Finkel

Question

A 5-year-old boy presents with mouth pain. His mother reports that he has required dental work for multiple caries. Over the last day, there is some worsening pain particularly when brushing his teeth.

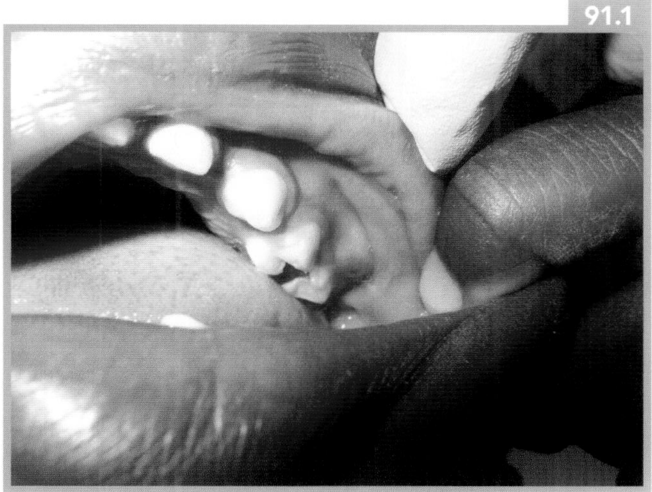

91.1

What do you see on examination and how do you manage this?

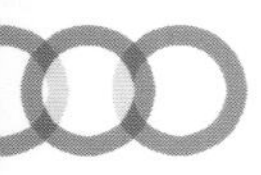

Answer

This patient has a dental abscess. On examination there is localized swelling of the gingiva with a fluctuant mass. There are often severe erosive dental caries as well as warmth and tenderness of the area. This is due to a collection of pus around or near a tooth. Many of these abscesses result from tooth decay or extensive periodontal disease. Patients usually present with extreme and worsening pain at the site of the abscess and occasionally local cellulitis. They may have anterior lymphadenopathy on the affected side and may present with headaches.

The incidence of dental abscess has decreased over the last 30 years due to fluoride in the water. Risk factors include certain tooth morphologies, infected buccal cysts, factors leading to caries, poor bone mineralization, and preceding dental trauma. The most common organisms involved include *Streptococcus viridans*, anaerobes (*Bacteroides*), *Prevotella* species, and *Fusobacterium* species. The diagnosis is primarily clinical and rarely requires imaging. Uncomplicated dental abscesses can be treated with needle aspiration and antibiotics. Ill-appearing children or children with evidence of invasive or systemic disease may require advanced imaging, parenteral antibiotics, additional investigations, and hospitalization. Patients should follow up with a dentist.

Keywords: dental, infectious diseases, head and neck/ENT

Bibliography

Seow, WK. Diagnosis and management of unusual dental abscesses in children. *Aus Dent J* 2003;48(3):156–68. http://onlinelibrary.wiley.com/doi/10.1111/j.1834-7819.2003.tb00026.x/epdf.

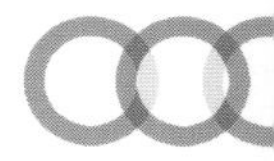

CASE 92

Timothy Ketterhagen

Questions

A 16-year-old male presents to the emergency department with right elbow pain. He was playing soccer when he tripped and fell onto an outstretched right arm. He reported immediate pain and deformity at the elbow. He denies any head trauma or loss of consciousness. No other injuries are reported.

Physical exam reveals a well-appearing young man holding his right arm in a semi-flexed position unable to move his elbow. There is swelling to the right elbow, and the right forearm appears shorter than the left. There is significant deformity of the right elbow with prominence of the ulna posteriorly. Sensation is intact distally. Distal radial and ulnar pulses are intact. Capillary refill is <2 s distal to injury. The patient is able to give a thumb's up, "OK" sign, touch his thumb to his fifth digit, and spread all his fingers apart on his right hand. There are no lacerations or bruising to the affected extremity. The physical exam is otherwise unremarkable. X-rays of the affected elbow are shown.

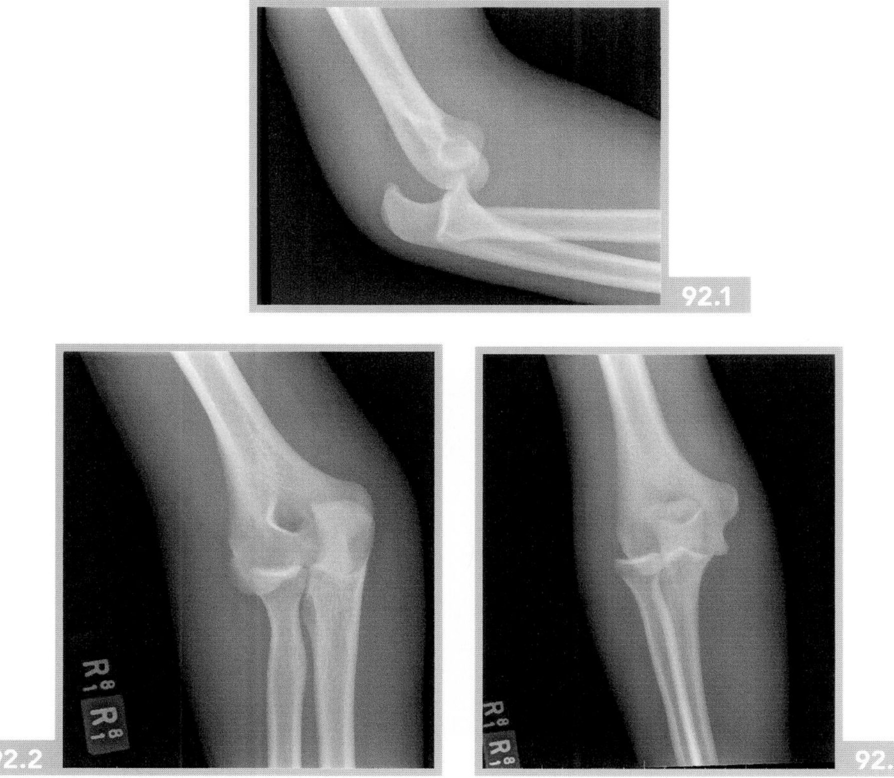

What is the diagnosis and what techniques may be used to correct the injury?

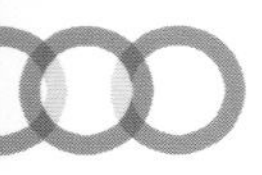

Answers

This patient has a sustained a right elbow dislocation. No fracture is appreciated. The majority of elbow dislocations are posterior. The brachial artery, median nerve, and ulnar nerve are all at risk of injury due to their relationship to the elbow. Prompt reduction of the elbow is crucial when there is risk of vascular compromise. Adequate analgesia and possible procedural sedation are indicated for reduction attempts.

Reduction techniques:

a. Sit the patient upright with the affected elbow held in 90° of flexion and hypersupination of the forearm. Apply posterior stabilizing force to the affected forearm, while simultaneously applying downward traction to the volar surface of the proximal forearm along the long axis of the humerus. This is followed by traction along the axis of the forearm to bring the coronoid process distal to the humerus. Flexion at the elbow with longitudinal traction and pressure on the volar aspect of the forearm are maintained to complete the reduction.
b. Place the patient in prone position with the affected forearm dangling over the examination table. Grasp the wrist and apply traction along the long axis of the forearm. Continue to apply traction until muscle relaxation is achieved, usually within 10 minutes. Grasp the olecranon with the thumb and forefinger, then guide it into position just distal to the humerus.

After successful reduction, assess range of motion and stability of the joint. Neurovascular assessment should be completed before and after reduction. Post-reduction radiographs should be obtained to ensure adequate reduction. Apply a posterior splint and sling. Multiple reduction attempts may result in further injury; therefore, orthopedic consultation may be required if initial efforts fail or if a fracture is present.

Keywords: orthopedics, extremity injury, procedures

Bibliography

Hoffman RJ, Wang VJ, Scarfone R. *Fleisher & Ludwig's 5-Minute Pediatric Emergency Medicine Consult.* Philadelphia: Wolters Kluwer Health/Lippincott Williams & Wilkins, 2012.

King C, Henretig FM. *Textbook of Pediatric Emergency Procedures.* 2nd ed. Philadelphia: Wolters Kluwer Health/Lippincott Williams & Wilkins, 2008.

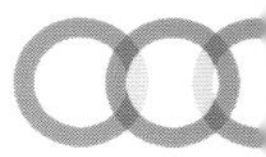

CASE 93

Timothy Ketterhagen

Question

A 15-year-old male presents to the emergency department due to right foot pain. He was at home earlier in the evening when he accidentally dropped a glass onto the ground and it broke into several small pieces. He was barefoot at the time and attempted to walk away but felt a sharp pain on the bottom of his right foot. He reports a small laceration where the pain is located that was bleeding initially, but has since stopped. He denies any other injuries. The patient's immunizations are up to date.

On physical exam he has a 1 cm superficial laceration to the sole of the right foot. The base of the wound is visualized and the edges are well approximated. Bleeding is controlled. No foreign bodies are visualized on initial examination. The patient is able to ambulate, but he does have a limp. His physical exam is otherwise unremarkable, and no other injuries are seen. X-rays of the injured foot with a piece of subcutaneous glass are shown.

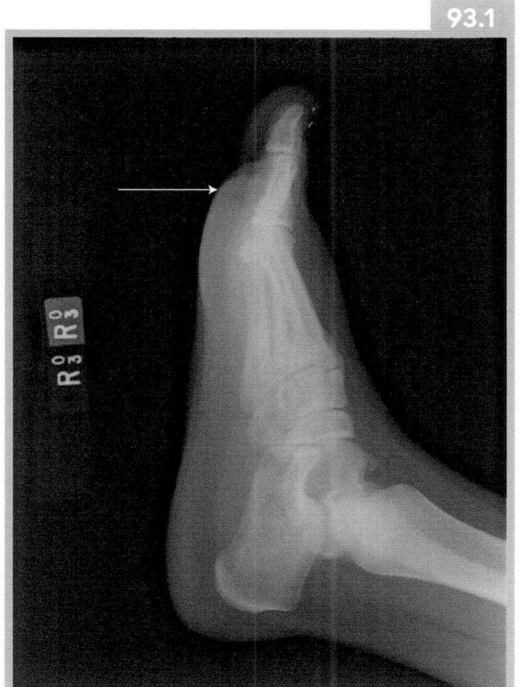

93.1

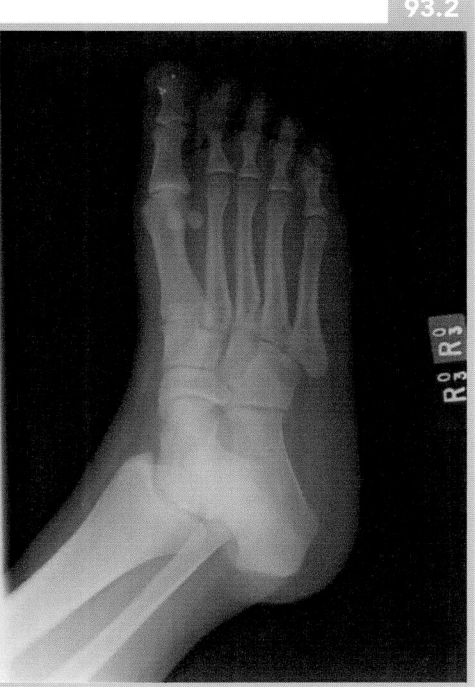

93.2

What is the management of subcutaneous glass in the foot?

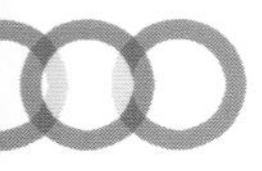

Answer

This patient has a piece of glass in the soft tissue in the sole of his right foot. Wounds that are suspicious for the presence of a foreign body should be radiographed. Surface markers and multiple radiographic views can aid in localizing the foreign body. The ability to inspect the bottom of the wound does not necessarily rule out the presence of a foreign body. The size, location, degree of reactivity of the material, and accessibility for removal with minimal risk of damaging surrounding structures should all be considered prior to extraction of a foreign body from a wound. Foreign bodies with a high risk of injury, infection, or toxicity should be removed.

Most types of glass are detectable on radiographs, and glass fragments as small as 0.5 mm may be visualized. Attempts to remove the foreign body should be made if the benefits outweigh the risks of removal. The patient's tetanus immunization status should be reviewed. Antibiotics are generally not required unless a foreign body is retained; there is heavy contamination; or the wound is over joints, bones, or tendons. Retained small foreign bodies composed of inert materials (glass, plastic, metal) in benign locations that are not able to be removed in the emergency department should be referred for surgical referral within 48–72 hours.

Keywords: foreign body, penetrating trauma, extremity injury

Bibliography

Fleisher GR, Ludwig S, eds. *Textbook of Pediatric Emergency Medicine*, 6th ed. Philadelphia: Lippincott Williams & Wilkins, 2010.

Hoffman RJ, Wang VJ, Scarfone R. *Fleisher & Ludwig's 5-Minute Pediatric Emergency Medicine Consult*. Philadelphia, PA: Wolters Kluwer Health/Lippincott Williams & Wilkins, 2012.

King C, Henretig FM. *Textbook of Pediatric Emergency Procedures*, 2nd ed. Philadelphia, PA: Wolters Kluwer Health/Lippincott Williams & Wilkins, 2008.

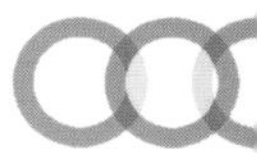

CASE 94

Diana Yan

Question

A 1-week-old baby boy presents to the emergency department after his mother noticed his tooth growing. The tooth was present at birth and is now causing his mother to have pain with breastfeeding, with associated abrasions and bleeding. There is no blood in the baby's mouth nor is there redness or drainage from the tooth. There are no fevers or increased fussiness. The baby is doing well with normal activity level and normal wet diapers. He was born full term, and there were no complications during pregnancy or at delivery.

Physical exam shows an alert and awake baby boy in his mom's arms. There is a small 5 mm protruding tooth on the anterior mandibular gum line. The tooth is firmly in place without any anterior or posterior subluxation. No other lesions are present, and the baby otherwise appears well hydrated.

94.1

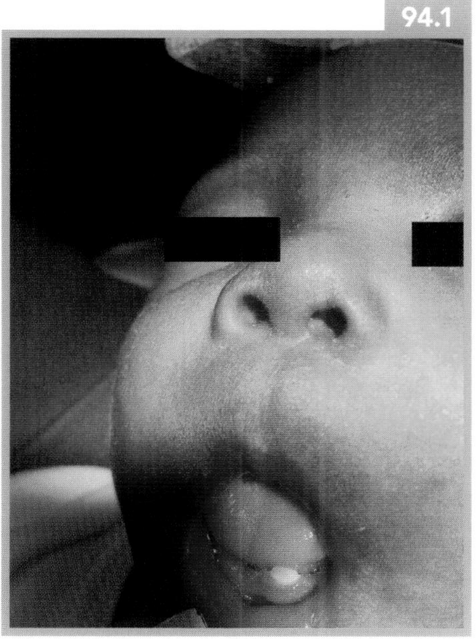

94.2

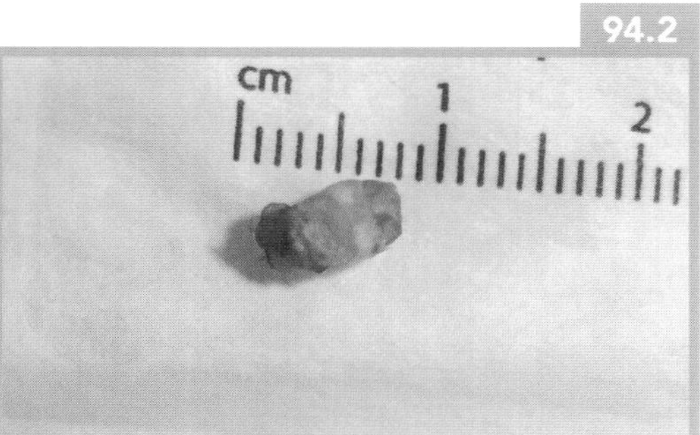

What is most appropriate treatment for this condition?

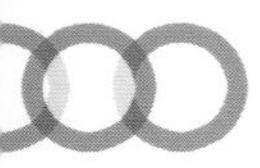

Answer

Extraction of the natal tooth. Normal eruption of the first primary teeth can occur as early as 6 months of age. A natal tooth is a tooth that is present at birth, whereas a neonatal tooth is one that erupts within the first 30 days of life. These teeth are usually in pairs and can look like normal teeth. However, more commonly they are small in size, yellow in color, conical, and have hypoplastic enamel and dentin. They usually have no or poor root formation. The most common location for a natal tooth is the lower central incisor. These teeth are thought to come from abnormal superficial migration of the tooth's germ line. The teeth can be classified into four categories based on where the tooth is located with respect to the gum line. These teeth can actually be left alone if they are determined to be part of the normal dentition through x-rays. However, complications can occur, including breastfeeding interference, sublingual ulceration, or aspiration of loose teeth. In such cases, a pediatric dentist should remove them after the age of 10 days. Removal will also avoid any future impaction or space issues.

Keywords: neonate, dental

Bibliography

Khandelwal V, Nayak UA, Nayak PA, Bafna Y. Management of an infant having natal teeth. *BMJ Case Rep* 2013. doi: 10.11136/bcr-2013-010049.

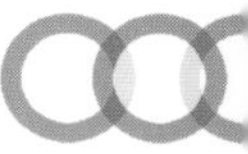

CASE 95

Michael Gottlieb

Questions

A full-term, previously healthy 8-month-old girl presents with a painful and swollen left fifth digit. There was no witnessed trauma and the mother denies any preceding fever or other swollen digits.

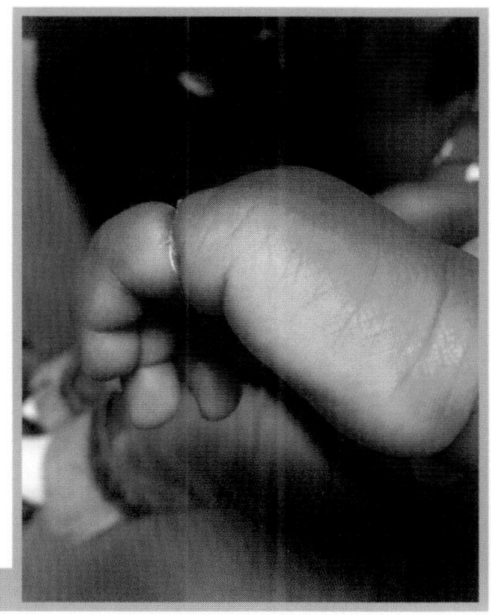

95.1

Initial presentation

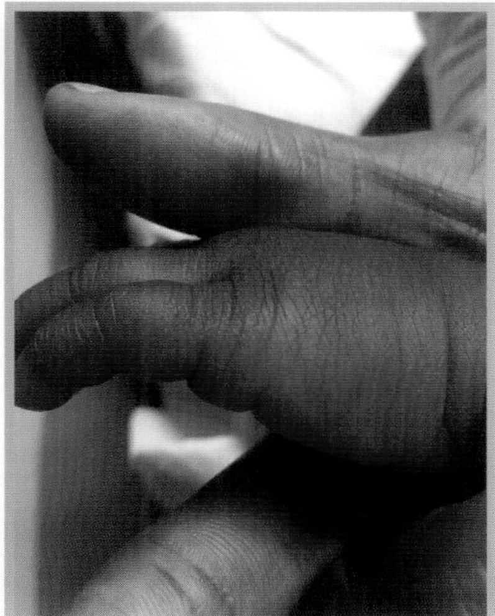

95.2

Post procedure

1. What is the likely etiology of the swollen digit in this patient?
2. What are the treatment options for this condition?

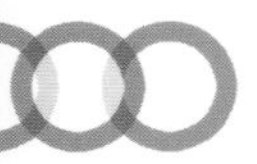

Answers

1. This patient is presenting with a hair tourniquet. This is a common medical condition, wherein a hair or thread becomes tied around a finger, toe, or penis, resulting in distal edema. This is considered a medical emergency, as prolonged compression can lead to ischemia and even loss of the affected digit.

2. When the etiology is known to be due to hair, a chemical depilatory agent may be attempted to dissolve the hair fibers. However, when there is significant edema or suspicion for an alternate tourniquet material, prompt excision of the constricting fibers should be performed (see Image 95.2). Excisions should be performed in a longitudinal direction over the area of skin depression. Often, it may be necessary to extend the incision down to the bone to ensure all of the fibers are released.

Keywords: hand injury, procedures

Bibliography

Barton DJ, Sloan GM, Nichter LS, Reinisch JF et al. Hair-thread tourniquet syndrome. *Pediatrics* December 1988;82(6):925–8.

Serour F, Gorenstein A. Treatment of the toe tourniquet syndrome in infants. *Pediatr Surg Int* October 2003;19(8):598–600.

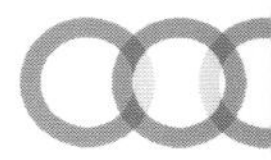

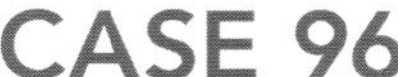

CASE 96

Leah Finkel

Question

A 7-year-old girl with no past medical history presents with swelling at the base of her mouth. Two weeks ago she fell on the playground and had some minor trauma to the mouth. On examination she is in no acute distress and has no increased work of breathing.

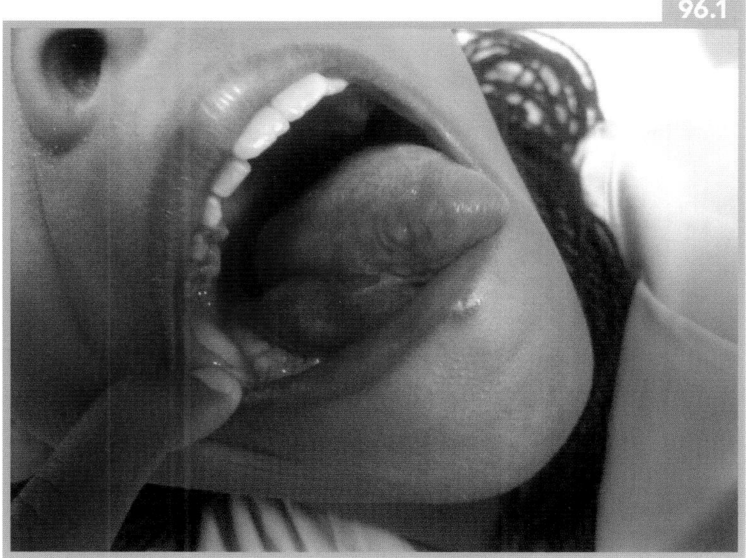

96.1

What do you see on examination, and how do you manage this?

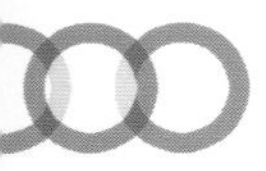

Answer

This is a ranula, which is a type of mucocele associated with the sublingual and submandibular ducts. Ranulas are fluctuant swellings lateral to the midline lower mouth and may have a bluish hue to them. They may congenital, secondary to trauma, or occur after incomplete drainage of the sublingual glands.

Diagnosis is clinical. Ranulas are mostly seen in young children or adolescents.

Large ranulas may present as neck masses. If small and asymptomatic, ranulas may be observed. Otherwise, oral surgery may be needed. Complete excision is usually the preferred management, though marsupialization and suturing of the pseudocyst wall may be effective.

Complications include infection, bursting and reformation, and dysphagia if the ranula is large.

Keywords: head and neck/ENT, congenital anomaly, mass

Bibliography

Patel MR, Deal AM, Shockley WW. Oral and plunging ranulas: What is the most effective treatment? *Laryngoscope* 2009 August;119(8):1501–9. http://www.ncbi.nlm.nih.gov/pubmed/19504549.

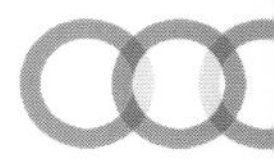

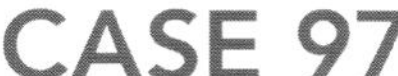

CASE 97

Michael Gottlieb

Questions

A 10-year-old obese boy presents with left knee and hip pain for the past 2 weeks. There was no preceding trauma, and he denies numbness or weakness. On exam, he has mild pain with hip range of motion and has a waddling gait. His sensation, strength, pulses, and capillary refill are normal in both extremities. A hip radiograph is demonstrated next.

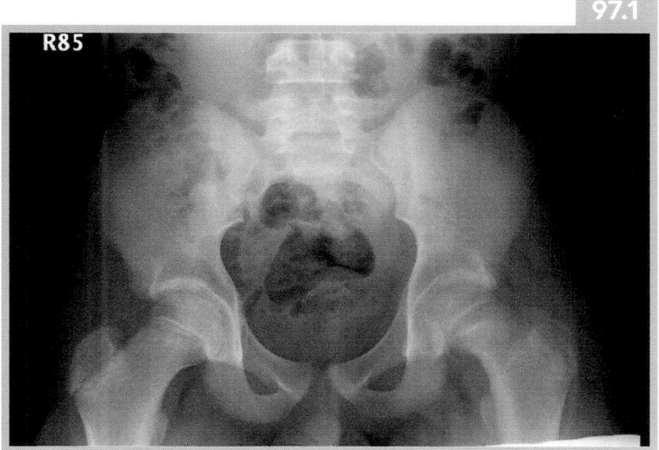

97.1

1. What is his diagnosis?
2. How is this diagnosed?
3. What is the treatment for this condition?

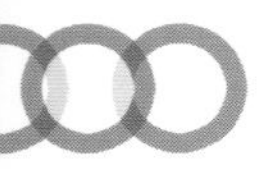

Answers

1. This patient has slipped capital femoral epiphysis (SCFE). SCFE is defined as the slippage of the proximal femoral epiphysis on the metaphysis (femoral neck) at the level of the growth plate. It is the most common hip disorder in adolescents, usually occurring between 8 and 15 years of age. It is more common in boys than girls and has a higher prevalence in overweight children. Patients typically present with subacute hip or knee pain with limited internal range of motion and an antalgic gait.
2. Radiography is the key to the diagnosis and should include both anteroposterior (AP) and frog-leg views of both hips. This can be diagnosed by drawing a line on the lateral edge of the femoral neck to the epiphysis (referred to as Klein's line). If the line does not intersect with the epiphysis, this suggests SCFE. Additional findings include loss of height of the epiphysis, widening of the epiphysis, and a double density at the proximal metaphysis on AP radiograph (referred to as the Steel sign).
3. Treatment involves open reduction and internal fixation with a single screw placed through the epiphysis and metaphysis. Patients should be admitted for strict non-weightbearing precautions while awaiting definitive management. Complications without proper treatment include avascular necrosis, chondrolysis, and early degenerative osteoarthritis.

Keywords: orthopedics, limp, do not miss, pitfalls

Bibliography

Georgiadis AG, Zaltz I. Slipped capital femoral epiphysis: How to evaluate with a review and update of treatment. *Pediatr Clin North Am* December 2014;61(6):1119–35.

Peck D. Slipped capital femoral epiphysis: Diagnosis and management. *Am Fam Physician* 2010 August 1, 2010;82(3):258–62.

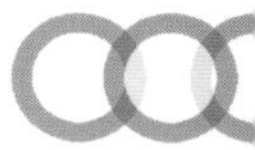

CASE 98

Catherine H. Chung

Question

A 3-year-old boy presents with a 2-day history of non-bloody, non-bilious vomiting, loose bloody stools, and occasional abdominal pain which seems to be intensifying and becoming more frequent. The patient otherwise is healthy without any surgical or travel history.

On physical exam his vital signs are normal and he is sitting in bed playing with blocks in no apparent distress. His exam shows mild dehydration with slightly dry oral mucosa but brisk capillary refill. He has a non-focal abdominal exam with slightly decreased bowel sounds. At the end of the exam, the patient starts holding his belly and cries for several minutes, and then resumes his activity.

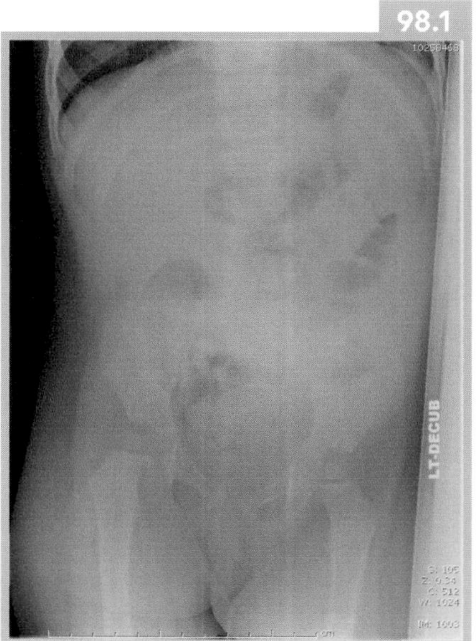

98.1

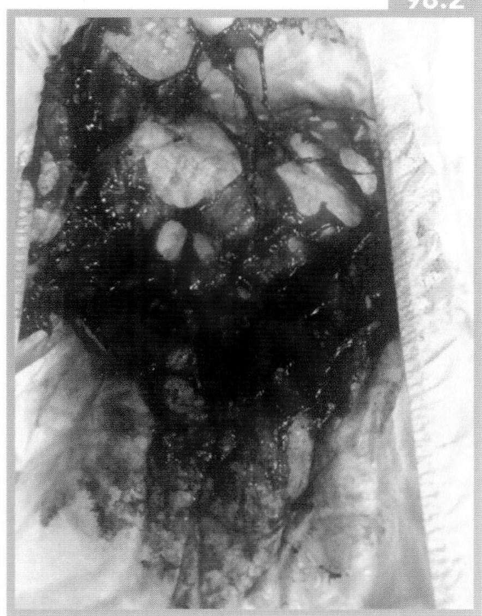

98.2

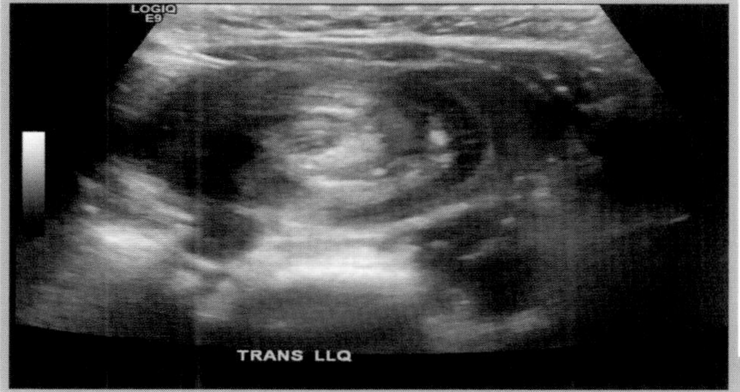

98.3

1. How will this diagnosis present in the early versus later stages?
2. What are notable findings on imaging studies you would you expect to see?

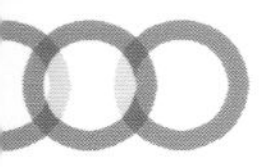

Answers

1. This patient has the classic signs of intussusception. Intussusception can distinguish itself from other acute abdomen pathologies by its waxing and waning episodes of severe abdominal pain. The etiology is due to proximal bowel being stuck inside the distal portion of bowel resulting in a bowel obstruction.

   In the beginning, patients may look very well and have no focal abdominal findings. These patients can easily be misdiagnosed as having gastroenteritis because clinicians will anchor on the vomiting and looser stools. It is prudent to ask parents about pain despite the child appearing well on initial evaluation. Over time, patients become more dehydrated and too lethargic to cry in pain. At this stage, they typically present with clinical signs of bowel obstruction and may have the classic currant-jelly stools (see Image 98.2). With delayed intervention, patients can develop bowel perforation and septic shock.

2. The initial workup is typically ultrasound, which is non-invasive and focuses on the right lower quadrant in the ileocecal region. The classic finding is the doughnut sign (see Image 98.3) which reveals the bowel within bowel.

   Plain radiographs may appear normal in the early stage of intussusception; only later in the course will signs of bowel obstruction including dilated small bowel loops and absence of air in the cecum be apparent.

   In some institutions, if the provider is highly suspicious, the patient may bypass an ultrasound and undergo an air or contrast enema, which is both diagnostic and therapeutic.

Keywords: surgery, abdominal pain, ultrasound, vomiting

Bibliography

Fleisher GR, Ludwig S, eds. *Textbook of Pediatric Emergency Medicine*. 6th ed. Philadelphia: Lippincott Williams & Wilkins, 2010.

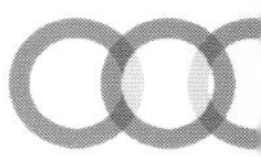

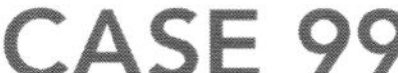

CASE 99

Emily Obringer

Question

A 10-day-old infant presents with a rash in the diaper area and inner thighs. The parents report that the rash started as red raised lesions but has progressed over the last 24 hours to large, fluid-filled blisters. Desquamated skin and crusting is present at the site of a ruptured blister. The child has been afebrile but has not been feeding as well. The rash appears painful when examined.

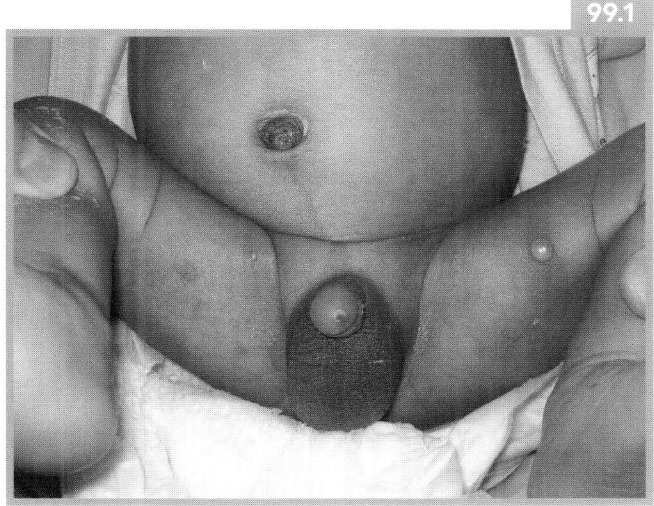

99.1

What is the most likely diagnosis and pathogenic organism?

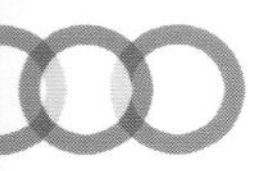

Answer

Bullous impetigo is a skin infection caused by toxin-producing strains of *Staphylococcus aureus* and is the localized form of staphylococcal scalded-skin syndrome. Erythematous vesicles rapidly progress to large flaccid superficial bullae. Systemic symptoms are uncommon. Bullous impetigo is most common in neonates and is often found in intertriginous areas, such as the diaper region, neck, and skin folds.

Non-bullous impetigo may be caused by *S. aureus* or group A streptococcus and is more common in children ages 2 to 5 years. The face and extremities are common sites of infection. Papules and vesicles evolve to pustules that rupture and leave a golden-colored crust on the skin over the course of a week.

Treatment of non-bullous and bullous impetigo includes topical antibacterial ointment. Mupirocin has been shown to be equivalent to oral systemic antibiotics and may be used in localized disease. When topical treatment is impractical or if disease is extensive, oral antibiotics should be considered. In such cases, particularly in the neonate, obtaining a blood culture and considering inpatient admission is prudent.

Keywords: skin and soft tissue infection, dermatology, infectious diseases

Bibliography

Cole C, Gazewood J. Diagnosis and treatment of impetigo. *Am Fam Physician* 2007;75(6):859–64.

Stanley JR, Amagai M. Pemphigus, bullous impetigo, and the staphylococcal scalded-skin syndrome. *N Engl J Med* 2006;355:1800–10.

Stevens DL, Bisno AL, Chambers HF, Everett ED et al. Practice guidelines for the diagnosis and management of skin and soft-tissue infections. *Clin Infect Dis* 2005;41:1373–406.

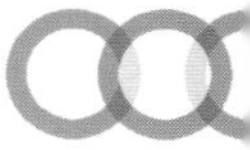

CASE 100

Michael Gottlieb

Questions

A 5-year-old boy was working with his father in the garage when he accidentally cut his finger on the circular saw. The father immediately brought him to the emergency department. The fingertip remains partially attached, but he has no sensation distally. There is exposed bone on exam.

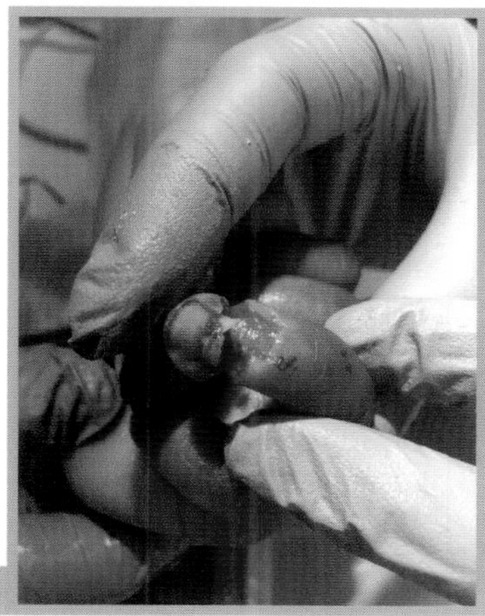

100.1

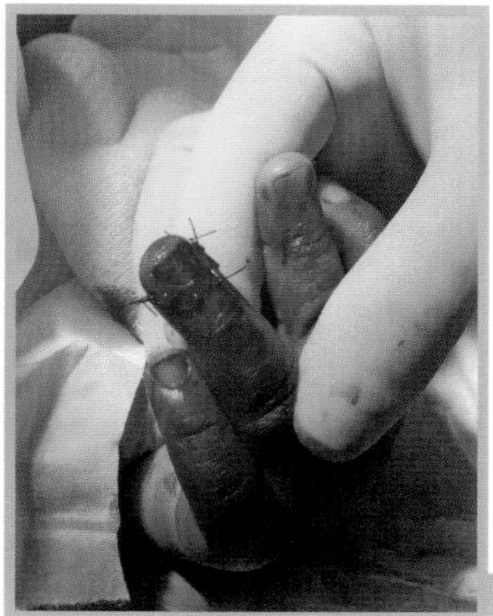

100.2

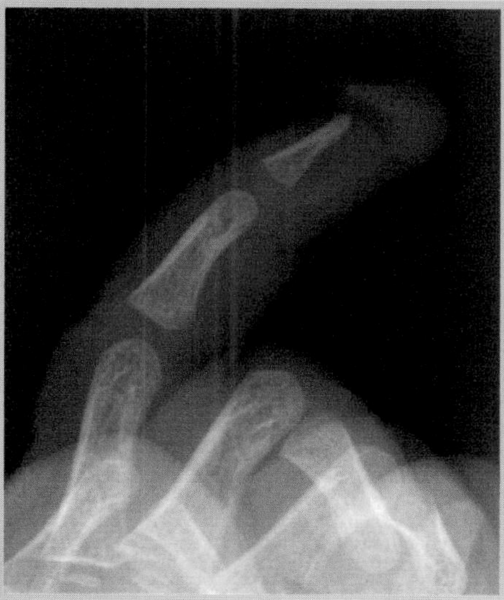

100.3

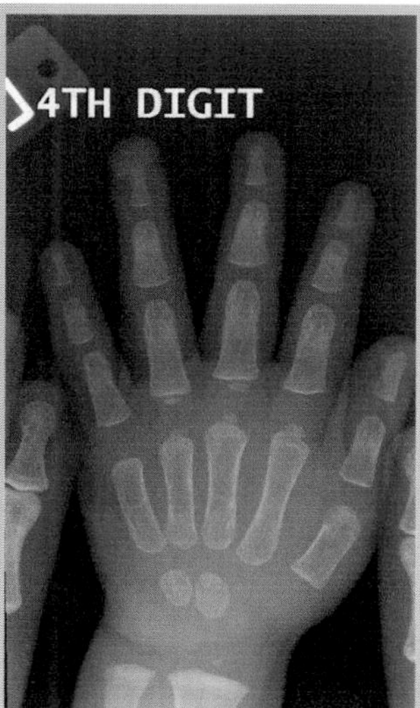

100.4

1. What is the appropriate management of this injury?
2. If this were a full amputation, what is the best method to preserve viability of the amputated digit?

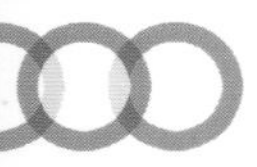

Answers

1. Given the significant degree of injury and loss of sensation in a pediatric patient, a hand surgeon should be consulted for consideration of repair. If repair is not feasible (i.e. the amputated part is not available), the finger should be anesthetized with a digital block, thoroughly irrigated, and closed. If there is exposed bone, the bone should be rongeured down to allow the skin to fully cover the exposed bone. Limited data are available to support antibiotic prophylaxis for open fractures of the distal phalanx, but should be considered in consultation with the hand surgeon.

2. The amputated digit should be covered with saline-soaked gauze and then placed inside of a watertight bag. The bag should then be placed in a container filled with a mix of water and ice. It is important not to place the digit directly on ice, as this can directly injure the tissue.

Keywords: penetrating trauma, hand injury, procedures

Bibliography

de Alwis W. Fingertip injuries. *Emerg Med Australas* June 2006;18(3):229–37.

Cheung K, Hatchell A, Thoma A. Approach to traumatic hand injuries for primary care physicians. *Can Fam Physician* June 2013;59(6):614–8.

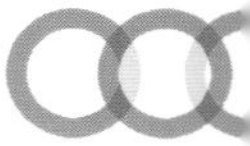

CASE 101

Diana Yan

Question

A 14-year-old male presents to the emergency room because of penile discharge. He has been complaining of abdominal and penile pain for the last 1–2 days. There has been no increase in urinary frequency, fevers, or redness of the penis. He has had a normal appetite and oral intake but did have decreased urine output for the last day. He reports today his urine stream is weak and it is taking him longer to urinate. He is otherwise healthy, and no one in the family has any kidney or urologic problems.

Physical exam shows an alert and awake teenager with suprapubic abdominal tenderness with some radiation into the groin. His abdomen is otherwise benign without any rebound or guarding. There is no penile discharge; however, a hard stone is visible and palpable at the meatus. There is no redness of the penis itself and no inguinal lymphadenopathy.

101.1

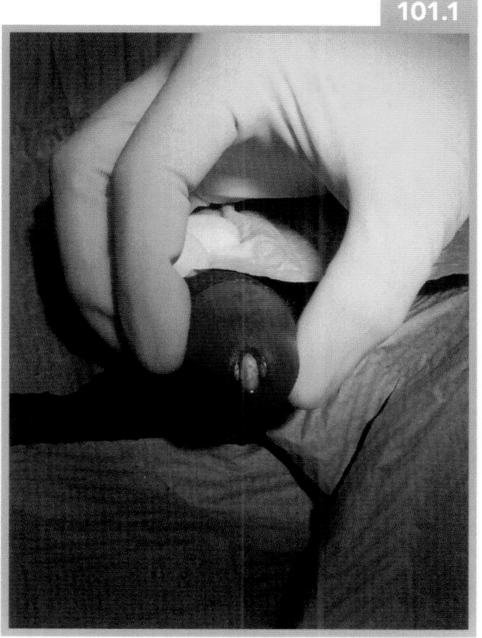

101.2

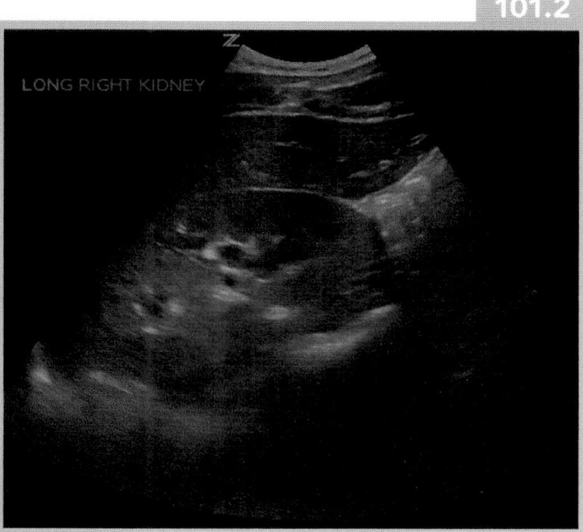

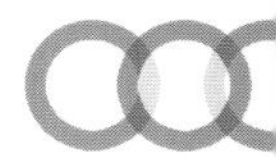

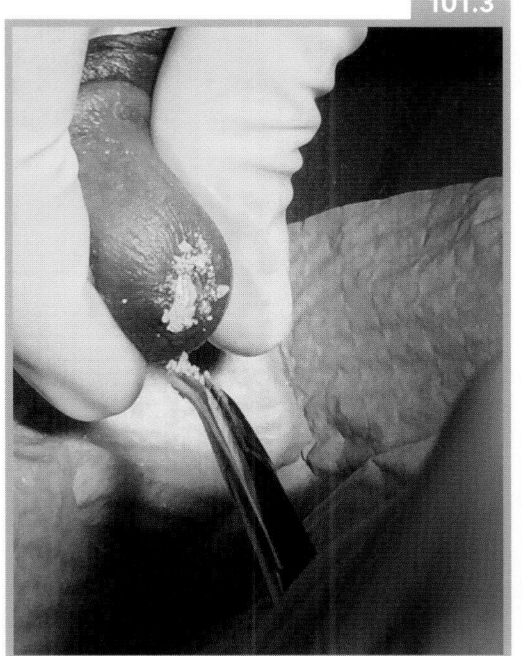

101.3

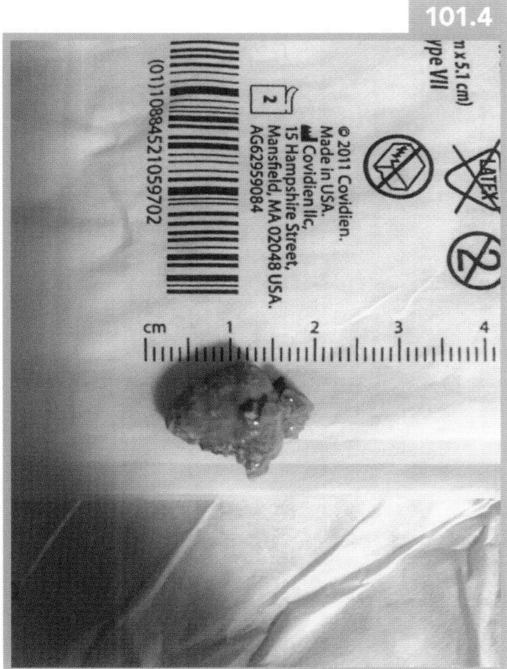

101.4

What are the major risk factors for developing bladder stones in children?

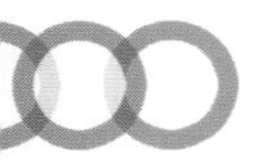

Answer

Hot climate, poor nutrition, or diarrheal diseases in underdeveloped countries and urinary tract infections or anatomic abnormalities in developed countries are the risk factors for developing bladder stones in children. In underdeveloped countries, diets low in animal protein or dietary phosphates and high in carbohydrates and chronic dehydration from diarrheal illness place children at risk. In developed countries, such as the United States, urinary stasis from a neurogenic bladder, megaureter, posterior urethral valves, extrophy, and other anatomic urologic abnormalities as well as infections are the biggest risk factors.

Bladder stones in low resource countries have a prevalence of as high as 15% in children under 15 years old, whereas in developed countries it is only 1% to 5%. There is also a male predominance. This is thought to be due to the non-tortuous anatomy in females, which allows for easier passage of small stone fragments. Patients present with abdominal pain, urgency, frequency, fevers, hematuria, and possibly urinary retention with associated kidney injury. Workup for these stones include a UA (urinalysis), urine culture, CBC (complete blood count), renal function panel, and imaging, which could include a abdominal radiograph or ultrasound. Treatment includes minimally invasive surgical removal like extracorporeal shock wave lithotripsy, dietary changes to prevent recurrence, pain management, and hydration.

Keywords: abdominal pain, genitourinary, child abuse mimicker, ultrasound

Bibliography

Rizvi SAH, Sultan S, Zafar MN, Ahmed B, Umer SA, Naqvi SAA. Paediatric urolithiasis in emerging economies. *Int J Surg* 2016;36:705–12.

Soliman NA, Rizvi SAH. Endemic bladder calculi in children. *Pediatr Nephrol* 2016. doi:10.1007/s00467-016-3492-4.

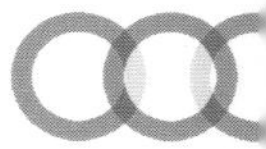

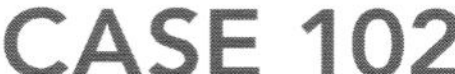

CASE 102

Emily Obringer

Questions

A 12-year-old boy presents to the emergency department with a rash on his right foot and leg. He denies trauma. He reports skin sensitivity and itchiness for 2 days before the rash appeared. He is well-appearing on exam with a unilateral rash as shown in a dermatomal distribution.

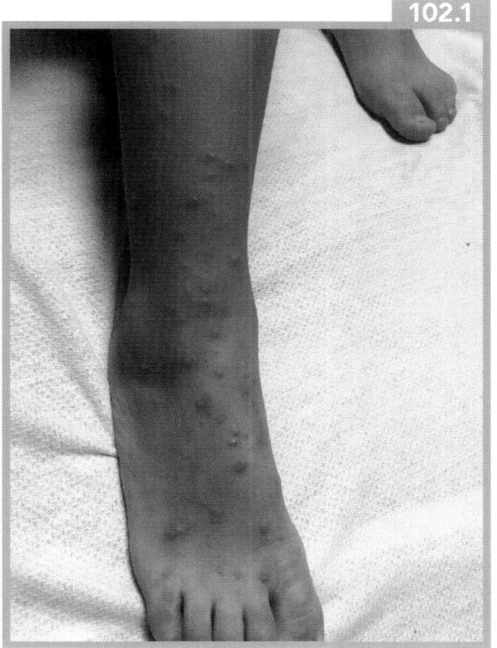

102.1

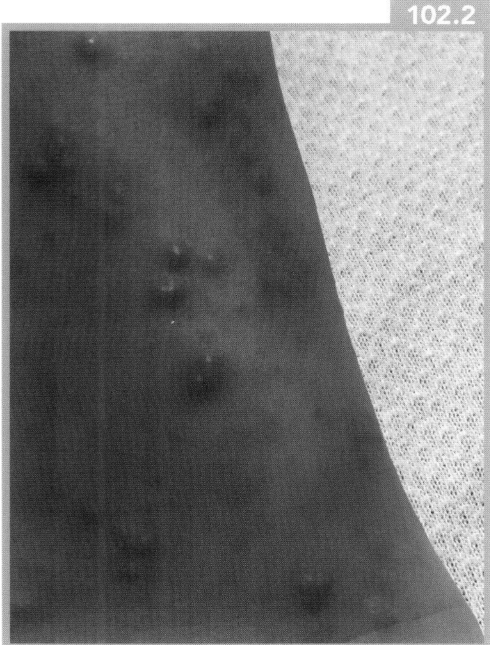

102.2

1. Painful papulovesicles in a dermatomal distribution are likely related to herpes zoster. What other disease mimics this pattern?
2. What infection control precautions should be utilized for a patient with suspected herpes zoster?

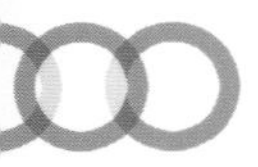

Answers

1. Many diseases can present with papulovesicles; however, only two are known to present in a dermatomal distribution. Herpes zoster, caused by varicella zoster virus, is the most common infection to present with painful papulovesicles in a dermatomal distribution. Another disease process that may present with similar symptoms is zosteriform herpes simplex virus. Approximately 13% of patients initially diagnosed with herpes zoster were found to have herpes simplex virus when lesions were cultured (Kalman and Laskin, 1986).

2. People with active herpes zoster lesions can spread varicella to susceptible individuals.

   For an immunocompetent patient with localized (no more than two contiguous dermatomes) herpes zoster, contact precautions should be implemented and the lesions should be covered (Kalman and Laskin, 1986).

   For an immunocompromised patient with localized disease or any case of disseminated herpes zoster, airborne and contact precautions should be instituted and the patient should be placed in a negative pressure room (Centers for Disease Control and Prevention, 2018). These precautions should remain in place until all lesions are dry and crusted.

   If a pediatric patient with herpes zoster requires hospitalization, regardless of immune status or extent of disease, hospital infection control should be contacted prior to transfer from the emergency department.

Keywords: infectious diseases, dermatology, rash, infectious

References

Centers for Disease Control and Prevention. Preventing varicella-zoster virus (VZV) transmission from zoster in healthcare settings. http://www.cdc.gov/shingles/hcp/hc-settings.html. Accessed on September 5, 2018.

Kalman CM, Laskin OL. Herpes zoster and zosteriform herpes simplex virus infections in immunocompetent adults. *Am J Med* 1986;81(5):775–8.

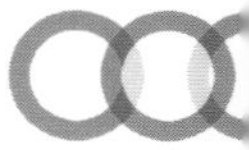

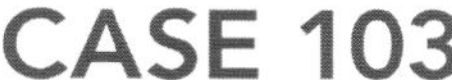

CASE 103

Michael Gottlieb

Questions

A 12-year-old boy presents to the emergency department with pleuritic chest pain after a recent URI (upper respiratory infection). The following ECG is obtained from triage.

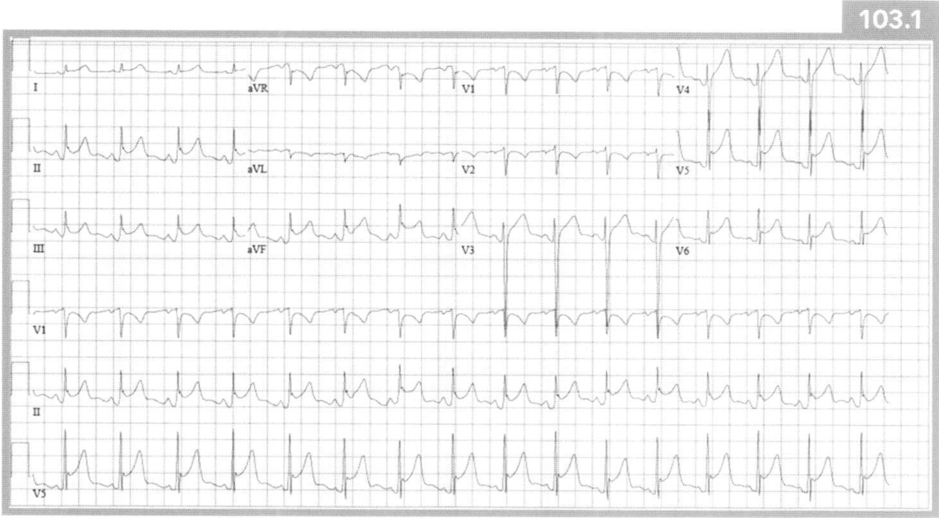

1. Based on this ECG, what is the most likely diagnosis?
2. What are some common underlying causes for this condition?
3. What is the recommended therapy for this condition?

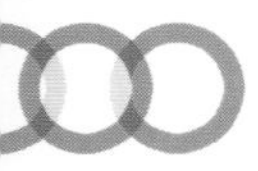

Answers

1. This ECG demonstrates a classic example of pericarditis. Note the diffuse ST segment elevations and PR segment depressions, as well as the localized ST depression with a PR elevation in augmented Vector Right (aVR). These are virtually pathognomonic for acute pericarditis.
2. Common causes include infections (viral, bacterial, and fungal), malignancy (leukemia, lymphoma, and melanoma), medications (procainamide and hydralazine), rheumatologic diseases (systemic lupus erythematosus [SLE], rheumatoid arthritis, scleroderma, polyarteritis nodosa, and dermatomyositis), radiation, uremia, and hypothyroidism.
3. Most cases of acute pericarditis are treated with bed rest and NSAIDs. Colchicine may also be added to this regimen. Avoid steroids when possible due to increased risk of recurrent pericarditis.

Keywords: cardiology, ECG, chest pain

Bibliography

LeWinter MM. Acute pericarditis. *N Engl J Med* December 18, 2014;371(25):2410–6.

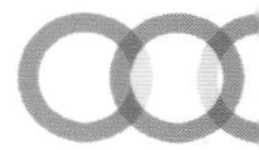

CASE 104

Catherine H. Chung

Question

A 10-year-old female presents with 4 days of worsening pain and redness to the anterior thigh. She was seen by her pediatrician 3 days ago and placed on an antibiotic for cellulitis. The affected area seems to be expanding with worsening pain. She is noted to have a slight fever but is otherwise well. Her exam reveals a 4 cm area of indurated skin with minimal fluctuance in the center. You are not sure if you should change her antibiotic regimen or perform an incision and drainage of the area.

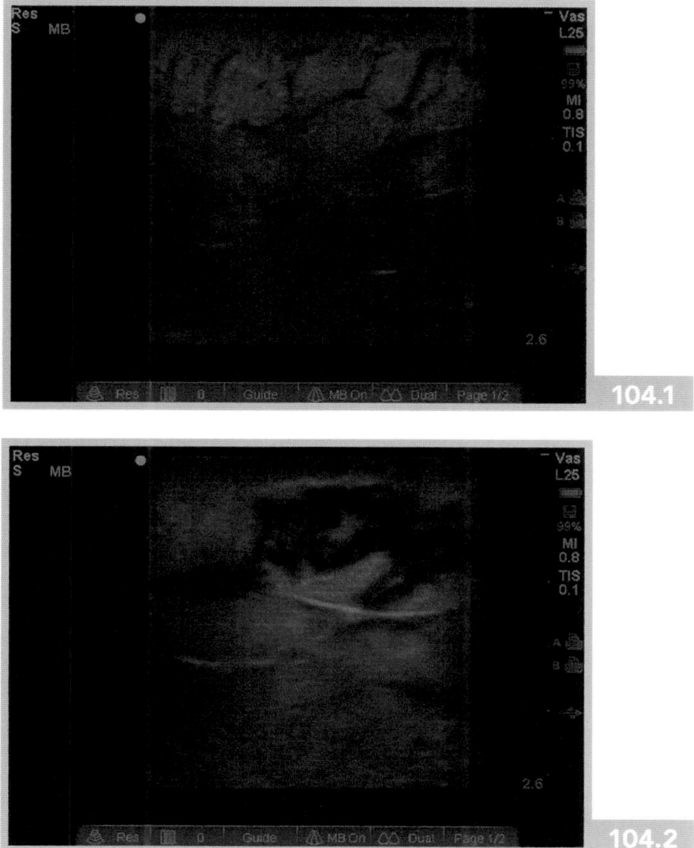

104.1

104.2

You perform a bedside ultrasound of the area (Image 104.1). What do you observe?

You change her antibiotic regimen and recommend close follow-up. She returns 2 days later and a repeat bedside ultrasound reveals the image above (Image 104.2). What do you observe?

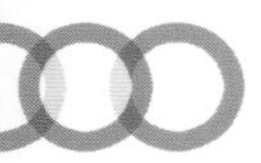

Answer

A bedside ultrasound exam can enhance your physical exam when evaluating skin infections. The first image reveals some edema of her skin, also referred to as "cobblestoning," which occurs in an inflammatory process. The second image reveals an abscess as noted by the dark multiloculated object that will require incision and drainage.

Keywords: infectious diseases, ultrasound, skin and soft tissue infection

Bibliography

Noble V. Ultrasound for procedure guidance. In *Manual of Emergency and Critical Care Ultrasound*. Cambridge: Cambridge University Press, 2007:230–2.

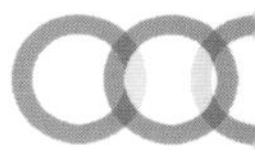

CASE 105

Catherine H. Chung

Question

A 7-month-old previously well child presents with a week of upper respiratory symptoms, low grade fevers, and increasing fussiness and poor oral intake. She has some tachypnea and capillary refill of 2–3 seconds. She has no abnormal lung sounds or murmurs on auscultation.

You perform a bedside ultrasound exam and see the following images.

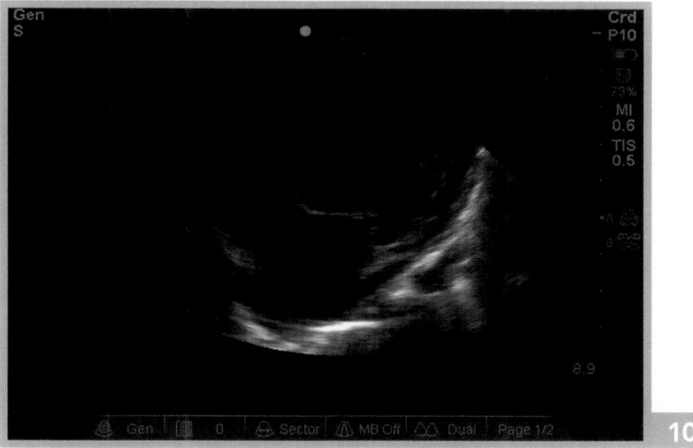

105.1

Subxiphoid view

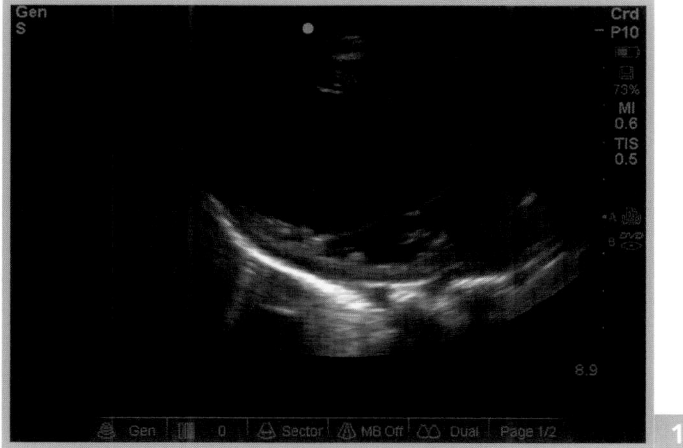

105.2

Parasternal long view

What abnormalities do you see and what is on your differential?

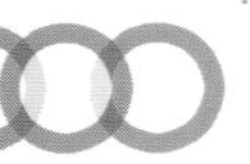

Answer

The cardiac bedside ultrasound exam reveals a grossly dilated heart with fair contractility. The ventricles are enlarged, and the septum is bowing into the right ventricle. The walls of the ventricle are noted to be thin.

Comparison of normal versus abnormal subxiphoid view.

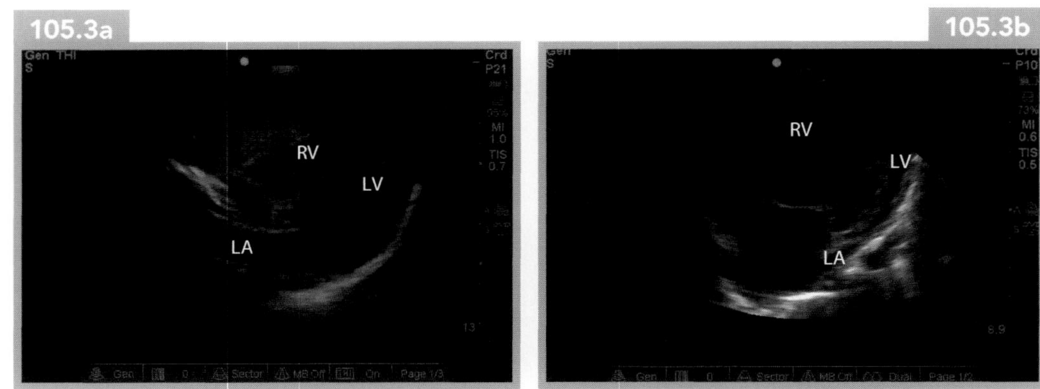

Normal subxiphoid — Abnormal subxiphoid

Comparison of normal versus abnormal parasternal view.

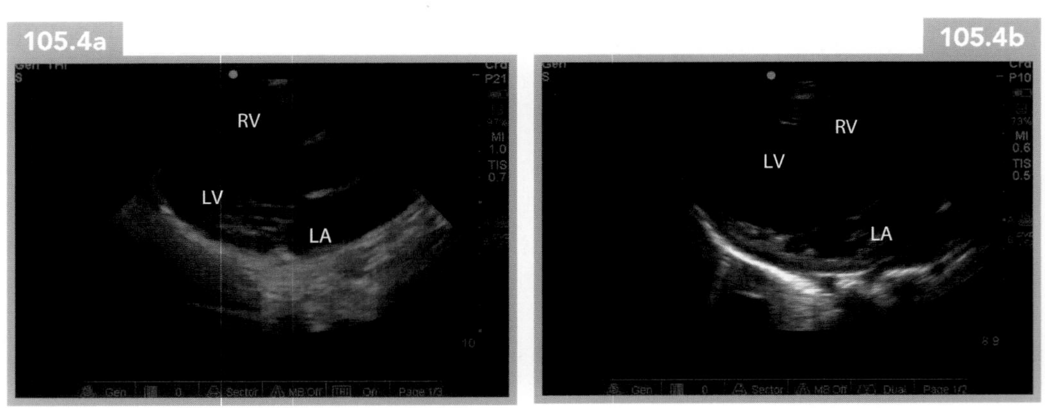

Normal parasternal — Abnormal parasternal

You can see dilated cardiomyopathy in this age group from infectious myocarditis, anemia, collagen vascular disease, anomalous left coronary artery from pulmonary artery, myocardial infarction, idiopathic, metabolic, or endocrine disorders.

Keywords: ultrasound, cardiology, infectious diseases, pitfalls, mimickers

Bibliography

Franklin, OM, Burch, M. Dilated cardiomyopathy in children. *Images Paediatr Cardiol* 2000;2(1):3–10.

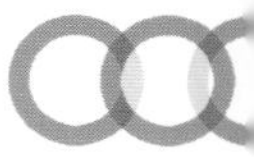

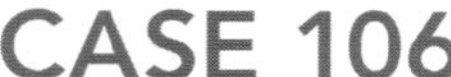

CASE 106

Catherine H. Chung

Question

A 15-year-old teenager presents with pain in her right buttock after sliding down a wooden plank earlier at school. She feels like there might be something in her skin, and her exam is noted to have some focal tenderness along her right buttock but no fluctuance or induration. X-rays are negative for foreign body.

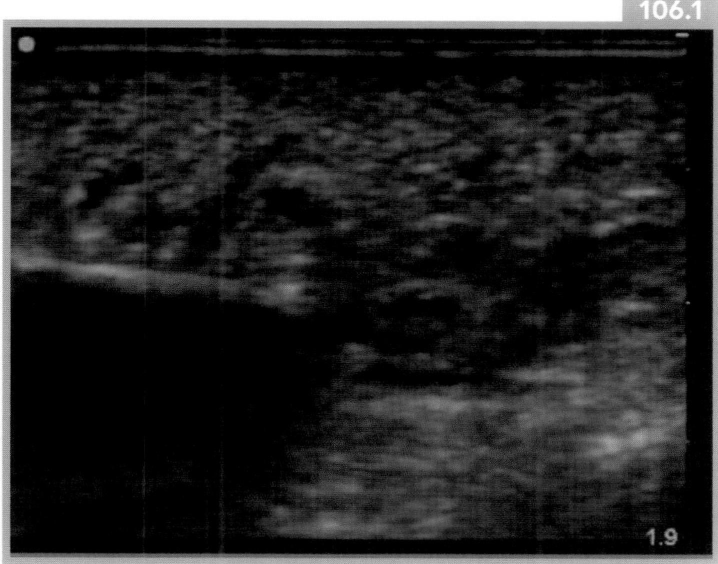

(Image courtesy Amie Woods.)

You perform a bedside ultrasound exam over the affected area. What do you observe?

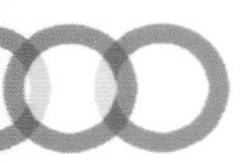

Answer

Bedside ultrasound reveals a foreign body in the skin as noted by the hyperechoic linear image with shadowing below it.

Non-metallic foreign bodies will often not show up on plain x-rays. Bedside ultrasound not only confirms diagnosis but allows visualization of the orientation of the foreign body and depth to help aid in its removal. This patient ended up having a 6 cm wooden splinter.

Keywords: foreign body, ultrasound, pitfalls

Bibliography

Noble V. Ultrasound for procedure guidance. In *Manual of Emergency and Critical Care Ultrasound*. Cambridge: Cambridge University Press, 2007: 224–30.

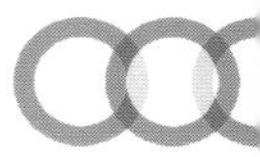

CASE 107

Catherine H. Chung

Question

A 4-year-old previously healthy child who attends day care presents with a limp for 3 days. His day care provider states they were at the park on the first day of symptoms and the child may have twisted his ankle, but she cannot recall any specific event. He also had some upper respiratory symptoms the week prior.

He is afebrile, well-appearing, and able to walk with a slight limp on his right leg. A more detailed exam is limited by his fear of health care providers and it is difficult to assess any point tenderness or if any manipulation causes pain. Otherwise, there is no fever, rash, or joint swelling.

You begin with x-rays of his tibia and fibula, which are negative. You perform a bedside ultrasound exam of his both his hips to evaluate for effusions.

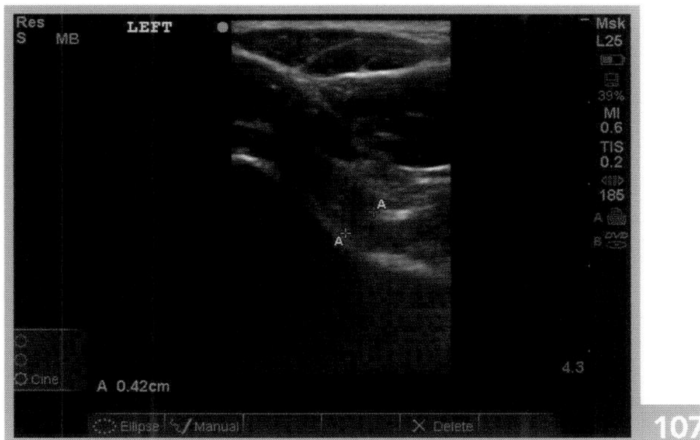

Asymptomatic left side

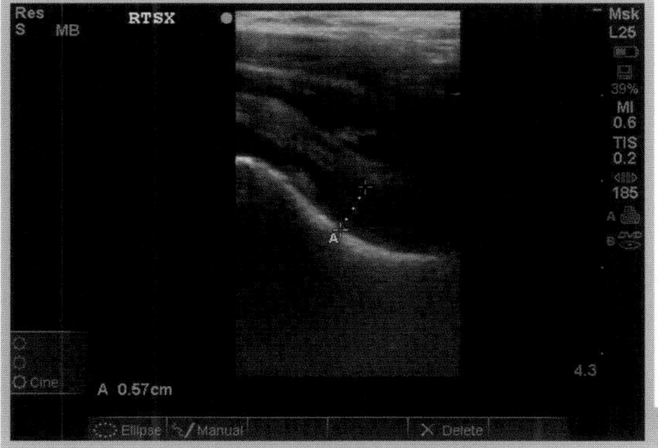

Symptomatic right side

Does the patient have an effusion? What is the differential for the etiology?

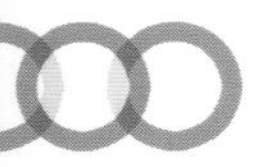

Answer

His hip ultrasound reveals an effusion. A hip effusion is diagnosed by the anterior synovial space of >5 mm or a 2 mm difference between the asymptomatic and symptomatic side.

The etiology can be from septic arthritis, transient synovitis, non-infectious arthritis, or Legg-Calvé-Perthes.

Keywords: orthopedics, ultrasound, limp

Bibliography

Donnelley L. Musculoskeletal. In *Pediatric Imaging: The Fundamentals*. Philadelphia: Elsevier Health Sciences, 2009:192–3.

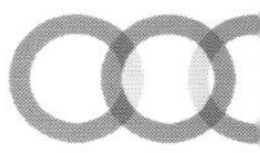

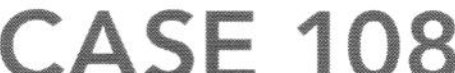

CASE 108

Alisa McQueen

Question

An almost 2 year old with asthma has had some trouble breathing and a persistent cough in the setting of an upper respiratory infection. Despite home treatment with inhaled albuterol every 4–6 hours, he is now getting a little worse.

On exam he's alert and playful but tachypneic with diffuse wheezes. After systemic steroids and several more hours of inhaled bronchodilator therapy, his wheezes are improved but he's still tachypneic. A chest radiograph is ordered.

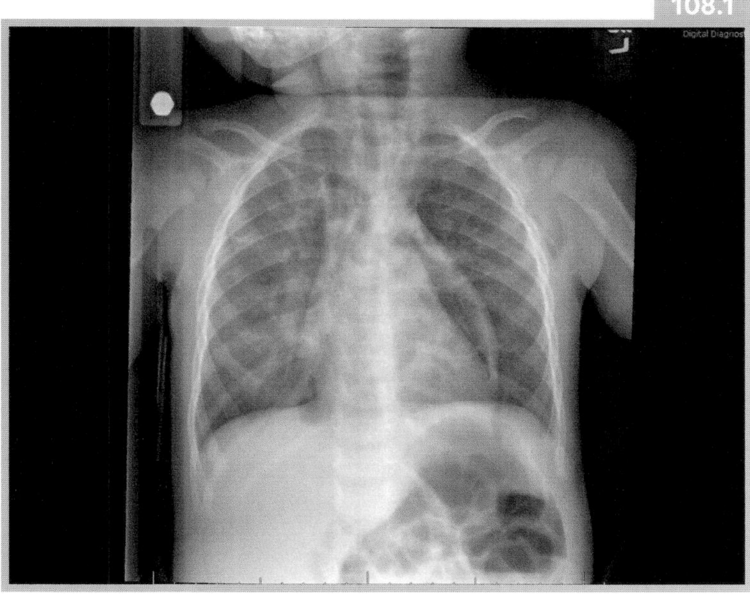

108.1

What does this radiograph display, and what additional physical exam findings might you expect?

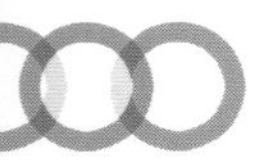

Answer

Pneumomediastinum occurs when gas tracks into the mediastinum from rupture of alveoli, laceration of the tracheobronchial tree, or rupture of the esophagus. In the absence of trauma, increased intra-alveolar pressure leading to rupture is the most common cause—either from an asthma exacerbation, foreign body, or Valsalva maneuvers including protracted coughing, exercise, or even childbirth.

Patients may be relatively asymptomatic, or may have sore throat or neck pain. Subcutaneous emphysema might be palpable on exam and "Hamman's crunch" may be auscultated in a small percentage of patients. Rarely, patients may develop pneumothorax or pneumopericardium. In spontaneous pneumomediastinum, treatment is supportive including analgesics and treatment of the underlying cause (asthma, forceful vomiting, etc.).

In the absence of history of blunt trauma or other potential surgical etiology, and with a plausible medical etiology (in this case, an asthma flare), how much additional workup is needed? In one of the largest series examining this question, a group of pediatric surgeons studied 53 children with pneumomediastinum and none had evidence of esophageal perforation. These authors conclude that in patients with idiopathic pneumomediastinum, it is still reasonable to investigate for esophageal perforation, but with an alternate explanation—in our case, an asthma flare—additional studies are not indicated. Conservative management can be carried out at home for otherwise well-appearing patients.

Keywords: pulmonary, respiratory distress, cough

Bibliography

Chapdelaine J, Beaunoyer M, Daigneault P, Bérubé D Bütter, A, Ouimet A, St-Vil D. Spontaneous pneumomediastinum: Are we overinvestigating? *J Pediatr Surg* May 2004;39(5): 681–4.

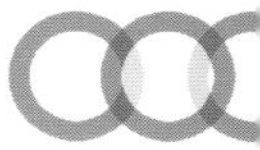

CASE 109

Nina Mbadiwe

Questions

A 4-year-old, previously healthy girl presents to the emergency department with one week of fever and cough. She has had a non-productive cough for the past 2 weeks and some decreased oral intake. The parents are concerned she has lost weight.

She is alert and non-toxic appearing. Her respiratory rate is 28, the pulse rate is 136, and the temperature is 38.8°C. The conjunctivae are pale. She has bilateral cervical lymphadenopathy with firm, non-tender nodes 1.5 cm. Lungs are clear to auscultation. There is hepatosplenomegaly. The hemoglobin is 6.8 g/dl with 50,000 white blood cells/microliter and platelet count of 30×10^3/microliter. There are blasts in the peripheral smear. The chest radiograph and CT scan are shown next.

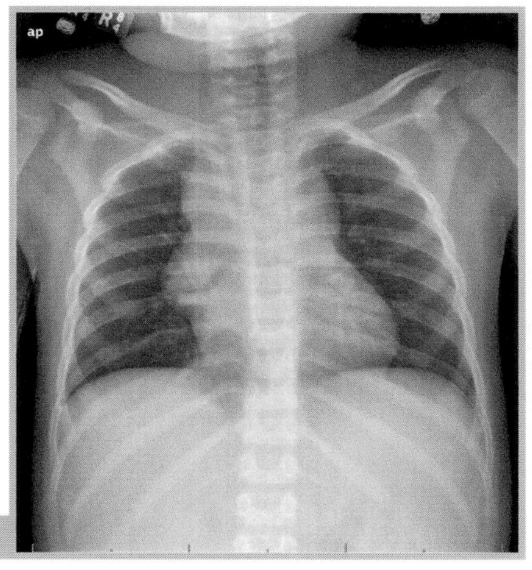

109.1

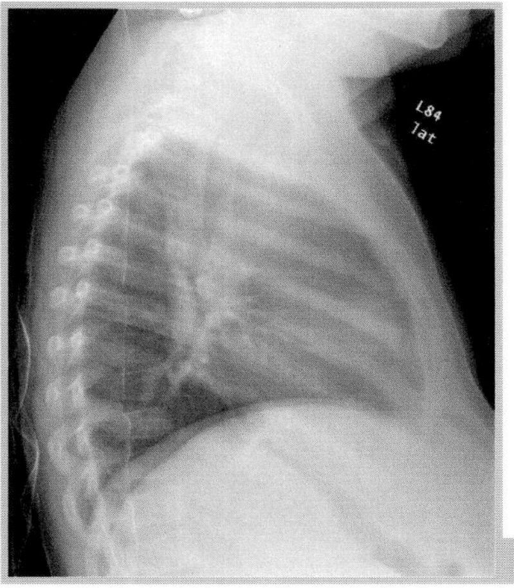

109.2

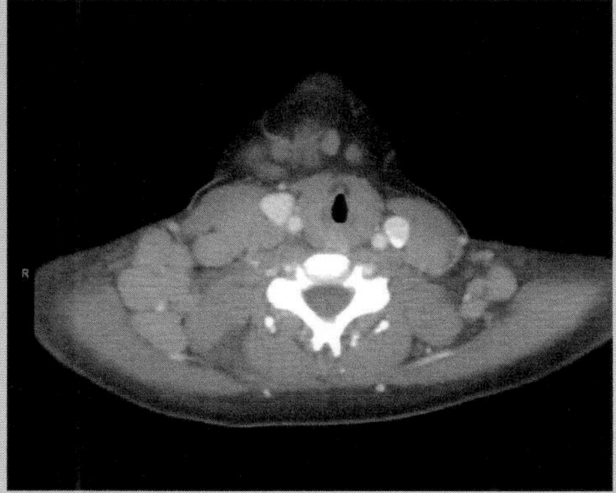

109.3

1. What does the chest radiograph show? What is the differential diagnosis?
2. What are the presenting signs and symptoms of a child with leukemia?
3. What are the oncological emergencies in a patient who presents with these signs and symptoms?

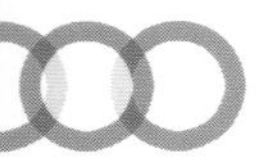

Answers

1. The chest radiograph shows a mediastinal mass. The differential diagnosis includes solid lesions (thymus, thymoma, lymphoma, teratoma), cystic lesions (thymic cyst, lymphatic malformation), fatty lesions (lipoma), vascular lesions (double aortic arch), nonvascular lesions (bronchogenic cyst), and lymphadenopathy (neoplasms primary, metastatic disease, infection).

2. Acute leukemia is the most common form of cancer in children. Children will usually have fever, pallor, hepatomegaly, splenomegaly, or unexplained bruising. Children may also have lymphadenopathy, musculoskeletal pain, headache, testicular enlargement, mediastinal mass, or abnormal peripheral blood counts.

3. A large mediastinal mass can narrow the trachea and cause respiratory distress. Use of medications for procedural sedation or/and anesthesia can lead to respiratory or circulatory collapse, even in the absence of respiratory symptoms.

   Massive tumor cell lysis with the release of nucleic acids, proteins, and intracellular metabolites can lead to tumor lysis syndrome. Tumor lysis syndrome is defined both by laboratory (elevation of uric acid, potassium, phosphate, calcium, creatinine) and clinical (cardiac arrhythmia, seizure) abnormalities, and can result in sudden death.

   Mechanical compression can lead to SVC syndrome (see Case 71).

Keywords: oncology, fever, mass, respiratory distress, do not miss, CT

Bibliography

Hammer GB. Anaesthetic management for the child with a mediastinal mass. *Pediatr Anesth* 14:95–7. doi:10.1046/j.1460-9592.2003.01196.x.

Hunger SP, Mullighan CG. Acute lymphoblastic leukemia in children. *N Engl J Med* 2015;373:1541.

Jones GL, Will A, Jackson GH, Webb NJA, Rule S and the British Committee for Standards in Haematology. Guidelines for the management of tumour lysis syndrome in adults and children with haematological malignancies on behalf of the British Committee for Standards in Haematology. *Br J Haematol* 2015;169:661–71. doi:10.1111/bjh.13403.

Ranganath SH, Lee EY, Restrepo R, Eisenberg RL. Mediastinal masses in children. *Am J Roentgenol* 2012;198(3):W197–216.

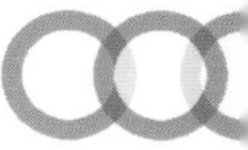

CASE 110

Michael Gottlieb

Questions

A 4-year-old girl presents with right knee pain after falling off the monkey bars onto her leg. She has no other injuries. On exam, she has focal tenderness and swelling of her right knee, and will not bear full weight on the right. She has good pulses, sensation, and strength distally.

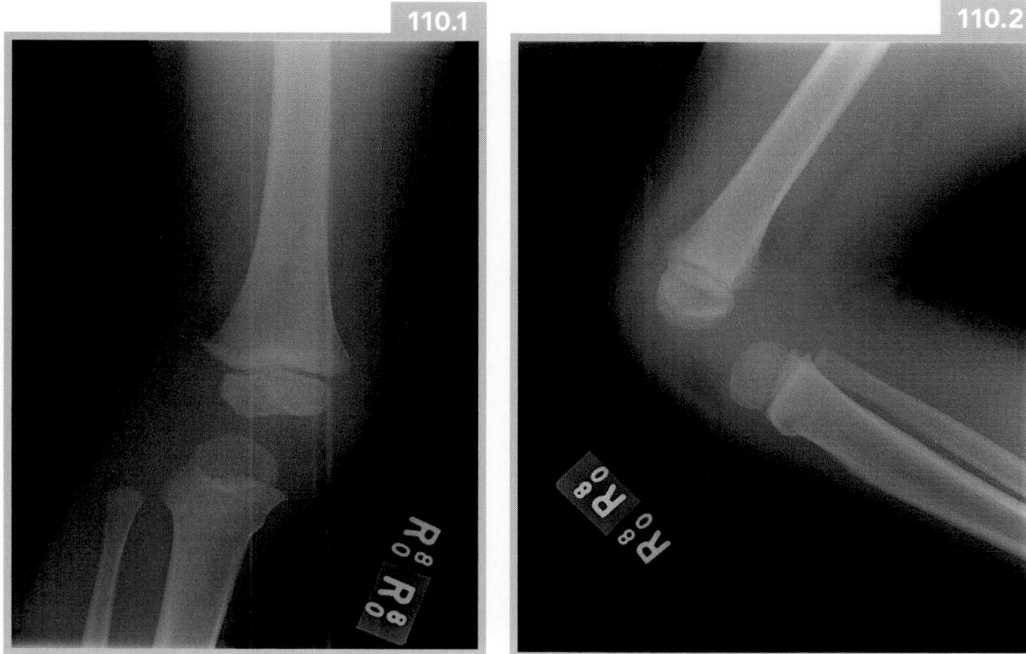

1. What type of fracture is demonstrated in this radiograph?
2. What is the management of these fractures?

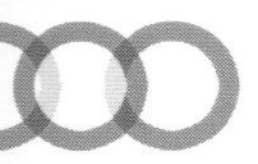

Answers

1. This patient has sustained a buckle fracture (also known as a torus fracture). This is a unilateral compression fracture commonly seen in children due to their relatively softer and more elastic bones. The most common etiology is axial loading of a long bone (typically, the radius or tibia).

2. Management of buckle fractures is typically conservative. The patient should be placed in a splint and be non-weight-bearing until seen by an orthopedic surgeon. These are stable fractures and rarely require reduction—even if mild to moderate angulation is present.

Keywords: blunt trauma, orthopedics, extremity injury

Bibliography

Boutis K. Common pediatric fractures treated with minimal intervention. *Pediatr Emerg Care* February 2010;26(2):152–7.

Chasm RM, Swencki SA. Pediatric orthopedic emergencies. *Emerg Med Clin North Am* November 2010;28(4):907–26.

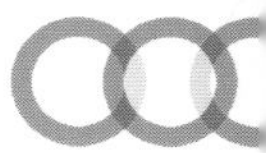

CASE 111

Emily Obringer

Question

A teenager presents to the emergency department with abdominal pain. As part of the workup, an abdominal CT with contrast is ordered. The patient returns from the radiology department with new onset edema, pain, and erythema to the left forearm. Plain films of the arm are shown.

111.1

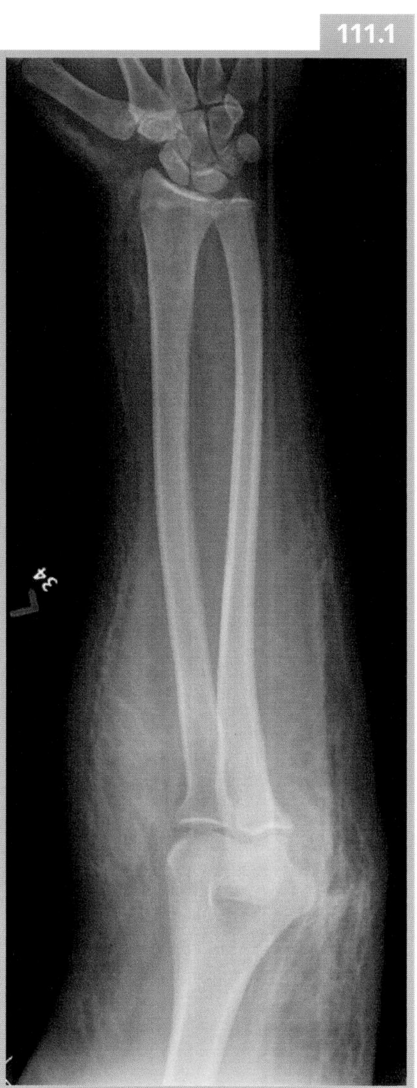

111.2

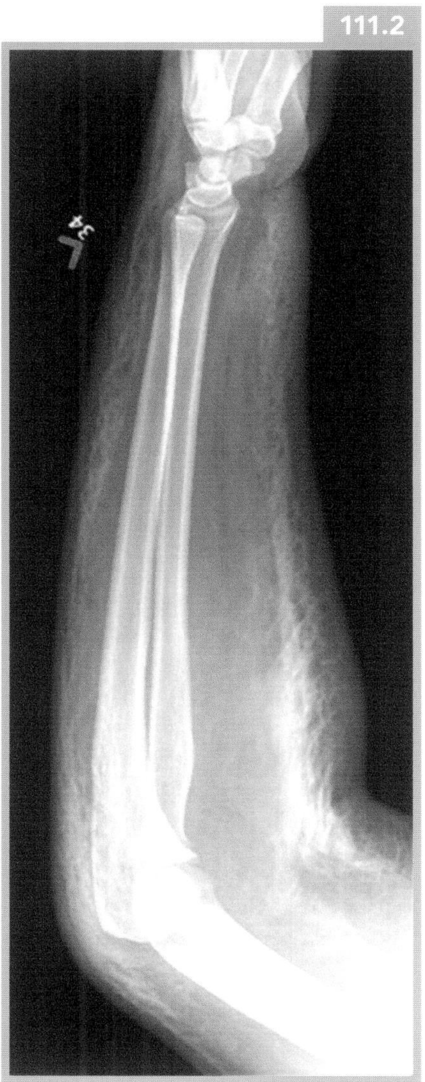

What happened? How should the patient be treated?

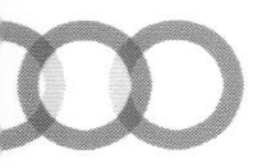

Answer

During the patient's abdominal CT, the IV displaced, resulting in accidental injection of contrast into the extravascular space. Extravasation into the subcutaneous tissue is a well-recognized complication of contrast use and occurs in less than 1% of all patients receiving contrast-enhanced CTs. Female patients and inpatients appear to be at increased risk of this complication. Common symptoms include pain and swelling at the injection site. Only rarely do severe complications, such as blistering, ulceration, and compartment syndrome, occur. Most extravasation events are self-limited and can be managed conservatively with ice packs and elevation. In moderate to severe cases, a plastic surgery consultation may be necessary. Long-term sequelae from contrast extravasation are rare.

Keywords: abdominal pain, iatrogenic complication

Bibliography

Shaqdan K, Aran S, Thrall J, Abujudeh H. Incidence of contrast medium extravasation for CT and MRI in a large academic medical centre: A report of 502,391 injections. *Clin Radiol* 2014;69(12):1264–72.

Wang CL, Cohan RH, Ellis JH, Adusumilli S, Dunnick NR. Frequency, management, and outcome of extravasation of nonionic iodinated contrast medium in 69,657 intravenous injections. *Radiology* 2007;243(1):80–7.

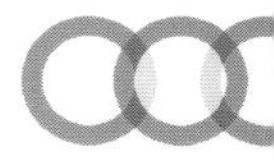

CASE 112

Emily Obringer

Question

A 5-year-old boy presents with worsening respiratory distress over the past 24 hours. He has had a persistent cough for several months and has been diagnosed with "asthma" and "pneumonia" on separate visits to the emergency department recently. He has been compliant with treatment but has had minimal change in symptoms.

His physical exam is significant for tachypnea, retractions, decreased breath sounds, and dullness to percussion over the left lung field. A chest x-ray is performed that shows worsening left-sided opacification. Given his lack of improvement with standard therapies, he is admitted to the hospital and a bronchoscopy is performed. Large, thick, branching casts are removed.

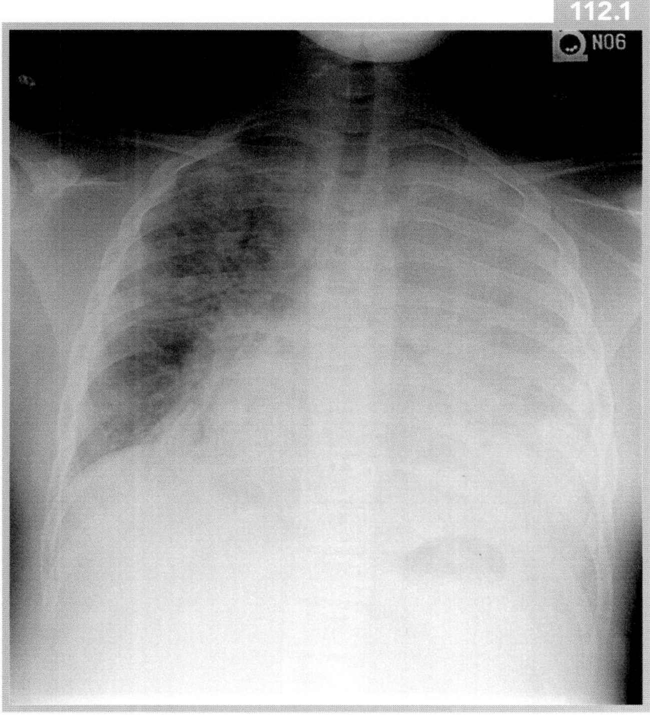

What is the patient's diagnosis, and what underlying disease is most commonly associated?

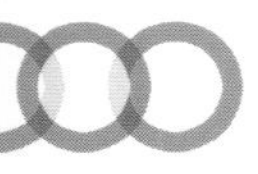

Answer

Reactive airway disease and pneumonia are common reasons for patients to present to the emergency department with pulmonary symptoms. However, when symptoms fail to respond to standard therapies or when other parts of the history or physical exam do not align, alternative diagnoses should be explored. In this case the finding of bronchial casts should lead to consideration of plastic bronchitis.

Plastic bronchitis is a rare disease that mainly occurs in children and is characterized by the expectoration or bronchoscopic removal of complex, branching bronchial casts. Unlike other diseases with mucous plugging such as allergic bronchopulmonary aspergillosis (ABPA) and asthma, these casts are large, rubbery, and branching on gross inspection and acellular on histopathology. The disease may be related to abnormalities in lymphatic drainage. Frequently patients with plastic bronchitis have an underlying systemic illness, with congenital heart disease, particularly after corrective surgery, being the most common (Dori et al., 2014). Patients present with cough, dyspnea, and airway obstruction and are often misdiagnosed initially as having reactive airway disease or pneumonia. Standard treatment for reactive airway disease and mucous plugging with albuterol, steroids, acetylcysteine, and dornase alfa are typically ineffective. Other therapies such as tissue plasminogen activator, and pulmonary vasodilators, such as sildenafil, have been used. Thoracic duct ligation and selective lymphatic collateral embolization have been shown to be curative (Caruthers et al., 2013). Acute bronchoscopic removal of casts causing airway obstruction may be lifesaving.

Keywords: mimickers, pulmonary, respiratory distress

Bibliography

Caruthers RL, Kempa M, Loo A, Gulbransen E, Kelly E, Erickson KR, Hirsch S, Schumacher KR, Stringer KA. Demographic characteristics and estimated prevalence of Fontan-associated plastic bronchitis. *Pediatr Cardiol* 2013;34(2):256–61.

Dori Y, Keller MS, Rychik J, Itkin M. Successful treatment of plastic bronchitis by selective lymphatic embolization in a Fontan patient. *Pediatrics* 2014;134:e590–5.

Panchabhai TS, Mukhopadhyay S, Sehgal S, Bandyopadhyay D, Erzurum SC, Mehta AC. Plugs of the air passages: A clinicopathologic review. *Chest* 2016;150(5):1141–57.

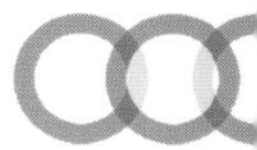

CASE 113

Michael Gottlieb

Questions

A 5-week-old boy with no significant birth history presents with persistent forceful, non-bilious, non-bloody vomiting after feeds for the past 3 days. He has not had any fever, respiratory symptoms, or diarrhea. The mother notes that he has had fewer wet diapers recently. He has no siblings or sick contacts. An ultrasound is obtained and is shown below.

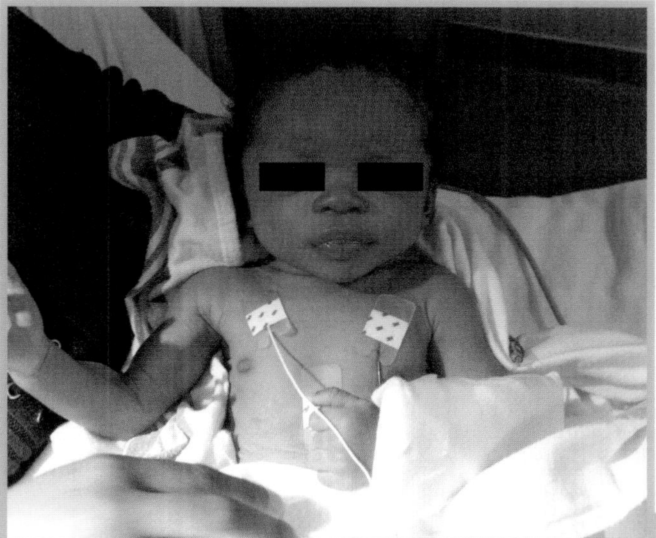

113.1

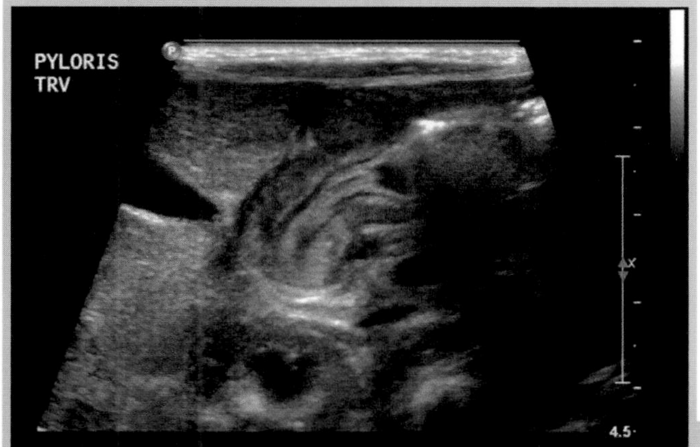

113.2

1. What is the diagnosis in this patient?
2. How is the diagnosis confirmed?

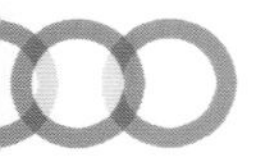

Answers

1. This patient has pyloric stenosis. This is hypertrophy of the pylorus with resulting narrowing of the pyloric sphincter that occurs most commonly in patients 4 to 6 weeks of age and is associated with males and firstborn children. Typically, patients will present with worsening, forceful, or projectile vomiting and failure to thrive. If labs are obtained, these patients can have a hypochloremic, hypokalemic, metabolic alkalosis, though this may be absent if they present early in the disease course.

2. Most cases are confirmed with ultrasound, which has sensitivities and specificities approaching 100%. Diagnostic criteria on ultrasound include a pylorus length greater than 14 mm or a single wall thickness greater than 3 mm. The diagnosis may also be confirmed with an upper gastrointestinal (GI) study, which will demonstrate either a string sign (i.e. a string of contrast through the elongated pyloric channel) or a double-track sign (i.e. several linear tracks due to redundant mucosa). An upper GI study may be valuable when the differential diagnosis includes midgut volvulus or malrotation.

Keywords: ultrasound, vomiting, mass, surgery

Bibliography

Leeson K, Leeson B. Pediatric ultrasound: Applications in the emergency department. *Emerg Med Clin North Am* August 2013;31(3):809–29.

Smith J, Fox SM. Pediatric abdominal pain: An emergency medicine perspective. *Emerg Med Clin North Am* May 2016;34(2):341–61.

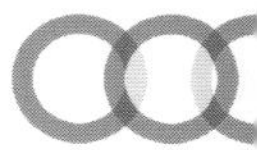

CASE 114

Michael Gottlieb

Questions

A 16-year-old, left-hand-dominant girl was slicing apples with her mother when she accidentally cut her right fifth digit. She denies numbness or paresthesias, but states she cannot move her finger. She is fully immunized and has no prior hand injuries. On examination, she has good capillary refill and intact sensation, but is unable to flex her left finger at the proximal or distal interphalangeal joint.

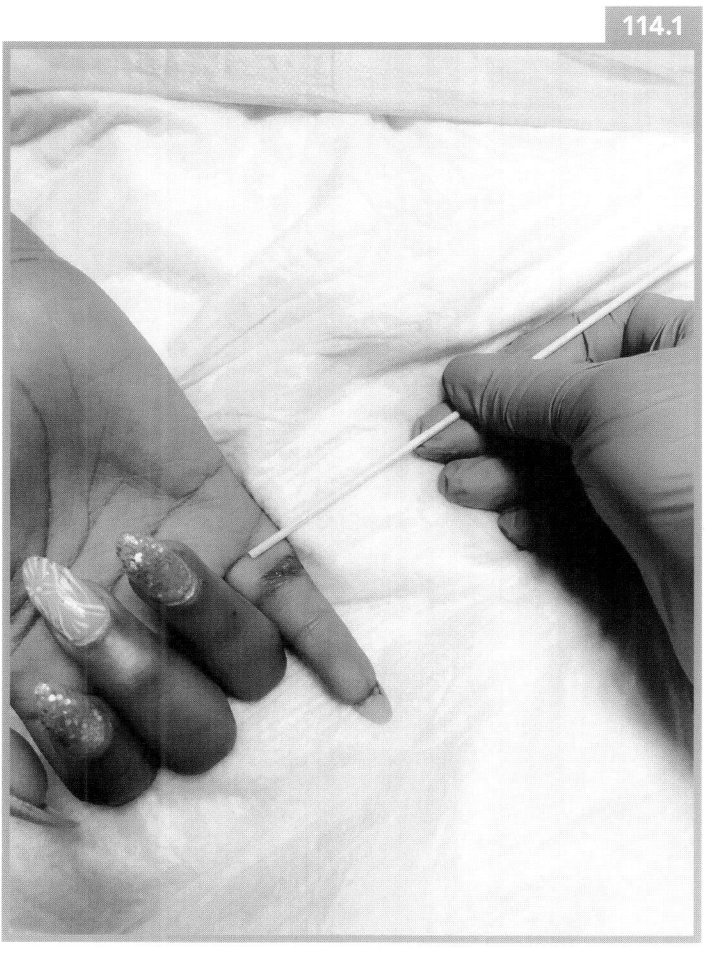

114.1

1. What structure(s) was/were likely injured in this patient?
2. What is the treatment and disposition for this condition?

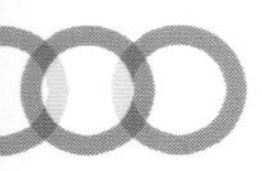

Answers

1. The inability to flex the digit at the proximal interphalangeal joint and distal interphalangeal joint suggests injury to both the flexor digitorum superficialis and flexor digitorum profundus, respectively. It is important to assess each joint independently, so as not to miss a potential tendon injury. While complete tendon injuries (as in this case) are relatively easy to diagnose on physical exam, partial tendon injuries can be more subtle. Clues to the diagnosis of a partial injury include pain with joint flexion, weak flexion against resistance, or a sensation of catching of the joint with flexion or extension. It may also be valuable to extend the wound and visualize the tendon through flexion and extension, examining for evidence of injury.
2. If there is any concern for flexor tendon injury, it is recommended to approximate the external wound, place the patient in a dorsal splint, and refer to a hand surgeon within 1–3 days. Splints should keep the wrist in 30° of flexion and the metacarpophalangeal joint in 70° of flexion to reduce the degree of tendon retraction.

Keywords: hand injury, penetrating trauma, pitfalls, do not miss

Bibliography

Harrison BP, Hilliard MW. Emergency department evaluation and treatment of hand injuries. *Emerg Med Clin North Am* November 1999;17(4):793–822.

Hart RG, Kutz JE. Flexor tendon injuries of the hand. *Emerg Med Clin North Am* August 1993;11(3):621–36.

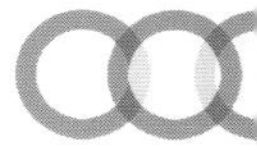

CASE 115

S. Margaret Paik

Question

An 11-month-old boy presents with a rash in the diaper region. The infant has been slightly fussier than usual but is eating normally. There is no history of fever. There is no change in the diet, detergent, soaps, or the brand of diaper or wipes used.

On physical exam, there is sharply demarcated perianal erythema. There are no external perirectal fissures or tags.

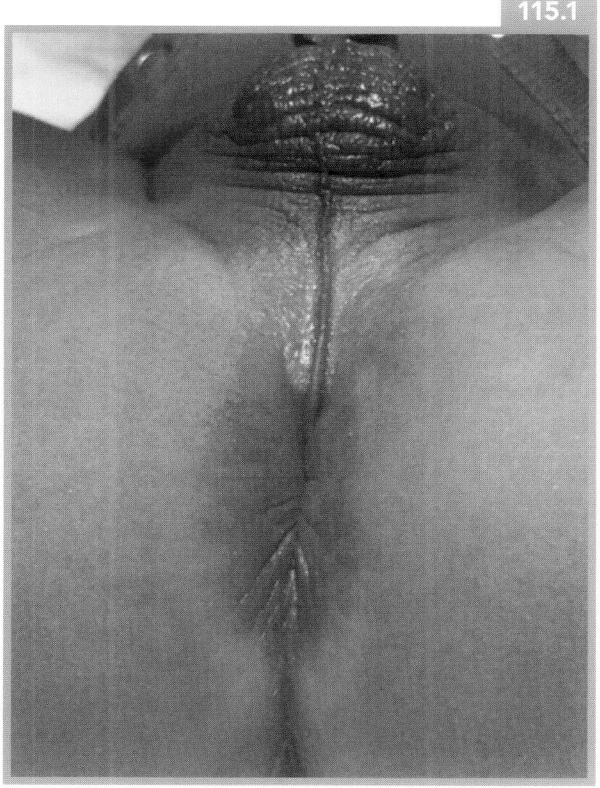

115.1

What does this child have? What is treatment of choice for this condition?

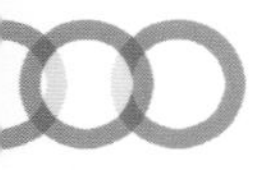

Answer

This is perianal streptococcal dermatitis or perianal cellulitis due to group A beta-hemolytic streptococci. Patients may present with incontinence, painful defecation with subsequent constipation, anal fissure, and blood-streaked stool. Balanitis and vulvovaginitis can also be seen. Bacterial culture can confirm the diagnosis. *Staphylococcus aureus* has been reported in some cases. The differential diagnoses include atopic dermatitis, seborrheic dermatitis, contact dermatitis, psoriasis, histiocytosis, candidiasis, scabies, and pinworms. Child abuse should be considered for severe or atypical presentations. Unless *Staphylococcus aureus* is strongly suspected, the treatment of choice is penicillin. A macrolide antibiotic can be substituted for penicillin-allergic patients. Topical therapy with antiseptic or antibiotic may accelerate clearance.

Keywords: child abuse mimicker, skin and soft tissue infection, dermatology

Bibliography

Barzilai A, Choen HA. Isolation of group A streptococci from children with perianal cellulitis and from their siblings. *Pediatr Infect Dis J* 1998;17(4):358–60.

Herbst RA. Perineal streptococcal dermatitis/disease: Recognition and management. *Am J Clin Dermatol* 2003;4(8):555–60.

Jongen J, Eberstein A, Peleikis H, Kaklke V, Herbst RA. Perianal streptococcal dermatitis: An important differential diagnosis in pediatric patients. *Dis Colon Rectum* 2008;51(5):584–7.

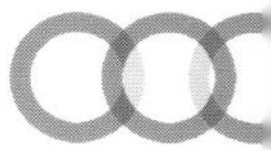

CASE 116

Nina Mbadiwe

Questions

A 6-year-old girl presents to the emergency department with pain of her left arm after falling off the balance beam onto her outstretched hand while she was at a gymnastics class.

On exam she is crying. Her left arm is in a sling. There is swelling at the left elbow with limited range of motion, but there is no gross deformity. The muscle compartments are soft. She has normal radial and brachial pulses, the capillary refill is less than 2 seconds, and she is able to oppose her thumb and index finger, cross her index and middle finger, and spread apart all five fingers. Two-point discrimination remains intact.

116.1

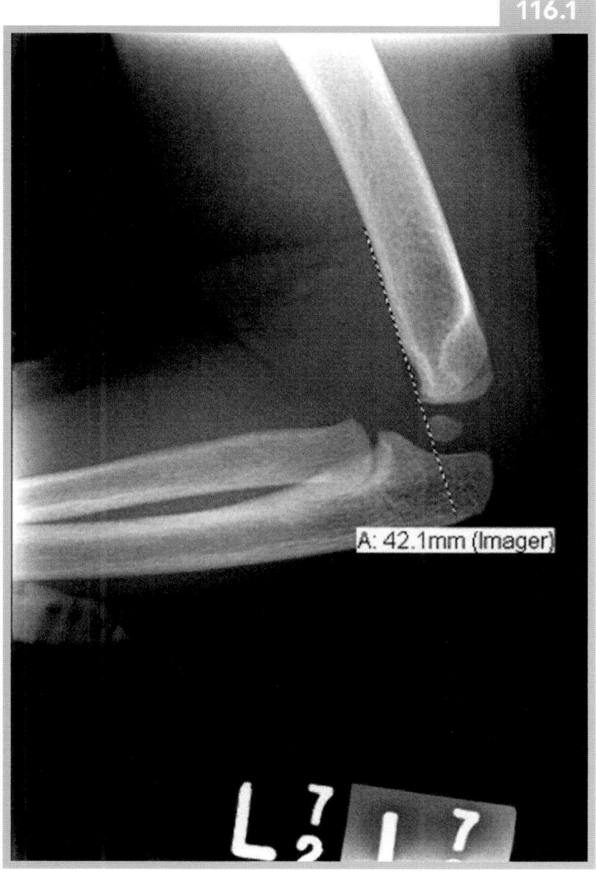

1. What does the radiograph indicate?
2. What are the different classifications of supracondylar fractures?

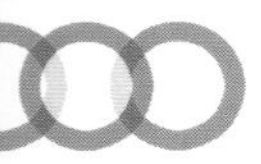

Answers

1. The anterior humeral line is anterior to the capitellum. In the normal elbow, a line drawn through the anterior cortex of the humerus intersects the capitellum in its middle third.

2. Type I fractures have no displacement or angulation and may have a displaced anterior fat pad or a posterior fat pad as the only radiographic finding. In type II fractures, the posterior periosteum is intact, but posterior displacement of the distal humerus occurs. The anterior humeral line passes through the anterior third of the capitellum or fails to intersect it and the anterior humeral line is displaced anteriorly. The humerus is displaced in type III supracondylar fracture with extensive tearing of the anterior and posterior periosteum (see Case 81).

Keywords: orthopedics, blunt trauma, extremity injury

Bibliography

Omid R, Choi PD, Skaggs DL. Supracondylar fractures on children. *J Bone Joint Surg Am* 2008;90:1121–32.

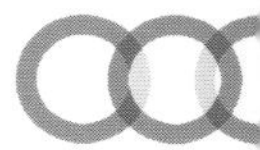

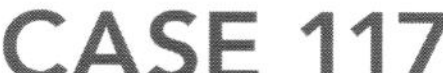

CASE 117

Catherine H. Chung

Questions

A 12-year-old female presents with 4 days of an area of redness on her inner thigh. She states it initially appeared to be a pimple, but then grew in size and became more tender and painful. She denies any history of trauma to the area, fevers, or history of skin infections in herself or her family.

Her vital signs are normal and her physical exam reveals a 5 cm × 7 cm well-circumscribed area of erythema and induration on her inner thigh. The rest of her physical exam is normal.

1. What would be your initial steps in management?
2. What considerations are there in antibiotic therapy?

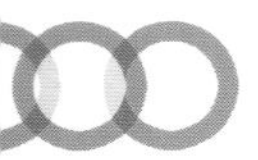

Answers

1. The affected area is a classic description of cellulitis with an abscess in the center. Cellulitis usually begins with minor insult to the skin, usually a small cut or bug bite. As the bacteria proliferate, causing tissue necrosis, an abscess is formed, which requires incision and drainage to allow alleviation of the swelling and pus. Without intervention, the infected area can grow deeper and wider with the potential to cause septicemia.

   In cellulitis, ultrasound images of the edematous overlying skin will show a "cobblestone" pattern (see Case 104). Ultrasound images of an abscess can be variable, including anechoic (black) to irregular hyperechoic (varying shades of lighter gray). Hyperechoic sediment and/or septae can also be seen.

   117.1

   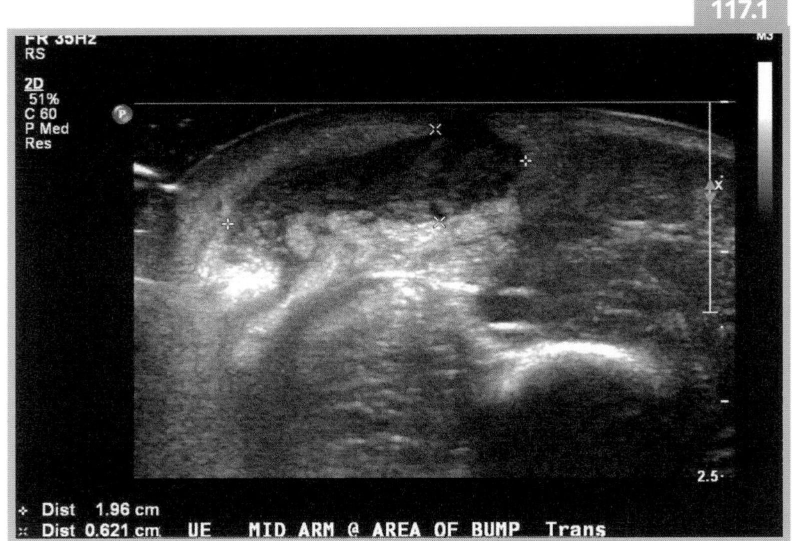

   This patient requires an incision and drainage to the 2 cm × 3 cm fluctuant area with the pus sent for culture to assess for antibiotic sensitivities in case the patient fails the first choice of antibiotics. The benefit of packing an abscess to keep the wound open is questionable, as recent literature has found no benefit in rate of recurrence or healing.

2. The most common organisms are group A streptococcus, methicillin-sensitive *Staphylococcus aureus* (MSSA), or methicillin-resistant *Staphylococcus aureus* (MRSA). Local microbial sensitives should be used to determine prevalence of the causative organisms and sensitivities to antibiotics. Commonly used antibiotics include cephalexin, amoxicillin/clavulanic acid, or dicloxacillan. If MRSA is suspected, trimethoprim/sulfamethoxazole or clindamycin should be considered.

Keywords: skin and soft tissue infection, infectious diseases, ultrasound

Bibliography

Bergstrom, KG. News, views and reviews. Less may be more for MRSA: The latest on antibiotics, the utility of packing an abscess and decolonization strategies. *J Drugs Dermatol* January 2014;12(1):89–92.

Fleisher GR, Ludwig S, eds. *Textbook of Pediatric Emergency Medicine*. 6th ed. Philadelphia: Lippincott Williams & Wilkins, 2010.

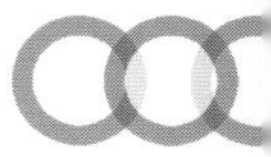

CASE 118

Diana Yan

Question

A 5-year-old girl presents to the emergency room with a cough for 3 weeks. She has not had any runny nose, congestion, fevers, vomiting, or diarrhea. She has no pain. She is still having good oral intake and normal urine output. Parents feel that the cough occurs all day without any factors that make it better or worse. No one is sick at home, but she does go to kindergarten. While talking about school, her parents do note that she doesn't seem to run around as much as the other children in class and wonder if she has asthma. They have never heard her wheeze. She is otherwise healthy without any hospitalizations. No family history of asthma.

Physical exam shows an alert and awake school-aged girl who is in no acute distress. She has a normal cardiovascular exam without murmurs, gallops, or rubs. On lung exam, she does have a focal decrease in aeration in the left middle and lower lobes. There is no increased work of breathing. No wheezing, crackles, or rhonchi are heard. The chest wall appears normal. There is no clubbing of the fingers. Otherwise her exam is normal. Imaging studies are presented next.

118.1

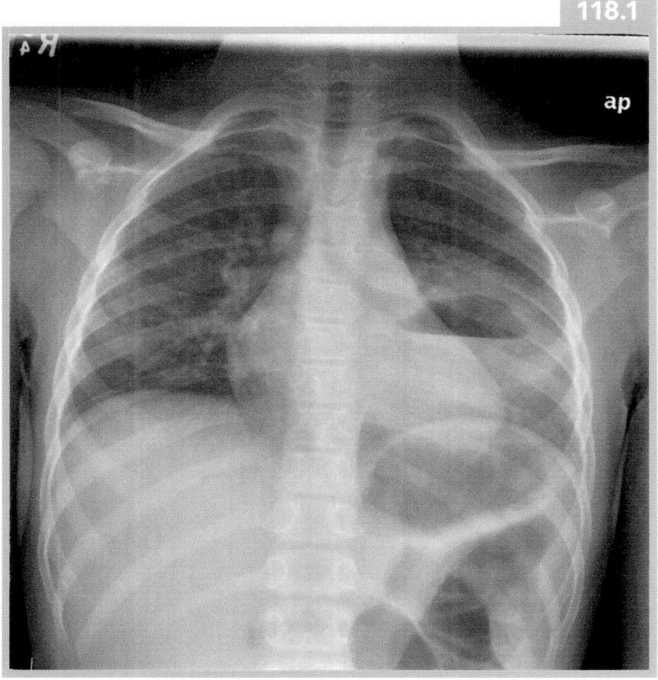

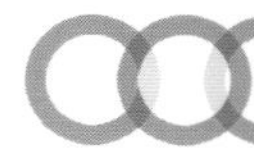

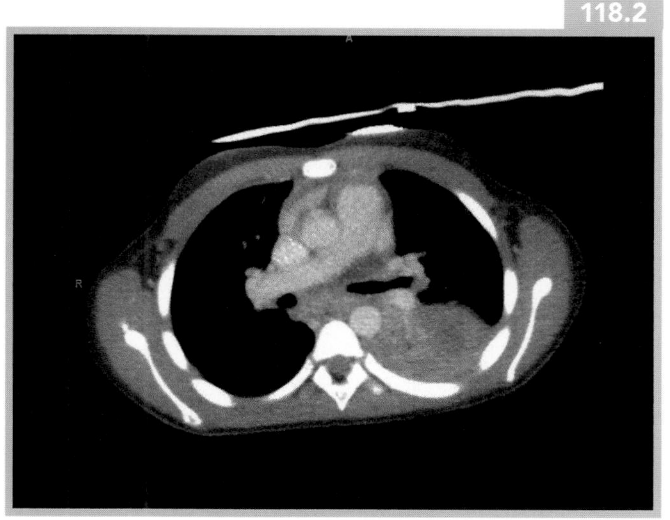

118.2

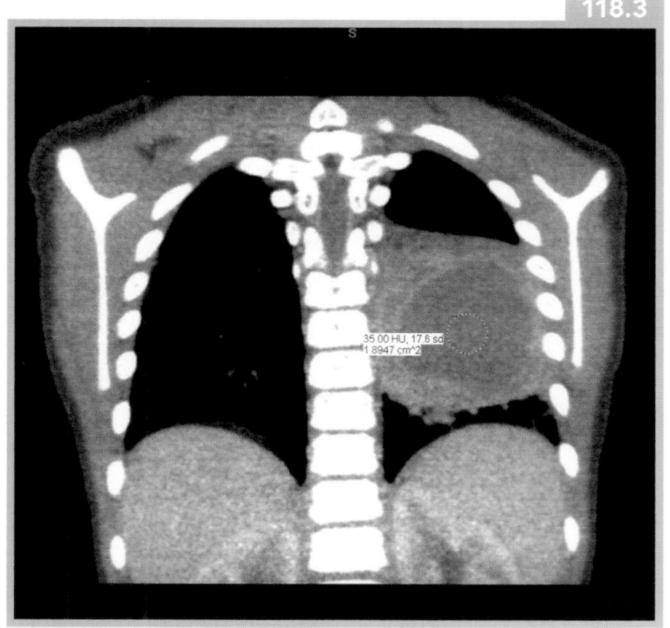

118.3

What is the diagnosis and treatment?

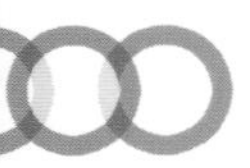

Answer

Congenital pulmonary malformation and resection. Congenital pulmonary malformations (CPMs) of the lung are present in 1:11,000 to 1:35,000 live births. In the neonate, they have a wide range of presentations from respiratory failure to a well-appearing infant. In children, they usually present with cough but can also present with dyspnea and fever. Hemoptysis is a rarer presentation. About 13% of children will present with a pneumonia or recurrent respiratory infections and 10% present with a pneumothorax. In children, congenital cystic adenomatoid malformations are the most common type of CPMs to convert into cancer with bronchogenic cysts (pictured earlier) as the second most common. In symptomatic patients, resection through lobectomy (versus segmentectomy or removal of cyst only) is the most common treatment. Controversy exists over the treatment of incidental or asymptomatic CPMs. Some surgeons recommend prophylactic surgery to prevent future infections, enhance compensatory lung growth, and to prevent development of malignancy. Most studies cite the lifetime malignant transformation rate of CPMs to be less than 5%. Pleuropulmonary blastoma is the most common cancer associated with CPMs in children and can develop from a cyst at any time. There is no consensus about surveillance of these cysts for malignancy as chest x-rays are not sensitive enough and repeated CT scans increase the risk for iatrogenic cancer. Other cancers that CPMs can evolve into include rhabdomyosarcoma, adenocarcinoma, squamous cell carcinoma, and mesenchymoma.

Keywords: pulmonary, cough, mass, oncology

Bibliography

Casagrande A, Pederiva F. Association between congenital lung malformations and lung tumors in children and adults: A systematic review. *J Thorac Oncol* 2016;11(11):1837–45.

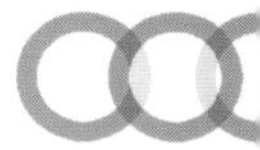

CASE 119

Timothy Ketterhagen

Questions

A 15-year-old boy is brought to the emergency department complaining of a headache. He reports a headache intermittently for the past few months, but it has been mild. Recently, his headaches have been occurring more frequently, waking him from sleep, and have become more severe. He has not been able to attend school and is not able to play with his friends due to his headache. He describes the pain as "aching" and located around his entire head. He was previously healthy and does not have a history of migraines. No head trauma is reported. He denies any fever, cough, rhinorrhea, neck pain, abdominal pain, tinnitus, sore throat, dizziness, blurry vision, difficulty ambulating, or numbness, tingling, or weakness of his extremities.

Physical exam reveals an uncomfortable but not toxic-appearing young man. Vital signs are within normal limits. Head and neck exam are unremarkable. A full neurologic exam is performed, which is unremarkable. The physical exam is otherwise unremarkable. An MRI scan of the head is shown next.

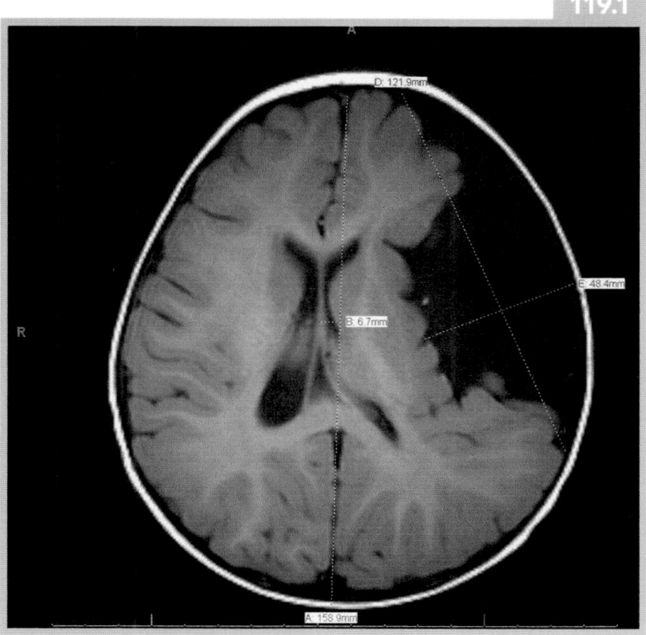

1. What is the diagnosis?
2. What is the treatment?

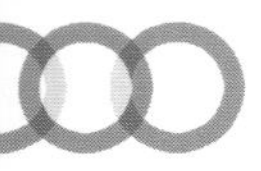

Answers

1. This patient has an arachnoid cyst. Arachnoid cysts are fluid-filled sacs around the spinal cord or (more commonly) inside the head. These cysts are often present at birth but can also be a secondary result of head trauma. Arachnoid cysts are diagnosed with a CT or an MRI.
2. Most arachnoid cysts never cause any symptoms. Rarely, symptoms may occur such as headache, nausea, vomiting, lethargy, seizures, visual changes, or other neurologic changes. If the patient is symptomatic, treatment may be required. Treatment options include fenestration (open the cyst) or shunt placement. If the patient is asymptomatic, MRIs may be performed in the future to monitor for cyst growth, but intervention is most likely not required.

Keywords: neurosurgery, headache, MRI

Bibliography

Seattle Children's Hospital. Arachnoid cyst. http://www.seattlechildrens.org/medical-conditions/brain-nervous-system-mental-conditions/arachnoid-cyst/. Accessed July 20, 2017.

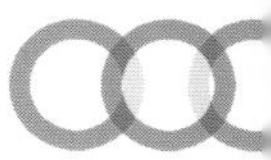

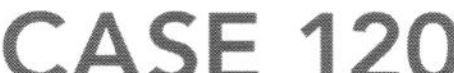

CASE 120

Nina Mbadiwe

Question

A 4-month-old girl presents to the emergency department with persistent crying and intermittent vomiting after falling out of her father's arms while he was standing. The fall occurred 4 hours previously. She lost consciousness for about 1 minute.

On exam she is persistently crying. She has a slightly bulging anterior fontanelle and a right temporal scalp hematoma. Otherwise, her exam is normal. A CT scan is obtained.

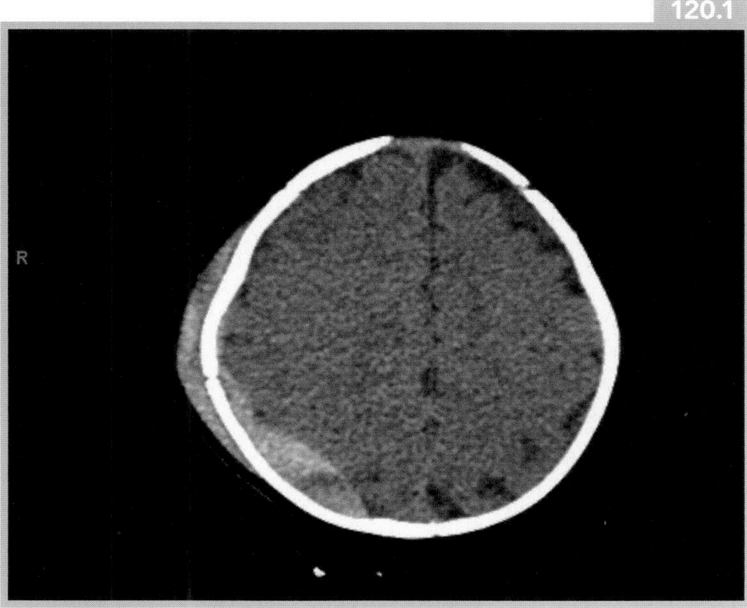

120.1

What is the most common cause of epidural hemorrhage in infants and young children, and what is the most common mechanism?

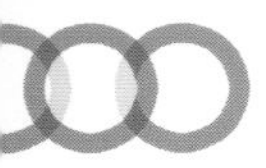

Answer

Epidural hematoma usually occurs after unintentional head trauma, with falls being the most common mechanism of injury. During impact, the skull is deflected inward and the dura is stripped from the undersurface of the bone, which results in blood accumulation. Head CT shows a biconvex mass that displaces the brain away from the skull. Children with closed sutures can present with symptoms of increased intracranial pressure, including lethargy, vomiting, hypertension, and bradycardia. Initial management should include assessment and stabilization of the airway, breathing, and circulation, as well as initiation of neuroprotective measures including elevation of the head of the bed, judicious fluid management, and consideration of mannitol or hypertonic saline infusion. Neurosurgical consultation is required.

Keywords: head injury, blunt trauma, child abuse, vomiting, altered mental status, CT

Bibliography

Bejjani GK, Donahue DJ, Rusin J, Broemeling LD. Radiological and clinical criteria for the management of epidural hematomas in children. *Pediatr Neurosurg* 1996;25:302.

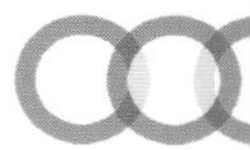

CASE 121

Diana Yan

Questions

A 15-month-old boy was found unresponsive at his uncle's home when his grandmother came home from the store. Emergency medical services found him apneic but with a pulse. He was intubated and transported to a pediatric trauma center where his primary survey showed an intubated toddler with equal breath sounds, peripheral pulses, and a heart rate of 80. On secondary survey, it is noted that he will withdraw from pain and a Glasgow Coma Scale (GCS) score of 6 is assigned E(1) V(1) M(4) (see Case 40). He has a large occipital hematoma with a palpable defect and some oozing blood from it. There is also bruising on his chest and lower extremities. His grandmother states that the child was well before she went to the store. She was gone for about 30 minutes and left the child with his uncle. The child is healthy and takes no medications. A CT of his head is shown next.

121.1

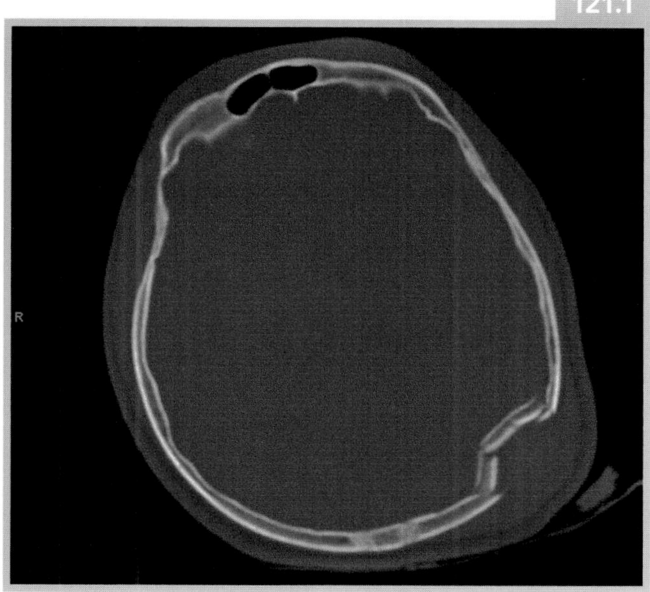

1. What is the overarching concern in this child?
2. What is the treatment for isolated pneumocephalus?

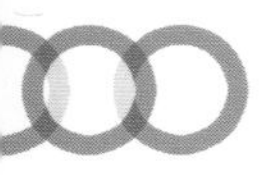

Answers

1. Non-accidental trauma (NAT). The CT head scan shows a depressed skull fracture with pneumocephaly, which, in the absence of a history of injury, very strongly indicates NAT. Children under 5 years of age are at the greatest risk of NAT and children under 3 are at the highest risk of fatal injuries, most commonly from head trauma. In 2014, there were 702,000 cases of confirmed child abuse/neglect in the United States, and 1580 of those cases ended in death. Twenty percent of these cases had a delay in diagnosis, which highlights the need for clinicians to consider NAT early in a patient's course. Risk factors for NAT include past abuse in the victim or perpetrator, intellectual disability in the child, a stressful home environment, and substance abuse. More than 80% of these cases are caused by a biological parent, whereas 12% are caused by a non-biological parent or partner. Patients with skull fractures can have concurrent intracranial hemorrhage and symptoms of lethargy, irritability, altered mental status, vomiting, headaches, and seizures. Other injuries include retinal hemorrhages and spinal cord injuries. The gold standard for the diagnosis of skull fractures and intracranial bleeding is a CT scan without contrast. MRI can be performed after initial resuscitation and treatment to assess for axonal injury and brain edema.

2. Conservative management. Pneumocephalus, or the presence of air in the intracranial cavity, is most frequently caused by trauma, but can also be caused by intracranial or spinal surgeries and infections. Symptoms can include nausea and vomiting, headaches, dizziness, and seizures. A tension pneumocephalus is created when the intracranial air causes increased intracranial pressure and neurological deterioration, which is fatal if untreated. Isolated pneumocephalus is usually conservatively treated and observed as the air will be absorbed without any complications. If there are concerns for increased intracranial pressure, then emergent surgical decompression may be required.

Keywords: child abuse, head injury, altered mental status, CT

Bibliography

Dabdoub CB, Salas G, Silveira EN, Dabdoub CF. Review of the management of pneumocephalus. *Surg Neurol Int* 2015;6:155.

Kim PT, Falcone RA Jr. Nonaccidental trauma in pediatric surgery. *Surg Clin N Am* 2017;97:21–33.

Paiva WS, de Andrade AF, Figueiredo EG, Amorim RL, Prudente M, Teixeira MJ. Effects of hyperbaric oxygenation therapy on symptomatic pneumocephalus. *Ther Clin Risk Manag* 2014;10:769–73.

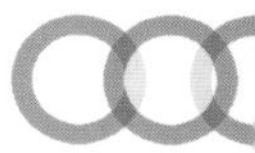

CASE 122

Michael Gottlieb

Questions

An 8-year-old boy presents to the pediatric trauma center with a laceration to his scalp. He was playing in the backyard when a ladder fell on his head. He is crying, but is consolable and has a Glasgow Coma Scale score of 15 without focal neurologic deficits. His examination reveals the following injury to his scalp.

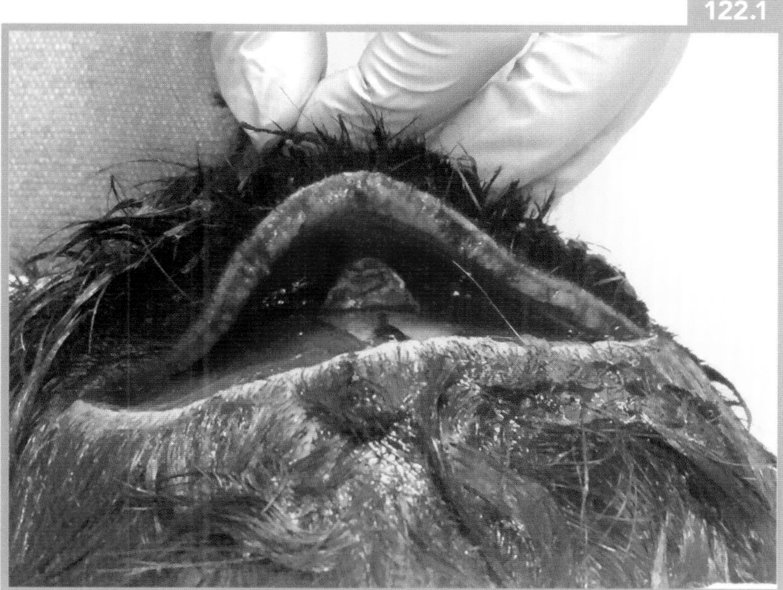

122.1

1. What is the galea aponeurotica, and why is it important to identify?
2. Describe three strategies for closing scalp lacerations.

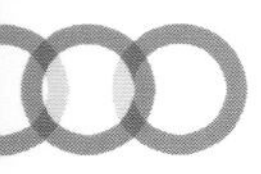

Answers

1. The galea aponeurotica is a dense, tendon-like structure that covers the skull. It connects to the frontalis muscle anteriorly and the occipitalis muscle posteriorly. It is important to evaluate this structure for lacerations, as failure to approximate lacerations of the galea aponeurotica can lead to cosmetic deformities due to asymmetric frontalis muscle elevation. Additionally, this serves as a layer to protect the skull from skin infections.
2. Scalp lacerations can be closed with suture, staples, or the hair apposition technique. When using sutures, it is important to use a different color than the patient's hair and leave the ends of the sutures long. The hair apposition technique is a newer strategy, where the hair is tied together, thereby approximating the skin. Adhesive glue may be used to facilitate this approach. The latter technique has been associated with improved patient satisfaction and fewer cosmetic problems.

Keywords: penetrating trauma, head injury, pitfalls, procedures

Bibliography

Atabaki SM. Pediatric head injury. *Pediatr Rev* June 2007;28(6):215–24.

Hollander JE, Singer AJ. Laceration management. *Ann Emerg Med* 1999;34:356.

Ozturk D, Sonmez BM, Altinbilek E, Kavalci C, Arslan ED, Akay S. A retrospective observational study comparing hair apposition technique, suturing and stapling for scalp lacerations. *World J Emerg Surg* July 2013;8:27.

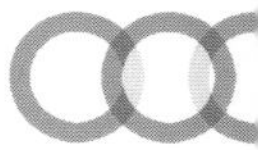

CASE 123

Jaimee Holbrook

Questions

A 6-month-old full-term boy presents to his pediatrician with thrush that has not improved with nystatin. His mother comments to the pediatrician that her pregnancy history is notable for a positive rapid plasma reagin (RPR) (1:32). She was initially referred to a specialist, but when confirmatory testing was negative, his mother cancelled the appointment. The infant's RPR is sent and is 1:2048.

Fluorescent treponemal antibody (FTA) is positive.

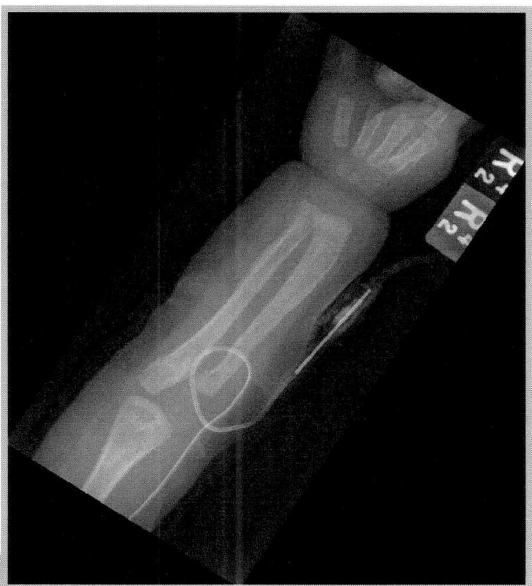

123.1

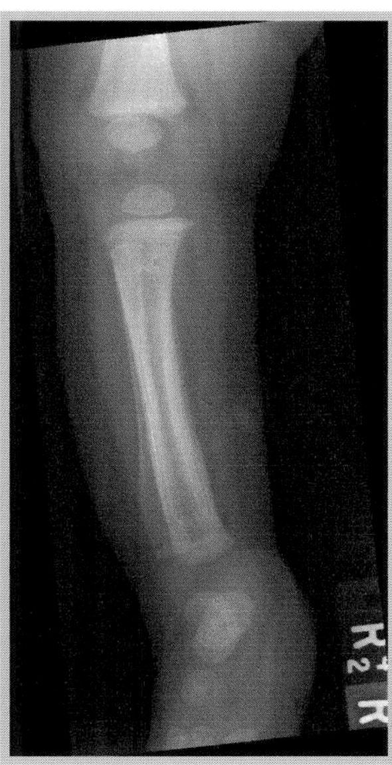

123.2

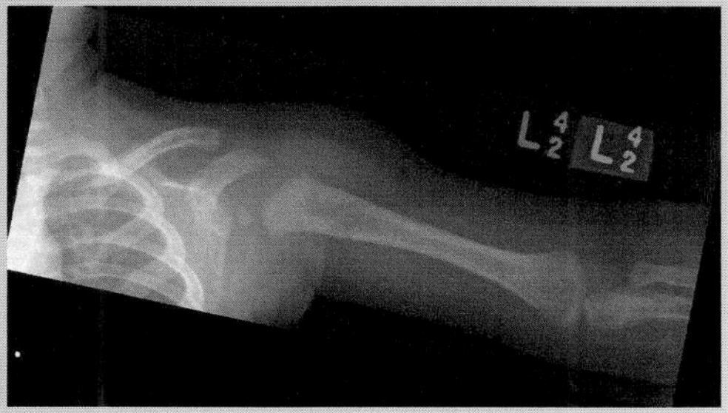

123.3

1. What is the diagnosis, and what additional workup is indicated?
2. What is Hutchinson's triad?
3. What do these radiographs show? What is the differential diagnosis?
4. What is the treatment?

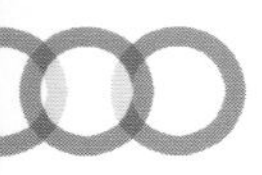

Answers

1. This infant has congenital syphilis, which results from transplacental transmission of spirochetes. After confirmatory testing, such as FTA testing, additional workup includes:
   a. Physical exam with common findings including persistent rhinitis ("snuffles"), generalized lymphadenopathy, hepatomegaly, and rash
   b. Laboratory studies including CBC (complete blood count), LFTs (liver function tests), CSF (cerebrospinal fluid), studies (protein, glucose, cell count, CSF Venereal Disease Research Laboratory [VDRL]), and HIV testing
   c. Long bone films to evaluate for periostitis and/or osteochondritis
   d. Ophthalmology evaluation for syphilitic ocular changes such as interstitial keratitis
   e. Auditory brainstem response (ABR) testing for sensorineural hearing loss

2. This classic triad has been described in infants with congenital syphilis, and includes interstitial keratitis, peg-shaped upper central incisors, and sensory deafness.

3. These long bone radiographs show classic changes associated with syphilis. This patient has diffuse periosteal reactions in the clavicle, radius and ulna, femur, and tibia. Note mild bowing of the distal right radius, and periosteal cloaking of the diaphysis of the tibia. These diffuse periosteal reactions at multiple sites could be accidentally misinterpreted as healing fractures in the setting of child abuse.

4. Treatment is penicillin G. In patients with positive CSF VDRL, prolonged therapy for neurosyphilis is indicated.

Keywords: infectious diseases, child abuse mimicker

Bibliography

Workowski KA, Bolan GA, Centers for Disease Control and Prevention. Sexually transmitted diseases treatment guidelines, 2015. *MMWR Recomm Rep* 2015;64:1.

American Academy of Pediatrics. Syphilis. In *Red Book: 2015 Report of the Committee on Infectious Diseases*, 30th ed., Kimberlin DW, ed. Elk Grove Village, IL: American Academy of Pediatrics, 2015:755.

Brion LP, Manuli M, Rai B et al. Long-bone radiographic abnormalities as a sign of active congenital syphilis in asymptomatic newborns. *Pediatrics* 1991;88:1037.

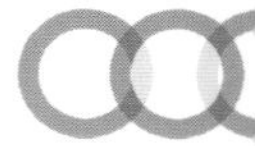

CASE 124

Michael Gottlieb

Questions

A 10-year-old boy presents to the emergency department with a left ear laceration. He has no other injuries and his immunizations are up to date. On examination, there is yellow material visible at the center of the wound.

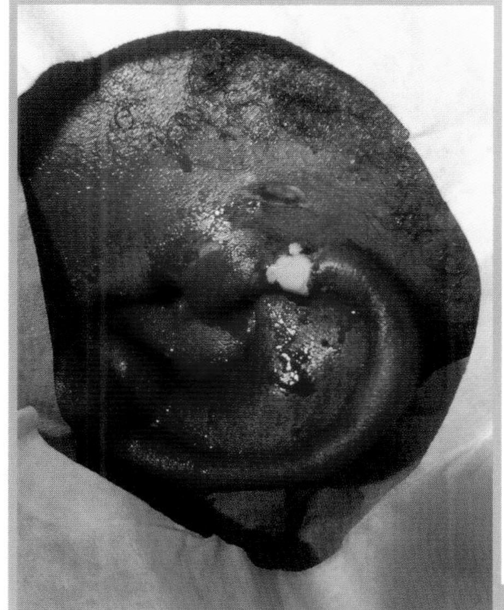

124.1

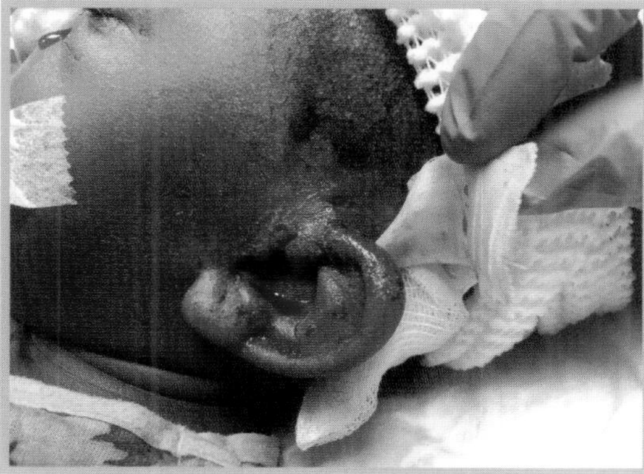

124.2

1. How should this laceration be repaired?
2. How should the wound be dressed after the repair?

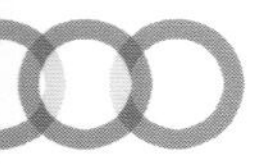

Answers

1. This patient is presenting with an ear injury with exposed cartilage. Cartilage is avascular and derives its blood supply from the overlying skin. Therefore, it must be fully covered with skin to reduce the risk of infection and avascular necrosis. First, approximate the cartilage with absorbable sutures. Then, place one suture at the helix to assist with alignment and suture the remaining areas until the cartilage is covered. It is important to minimize wound debridement in case wound revision is necessary.

2. These wounds are at risk of developing auricular hematomas, which can lead to cartilage damage and external deformity, commonly referred to as "cauliflower ear." This can be prevented by using petrolatum-impregnated gauze and a compressive dressing to prevent hematoma development and expansion.

Keywords: head injury, pitfalls, do not miss, procedures, penetrating trauma

Bibliography

Coates WC. Face and scalp lacerations. In *Tintinalli's Emergency Medicine: A Comprehensive Study Guide*, 8th ed., Tintinalli JE, Stapczynski J, Ma O, Yealy DM, Meckler GD, Cline DM, eds. New York: McGraw-Hill, 2016:chap. 42.

Mayersak RJ. Facial trauma. In *Rosen's Emergency Medicine*, 8th ed., Marx JA, Hockberger RS, Walls RM, eds. Philadelphia: Elsevier, 2014:chap. 42.

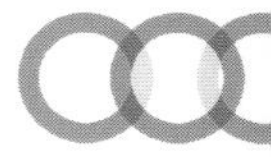

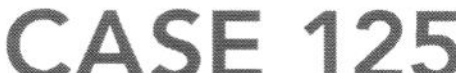

CASE 125

Veena Ramaiah

Question

An 8-month-old was placed on the bed while his mother was cleaning out the crib. He fell off the bed onto the radiator that was between the bed and the wall. Upon seeing a wound developing, she brought him immediately to the emergency room. Due to the appearance of the burn and the pattern mark seen, a report was made for child welfare and police to investigate.

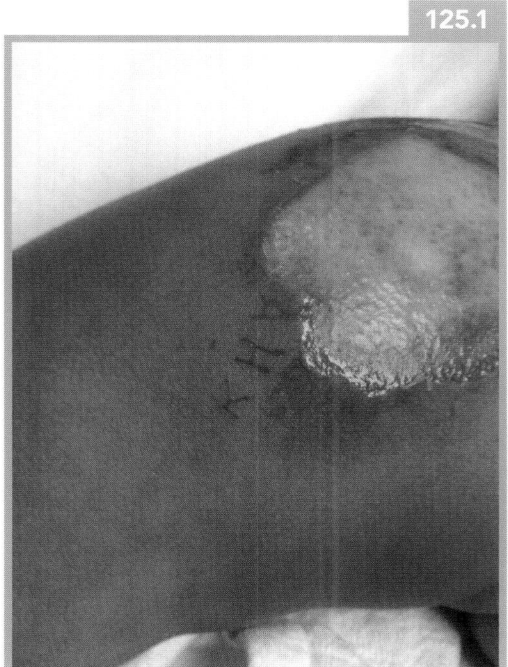

125.1

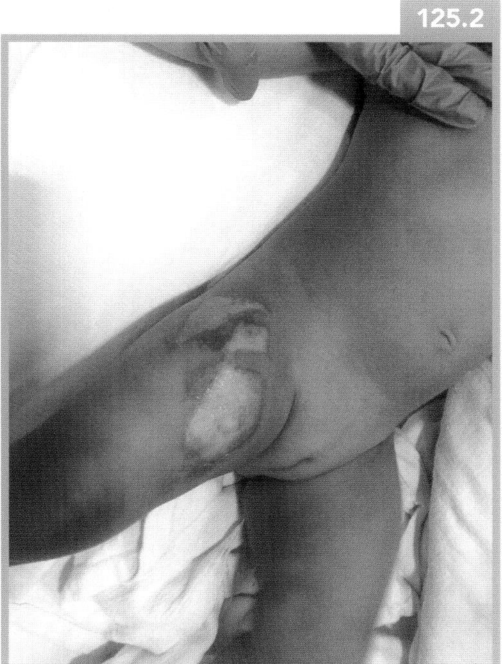

125.2

What characteristics would prompt an investigation? How is the investigation helpful?

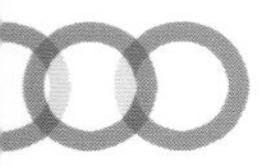

Answer

Contact burns with a very distinct pattern can be concerning for inflicted injury, especially in a non-verbal child. Confirming the mechanism of injury or determining manner of injury often requires a multi-disciplinary approach. Physicians may not be able to make these determinations at the bedside without other input or investigation. Reports to investigative agencies may be an integral component of the workup in order to provide additional information such as scene re-creation and interviewing of other corroborating witnesses.

During the scene investigation, the lettering from the radiator pipe was found that matched the imprint on the child's leg. Based on the young age of the infant, ability to roll off bed, scene re-creation with the parents as to the position he was found in, and home investigation, the event was ruled accidental. The radiator did not have a cover and was "scalding hot" to the touch.

Contact burns are burns from a hot surface. This type of burn can be accidental or inflicted and distinguishing between the two is often difficult. In general, accidental burns are described as glancing, more superficial, on exposed areas of the body, and not patterned. In general, abusive burns are described as uniform, deeper, on covered areas of the body, and patterned. These are sometimes referred to as "branding" injuries. Movement of the child at the time of contact can create an unusual appearance if the child is struggling to get away and cannot.

This case illustrates a contact burn with a pattern to it that resulted from short contact with the object. This can occur depending on how hot the surface is. Investigation by child welfare and police including scene investigation is vital to elucidating the manner of injury.

Keywords: child abuse, mimickers, environmental

Bibliography

Hodgman EI, Pastorek RA, Saeman MR, Cripps MW, Bernstein IH, Wolf SE, Kowalske KJ, Arnoldo BD, Phelan HA. The Parkland Burn Center experience with 297 cases of child abuse from 1974 to 2010. *Burns* June 3, 2016; pii: S0305-4179(16)00071-1.

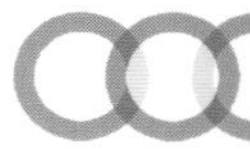

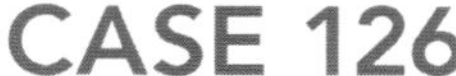

CASE 126

Veena Ramaiah

Question

A 2 year old presents to the emergency department with these burns.

126.1

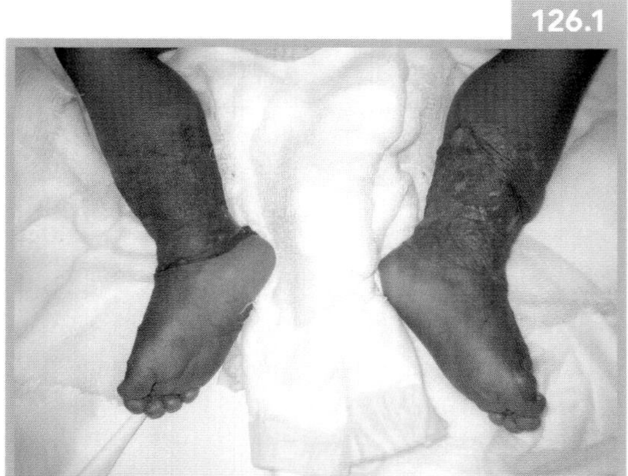

126.2

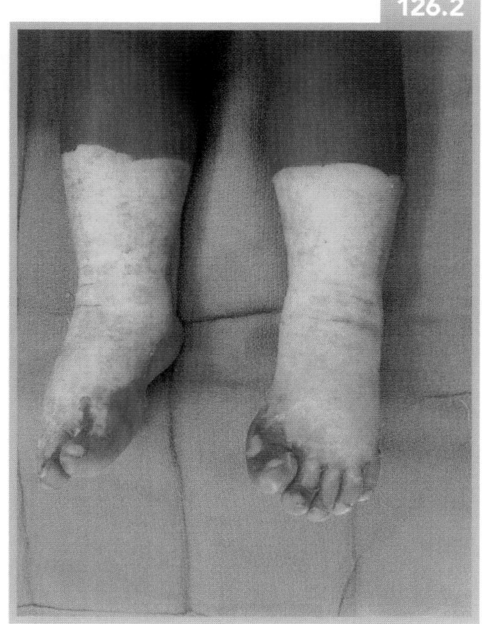

Is this burn abusive or accidental?

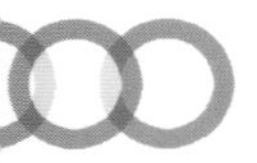

Answer

This is actually a trick question! Before making any determination about manner of injury a history of the injury must be obtained. Clinicians should avoid making rapid judgments based on an appearance, photo, or x-ray. Many injuries can have an accidental explanation or an abusive explanation, and jumping to conclusions prematurely can do harm to a patient or their family. This is the purpose of child welfare or police investigation. In a busy emergency department, there may not be time or ability to elucidate all the details of an event, or the caretaker during the event may not be present so the history is secondhand. It is important, however, to recognize when something is suspicious and warrants an investigation.

Per the father, he went to give the patient a bath, turned on the water, put the stopper in, and placed the patient in the tub. He did not think the water was hot but did not check it, and the patient did not scream or cry immediately. He starting whining and the father took him out of the water. He was in the water for about 2 minutes. The father denies that the water felt hot after he took him out. The father denies leaving the bathroom. He then noticed the skin looking dark and wrinkled. He called the patient's mom to ask what to do and she advised him to go to the emergency room.

On arrival, he was tachycardic, afebrile, and normotensive. He was quiet if left alone but began crying with any movement of his feet or exam on his feet. After IV access is obtained and he is given pain medicine, a thorough skin examination is done that is negative for bruises, marks, scars, or other burns aside from those pictured. He receives IV fluids and is admitted to the burn unit for burn care.

There are a few things that are concerning: the pattern, the absence of crying or screaming even after being in the water for about 2 minutes, and the father denying that the water felt hot. The pattern of the burn is an immersion pattern. This is indicative of someone being placed or immersed in hot water. The absence of any splash or spill pattern is concerning in that a child this age would be moving or kicking to attempt to get out of the water. There are no splash burns or irregular edges of the burn to indicate movement. In addition there is sparing of the soles. This particular pattern is often seen when the feet are against the bottom of the tub sparing the soles from being burned at all or burned as deeply. Burns cause pain. In a neurologically normal child, he would be crying or screaming in response to being burned.

There is a well-documented freeze response that sometimes children have in response to pain or heat but that lasts a few seconds before they react. Last, the water was hot enough to burn the child which means an adult who is neurologically intact would be able to feel the heat. This part of the history is obviously false as you have evidence of an injury since the patient is burned.

This patient's feet were debrided as shown in Image 126.2.

It is important to recognize when seeing injuries that as a mandated reporter it is required to have a reasonable suspicion of abuse, not to know that abuse has occurred. A manner of abuse often cannot be determined without a thorough investigation that may include a scene investigation. Determining the manner of injury without enough information can be detrimental to the patient and the family. Immersion pattern burns can be accidental; however, that is much less common and again would warrant a full investigation in order to corroborate an accidental mechanism being provided.

Keywords: child abuse, dermatology, environmental

Bibliography

Pawlik M-C, Kemp A, Maguire S, Nuttall D, Fedlman KW, Lindberg DM, ExSTRA Investigators. Children with burns referred for child abuse evaluation: Burn characteristics and co-existent injuries. *Child Abuse Negl* 2016;55:52–61.

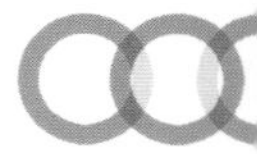

CASE 127

Veena Ramaiah

Question

A 5-month-old infant presents with right leg swelling. Per the mother, the baby rolled off of the bed while she was in another room. She did not witness the fall but heard a cry. The bed is a box spring and mattress on a frame and the floor surface is hardwood. She cannot recall the position the baby was in when she got to him. There are several caretakers at home including the father and maternal grandmother. Mom reports both were at home; however, they are not present in the emergency room (ER) to interview.

On exam, his vital signs are stable, and he is alert and quiet. He is in no apparent distress until the extremity exam. His head shows no signs of injury and his skin exam has no marks or bruises. His extremity exam shows swelling to the mid-thigh area. He cries and is very tender to palpation of the mid-thigh area and has apparent pain with any range of motion of the leg. He does not cry with palpation of the right foot and lower leg. He cries with flexion of the right knee.

An x-ray of his right femur is shown next.

127.1

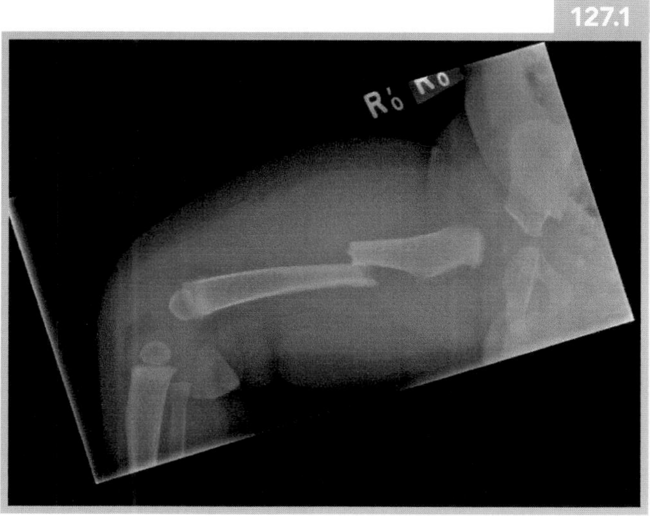

Is this fracture morphology concerning for abuse? Does the history provided adequately explain the fracture seen here?

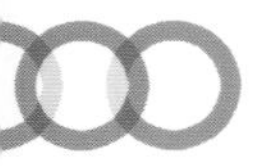

Answer

Yes, this fracture morphology is concerning for abuse. It is a commonly held misconception that spiral fractures are the most concerning for abuse. However, recent studies have identified that the most common morphology of abusive fractures is transverse.

Ultimately, any fracture morphology can be from an accidental or abusive manner. The key to determining which one lies in the history, the level of suspicion, and the investigation to corroborate or refute the history given. Non-ambulatory infants are at highest risk of abusive injury, and their injuries often warrant further medical evaluation and child welfare and police investigation. Even when a history is provided, it is not possible to determine the truthfulness of that history oftentimes without an investigation. Many explanations are plausible; however, determining the truth is often beyond the resources of the ER or a clinic.

Due to concerns about the history provided, the patient's age and developmental level, and the need to corroborate the history, a report was made to police and child welfare for an investigation. While in the ER, the child underwent a skeletal survey, head CT, and trauma labs. The skeletal survey revealed three healing rib fractures to the posterior right ribs. On further investigation, it was discovered that his mother was home alone with the baby. There were no other adults present as originally reported. In addition, there was no prior history of trauma to explain the rib fractures. In spite of an in-depth investigation, no other history was obtained to explain the femur fracture; however, the rib fractures remained unexplained. There was not enough evidence for criminal charges; however, child welfare indicted the mother for abusive injury and the child was placed in a safe environment while the mother underwent services and intervention.

Keywords: extremity injury, child abuse, orthopedics

Bibliography

Murphy R, Kelly DM, Moisan A, Thompson NB et al. Transverse fractures of the femoral shaft are a better predictor of nonaccidental trauma in young children than spiral fractures are. *J Bone Joint Surg* January 2015;97(2):106–11.

Pierce MC, Bertocci GE, Janosky JE, Aguel F et al. Femur fractures resulting from stair falls among children: An injury plausibility model. *Pediatrics* June 2005;115(6):1712–22.

Scherl SA, Miller L, Lively N, Russinoff S et al. Accidental and non-accidental femur fractures in children. *Clin Orthop Relat Res* July 2000;376:96–105.

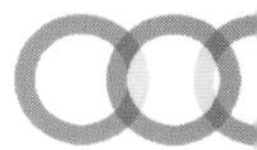

CASE 128

Veena Ramaiah

Question

A 7-month-old boy is brought to the emergency department for a scald burn. His mother states she was bathing him in the sink, using both hot and cold water faucets with an appropriate water temperature. She stated she left the room with the child in the sink under running water to get a towel. While out of the bathroom, she heard a scream and rushed back into the bathroom. She said she immediately took the baby out of the sink and felt the water. It was scalding hot to the touch as only the hot water faucet was on. The skin was red initially. Blistering and peeling of the skin was noted after an hour and prompted the mother to bring him immediately to the emergency department.

The burn is as pictured next.

128.1

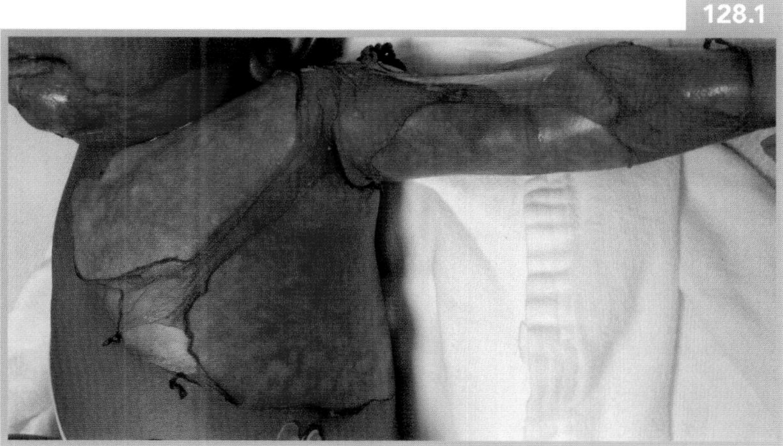

There is a partial-thickness scald burn involving 20% BSA to left face, neck, chest, arm, and back. The burn is a combination of superficial partial thickness and deep partial thickness. The pattern is consistent with a flow pattern. The patient is well-developed, well-nourished, and has no other marks or bruises on exam. By report, he is developmentally normal including normal tone and motor strength in all extremities. On exam, he has a normal neurologic exam for a 7-month-old infant.

Is this burn consistent with the history provided? Would you expect this pattern and depth of injury from the mechanism described?

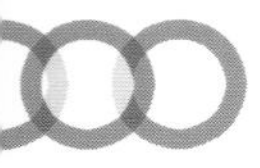

Answer

Scald burns are a type of thermal burn involving hot liquid or hot steam. There are generally two different patterns of injury seen with scald burns: splash/spill or flow pattern, and immersion pattern. A single burn event can have separate patterns or combinations of both. In general, splash/spill patterns are produced by the flow of hot liquid as it travels down or over a certain plane of the body. The point of deepest burn is often the area of initial contact; the burn depth lessens as the hot water flows and the liquid cools. Irregular edges and possibly even discrete areas of splash would indicate splashing water as the child is trying move or flail around in response to the heat of the liquid. There may not be significant splash if the child is in a situation where he or she cannot move away or move around much. Immersion pattern burns, on the other hand, are often more uniform in depth and result from that part of the body being submerged or immersed in standing water. Neither of these patterns are pathognomonic of abusive injury; however, splash/spill pattern burns are highly correlated with an accidental manner of injury and immersion pattern burns are highly correlated with an abusive manner of injury. The pattern seen in this child is a splash/spill or flow pattern which would be consistent with water flowing from a sink faucet.

Depth of burn is dependent on the temperature of the liquid and time of contact with the liquid. Based on studies done in the 1940s, time to burn depth of full-thickness in adult skin was found to be 10 minutes at 120°F. This time decreased rapidly as temperature rose culminating in deep partial-thickness burn in 1 second at 158°F. This time is shorter in children. Temperatures greater than 130°F can result in significant burns within the reaction time.

This case was reported to child welfare for investigation because of the young age of the infant and the severity of the burn. It was discovered that the water temperature with only hot water running reached 130°F at 17 seconds and 140°F at 30 seconds. The patient's mother estimated that she had left the bathroom for about 15–20 seconds when the police had her re-enact the events of that day. The handles on the bathroom sink were the lever type with hot and cold each having its own handle. When the water is on, the levers are turned toward the basin. With an active, vigorous, and developmentally normal infant who kicks, it was speculated that he kicked the cold water handle off leaving only scalding hot water running down his body. The mother did not realize that water from her tap could cause this extent and depth of burn so rapidly.

Based on the information provided by the scene investigation, the final manner of injury was accidental.

The secondary teaching point to this case is anticipatory guidance for injury prevention for parents of infants. Infants should not be bathed in running water as the temperature can fluctuate unexpectedly resulting in significant burn injury. The convenience and rapidity of bathing a child in running water is often a strong motivator for families.

Keywords: child abuse, dermatology, environmental

Bibliography

Baggott K, Rabbitts A, Leahy NE, Bourke P et al. Pediatric sink-bathing: A risk for scald burns. *J Burn Care Res* November/December 2013;34:639–43.

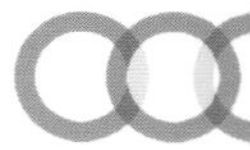

CASE 129

Barbara Pawel

Question

A 15-year-old male presents to the emergency department with a gunshot wound (GSW) to the left thigh. He is complaining of left thigh and groin pain.

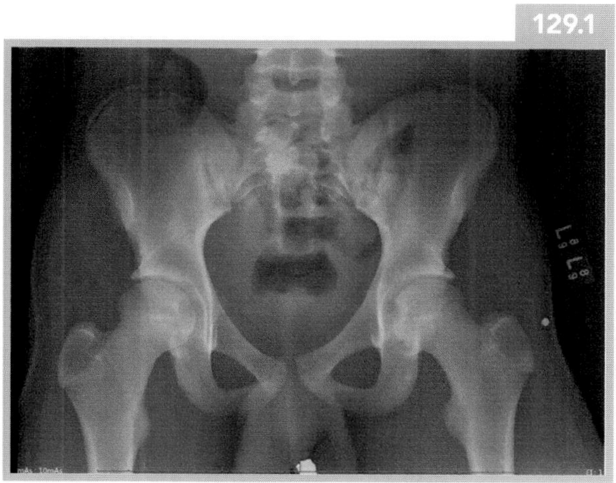
129.1

129.2

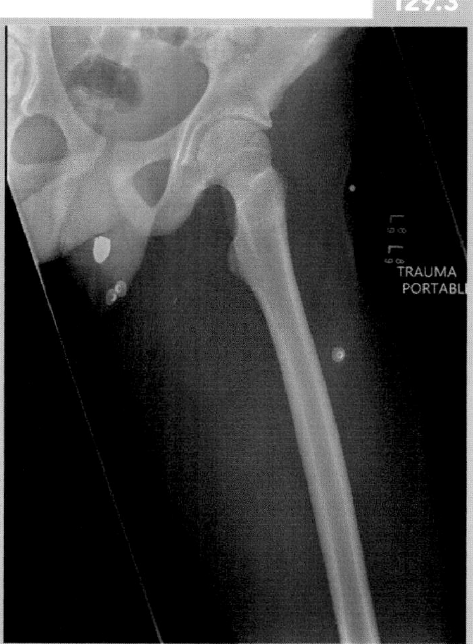

129.3

What are the mechanisms of injury that present with penetrating scrotal trauma?

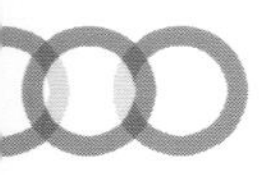

Answer

Bicycle handlebars, falls with impalement, animal bites, stab wounds, and GSWs can all result in penetrating trauma to the scrotum and testes.

Penetrating wounds to the lower abdomen, pelvis, penis, rectum, and upper thighs may involve the scrotum due to anatomical proximity. GSWs to the lower extremities are commonly associated with scrotal wounds. A thorough examination to determine entrance and exit wounds in addition to careful inspection of the scrotal skin for lacerations and ecchymosis is necessary. Any penetrating trauma through the dartos layer has a high association of testicular injury. Significant pain with marked edema localized to the testicle or scrotum requires early surgical consultation. Assess the testicular lie and tenderness, the cremasteric reflex, and quality of the femoral artery pulses. The presence of a hematocele (blood within the tunica vaginalis but outside of the tunica albuginea) is concerning for a testicular rupture and ultrasound is recommended. Scrotal edema/ecchymosis may also be caused by blood tracking from an intra-abdominal injury through a patent processus vaginalis.

Keywords: penetrating trauma, GU trauma, urology

Bibliography

American College of Surgeons Committee on Trauma. *Advanced Trauma Life Support (ATLS) Student Course Manual.* 9th ed. Chicago: American College of Surgeons, 2012.

Simhan J, Rothman J, Canter D, Reyes JM, Jaffe WI, Pontari MA, Doumanian LR, Mydlo JH. Gunshot wounds to the scrotum: A large single-institutional 20-year experience. *BJU Int* 2012;109(11):1704–7.

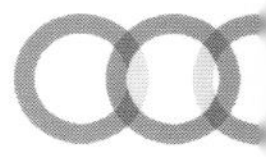

CASE 130

Veena Ramaiah

Question

A 6-month-old presents to the emergency department for coughing and congestion. The child is happy, smiling, playful, and in no distress, with mild URI symptoms but otherwise appears well. On full skin exam, red marks are found as shown. There is mild tenderness over the red marks but no pain or marks anywhere else on the body. When asked, the mom reports "blowing kisses" on the child's back. The resident is very concerned as these bruises do not blanch and are not fading.

130.1

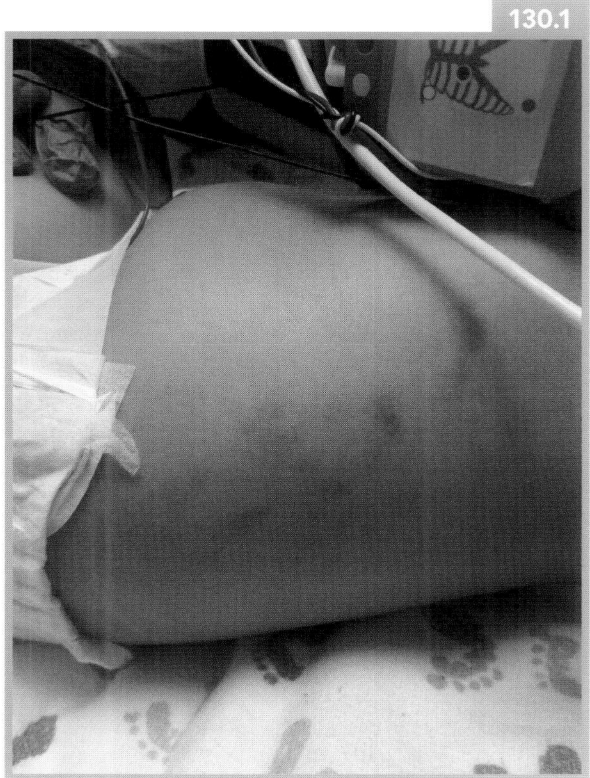

What factors trigger the most concern in this child with bruising?

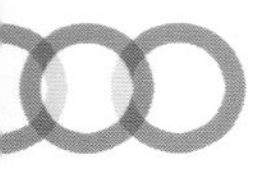

Answer

The age and developmental level of this child is the key to the concern. Unexplained bruising in a non-ambulatory infant is very concerning and should precipitate further workup.

Trauma labs, skeletal survey, and head CT are done. Upon return from radiology, her labs reveal elevated liver enzymes. Abdominal CT is performed and the child is found to have a moderate-sized liver laceration. Mom has no explanation for this.

In light of unexplained bruising and unexplained liver laceration—two significant indicators of trauma—child welfare and police are called and the child is placed in a safe environment.

Bruising in infants is rare, especially in non-mobile infants. In 1999, Sugar et al. published a study looking at bruising in healthy children from 0 to 36 months presenting for well-child visits. Of 973 children, 203 (20.9%) had bruises. They divided the children into three groups: pre-cruisers, cruisers, and walkers. Age was associated with bruising as 2.2% of pre-cruisers, 17.8% of cruisers, and 51.9% of walkers had bruises. The pre-cruisers group had the largest number of patients. Based on this data, the authors created the phrase "Those who don't cruise rarely bruise."

Building on this, in 2010, Pierce et al. published a study proposing a clinical decision rule for predicting abusive trauma called the TEN-4 BCDR. This was a body region–based and age-based bruising clinical decision rule. This study compared children 0–48 months who were victims of abuse with controls who sustained known accidental trauma. TEN-4 represents bruising found on the thorax, ears, and neck in a child <4 years old or bruising found anywhere on the body of a child <4 months old. Their data showed that bruising in the TEN region or bruising in a young infant in the absence of a verified or corroborated accidental injury was highly sensitive (97%) and specific (84%).

Bruising in infants, especially pre-mobile ones, is extremely concerning. Infants are at highest risk of death by inflicted injury as they cannot escape from the perpetrator. Even a single bruise in an infant that is unexplained or inadequately explained should raise suspicion for abuse and trigger further workup or reporting.

Keywords: child abuse, dermatology

Bibliography

Pierce MC, Kaczor K, Aldridge S, O'Flynn J, Lorenz DJ. Bruising characteristics discriminating physical child abuse from accidental trauma. *Pediatrics* January 2010;125(1):67–74.

Sugar NF, Taylor JA, Feldman KW, Puget Sound Pediatric Research Network. Bruises in infants and toddlers: Those who don't cruise rarely bruise. *Arch Pediatr Adolesc Med* 1999;153(4):399–403.

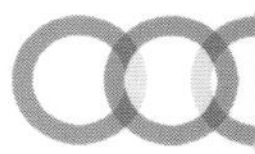

CASE 131

Veena Ramaiah

Question

A 2-year-old male was noted to have right forearm swelling this morning. No swelling was noted the day before. He went to the park with his mother. There was no history of a known fall, trauma, or insect bite. He has been using his right arm normally without any signs of pain. There is no history of any recent illness, fever, chills, or weight loss. He lives with his mother and visits his father on the weekends.

On physical exam, he has no fever, tachycardia, tachypnea, or hypertension. His exam is normal except for his right forearm with non-tender swelling with no erythema. There is no tenderness to the wrist or elbow and he has normal range of motion of wrist and elbow. His pulses and perfusion are normal and he has no other marks or bruises on his body. No rash or lesions are noted. His family history is only positive for type 2 diabetes.

X-rays were obtained and are presented next.

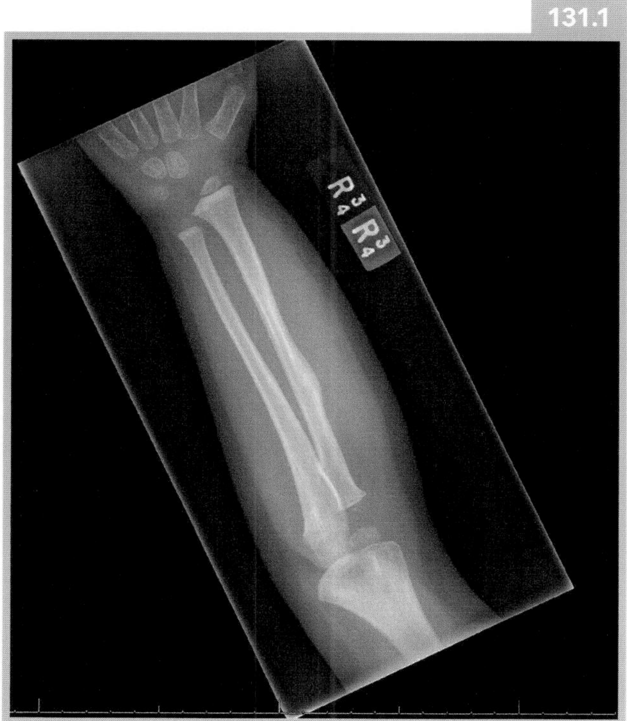

131.1

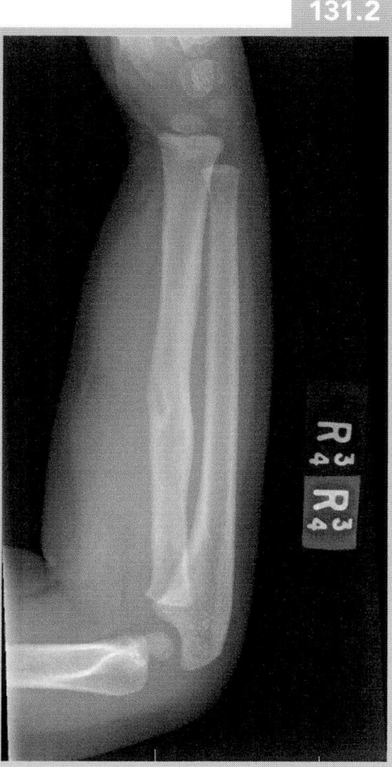

131.2

What is in your differential diagnosis?

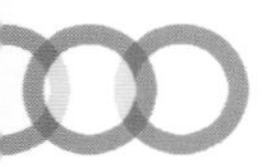

Answer

The x-rays show a sclerotic lesion with a lucent center in the mid-shaft of his right radius with significant soft tissue swelling. The differential includes Brodie's abscess, osteoid osteoma, Langerhans cell histiocytosis (LCH), osteomyelitis, and healing fracture.

Osteomyelitis is less likely based on the history. Fractures are common in active children, but the absence of an identified trauma would raise the concern for physical abuse. This appearance is not typical for a healing fracture. A skeletal survey was done to assess for other occult injuries or bone disease. There were no other lesions or fractures identified.

He was admitted to the hospital for further workup including MRI, orthopedic consultation, and lab testing. Initial screening lab work including electrolytes, CBC (complete blood count), liver function tests, blood cultures, ESR, and CRP was unremarkable.

The MRI of the forearm is shown in the following.

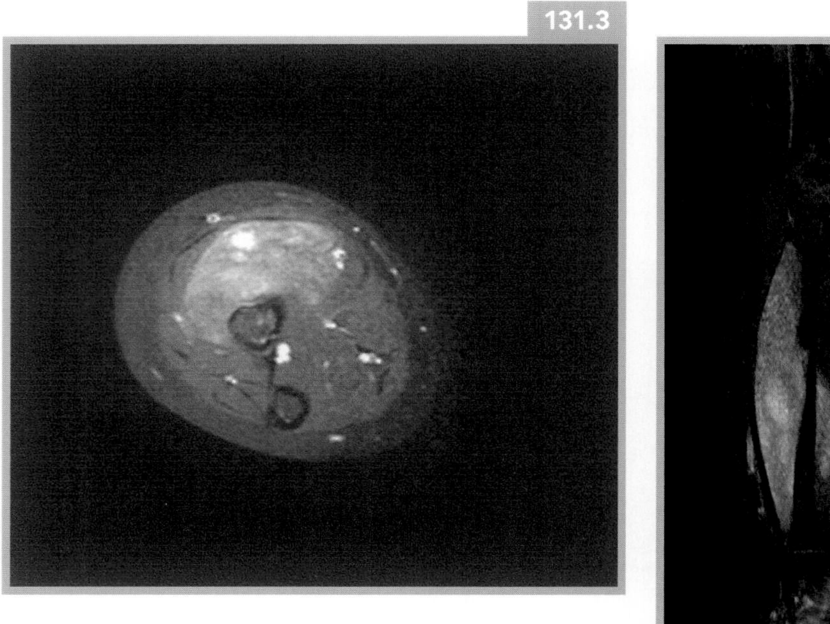

131.3

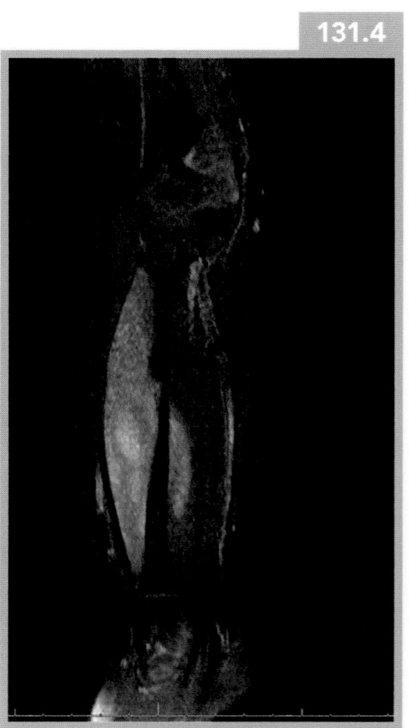

131.4

The MRI reading indicated a soft tissue mass described as "heterogenous, avidly enhancing, well-circumscribed soft tissue mass with focal disruption of the cortex of the radius and surrounding thickening of the cortex indicating osseous remodeling with small amount of extension of the mass into the cortex."

On biopsy, the final diagnosis was plexiform schwannoma.

Plexiform schwannoma is a benign nerve sheath tumor that develops from Schwann cells. There are seven types of schwannoma, and plexiform accounts for only 5%. They are made up entirely of Schwann cells and the characteristic pattern of growth is plexiform or multinodular. They can be sporadic lesions but are commonly associated with neurofibromatosis type 2. It is important

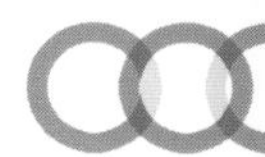

to distinguish them from plexiform neurofibroma that is associated with neurofibromatosis type 1. Plexiform neurofibroma carries a risk of malignant transformation, whereas plexiform schwannoma is strictly benign.

These are rare in children and a workup for neurofibromatosis is warranted. In adults, the treatment is complete excision with best attempt to preserve nerve function. This patient's mass was surgically removed and the final pathology confirmed plexiform schwannoma. Post-operatively he had no loss of motor or nerve function.

Keywords: oncology, benign, extremity injury, MRI

Bibliography

Jacobson JM, Felder JM, Pedroso F, Steinberg JS. Plexiform schwannoma of the foot: A review of the literature and case report. *J Foot Ankle Surg* 2011;50(1):68–73.

Li XN, Cui JL, Christopasak SP, Kumar A, Peng ZG. Multiple plexiform schwannomas in the plantar aspect of the foot: Case report and literature review. *BMC Musculoskelet Disord* 2014;15:342.

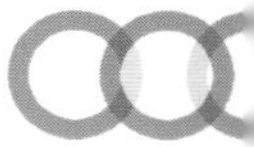

CASE 132

Veena Ramaiah

Question

A 15-month-old boy is brought to the emergency department for lesions to the trunk. The lesions seem mildly painful, and the child is rubbing and scratching them occasionally. His parents report the lesions appeared 48 hours ago and more lesions are appearing in the areas he has been scratching. The child has been well otherwise and there is no history of fever. He has no other medical problems and has never had these lesions before. There is no history of previous dermatologic conditions.

On arrival to the emergency department, the triage nurse alerts the physician about a concern for cigarette burns. The boy's vital signs are T 37.9°C, HR 128, RR 22, BP 105/85. He is well-appearing and interactive on exam. He occasionally scratches his trunk and cries but is easily consolable. There are several circular ulcerated lesions to his trunk and lateral neck ranging in size from 0.5 cm to 1.5 cm wide. Some lesions have central-thickened hyperpigmented keratotic plaque. Some of the lesions have a small rim of surrounding erythema. There is no fluctuance. Yellow discharge is expressed with removal of the overlying plaque of a lesion. The patient has no pattern marks, bruising, or petechiae to the rest of his body.

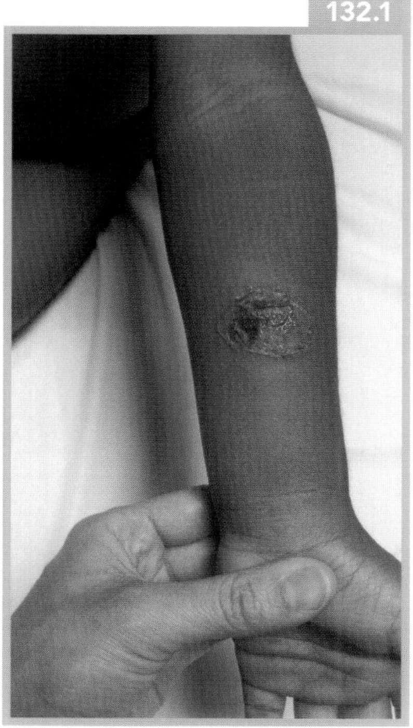

132.1

Are these traumatic lesions or infectious? How do you distinguish?

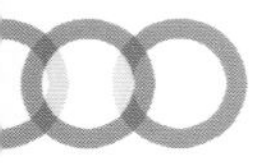

Answer

This is an infectious condition called ecthyma. Ecthyma is a deeper form of impetigo extending down into the dermis. It is characterized by small punched out ulcers often with a thick brown-black crust or plaque. There may also be surrounding erythema. The lesions spread on the body via scratching or direct contact. The bacterial etiology is *Streptococcus pyogenes* (GAS) or *Staphylococcus aureus.*

The treatment is usually a beta-lactamase penicillin or cephalosporin. Warm soaks to remove the crusting and topical mupirocin are helpful adjuncts to treatment. Localized ecthyma can be treated topically but more widespread lesions require systemic antibiotics.

The ulcerated appearance can be mistaken for cigarette burns. However on closer inspection, the varying sizes, the overlying crust or plaque, and the evolving progression of the lesions point more toward an infectious cause. It is important to completely undress the patient for a thorough skin exam. The quantity and location of the lesions may be more indicative of an infectious etiology. In addition, cigarette burns often have a deep central crater as this is the hottest part of the cigarette. As with any concern of abuse, children with medical conditions can also be abused and children with a concern of abuse can have a medical condition. This can cause difficulty in distinguishing. Ecthyma can also have the appearance seen in these subsequent photos, which makes them easier to distinguish from cigarette burns.

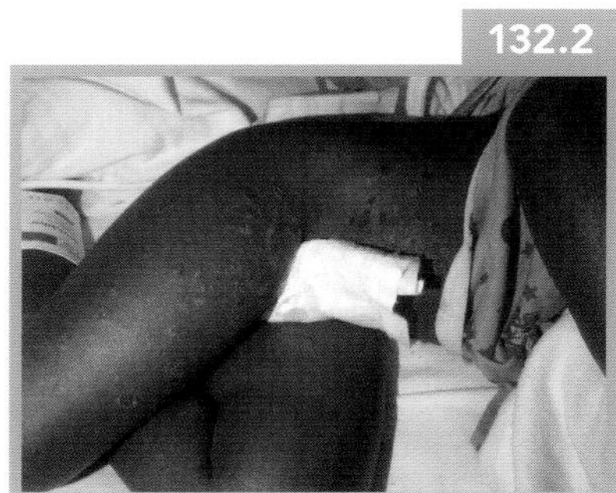

132.2

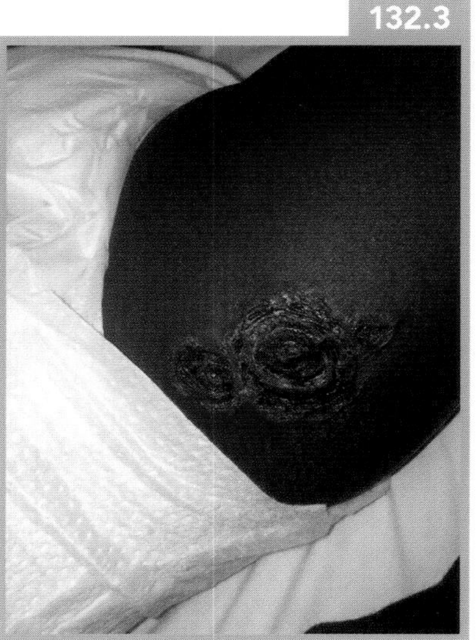

132.3

Keywords: skin and soft tissue infection, child abuse mimicker, dermatology

Bibliography

Millett CR, Heymann WR, Manders SM. Pyodermas and toxin-mediated syndromes. In *Harper's Textbook of Pediatric Dermatology*, 3rd ed., vol. 1, Irvine AD, Hoeger PH, Yan AC, eds. Hoboken, NJ: Wiley Blackwell, 2011:chap. 54.

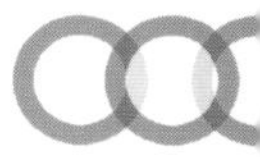

CASE 133

Timothy Ketterhagen

Question

A 15-year-old girl presents to the emergency department with left flank pain which has been present for the past few weeks. The patient describes the pain as a "constant aching" and increasing in severity recently. The pain is worse with deep inspirations and twisting movements. She denies any trauma and is not sexually active. She has no significant medical or surgical history. There are no reported fevers, night sweats, cough, vomiting, diarrhea, rashes, joint swelling, dysuria, vaginal bleeding, or discharge.

Physical exam shows a well-appearing young woman. Vital signs are normal. Her abdomen is soft, non-distended, with normal bowl sounds, and no rebound or guarding. The patient is minimally tender in the left upper quadrant and also has point tenderness on the left flank overlying the distal ribs. No hepatosplenomegaly or lymphadenopathy is appreciated. The physical exam is otherwise unremarkable. Images of the patient are shown next.

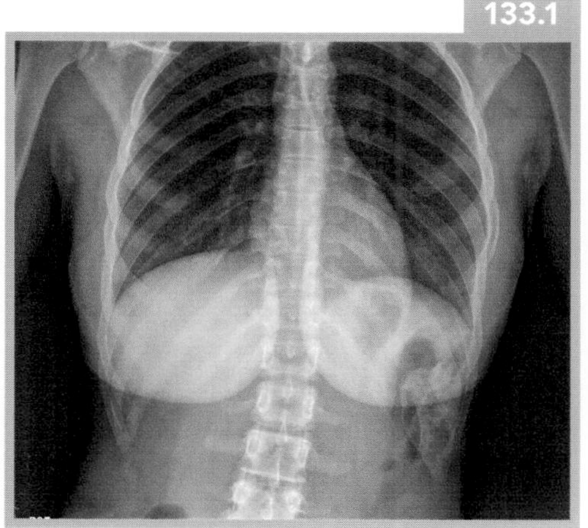

133.1

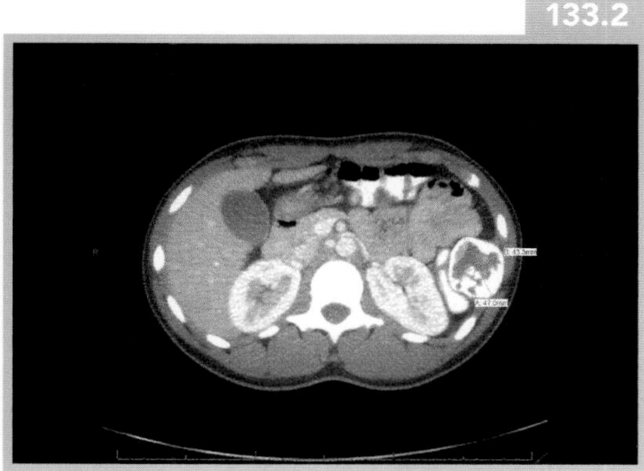

133.2

What is the diagnosis?

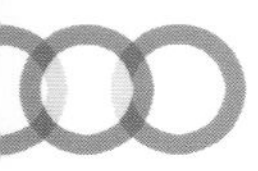

Answer

This patient has fibrous dysplasia. Fibrous dysplasia is a bone disease that replaces normal bone with a fibrous-type tissue (as seen in the left upper quadrant on these images). This tissue is not as hard as normal bone and therefore more susceptible to fracture. One or multiple bones may be affected, most commonly the femur, tibia, or humerus. However, any bone may be affected. Fibrous dysplasia usually occurs between 3 and 15 years of age. Fibrous dysplasia is also a feature in McCune-Albright syndrome, a genetic disorder affecting bone, skin, and endocrine systems.

Symptoms of fibrous dysplasia include bone pain, fractures, or localized symptoms depending on the bone that is affected. Treatment options include medications, such as bisphosphonates, or surgical intervention. Prognosis is good, but long-term monitoring for recurrence may be required.

Keywords: abdominal pain, mass, CT

Bibliography

Children's Hospital of Philadelphia. Fibrous dysplasia. http://www.chop.edu/conditions-diseases/fibrous-dysplasia. Published February 23, 2014.

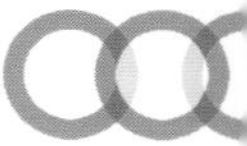

CASE 134

Michael Gottlieb

Questions

A 4-year-old girl presents to the pediatric trauma center after a motor vehicle collision. She was in the front seat when her vehicle was involved in a high-speed collision. She was placed on a backboard and cervical collar, then brought to the trauma center. On arrival, a lateral cervical spine film and cervical spine CT demonstrated the following injury.

134.1

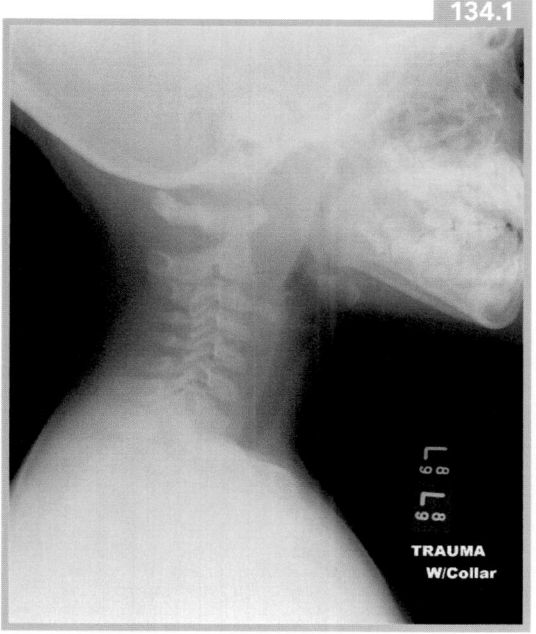

134.2

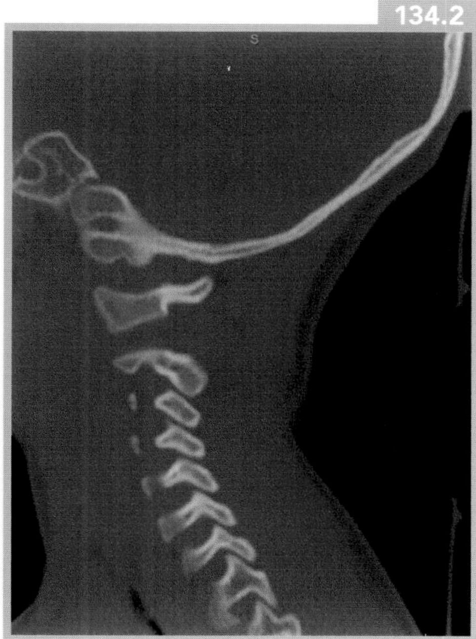

1. What is the injury demonstrated in the images?
2. What is the prognosis with this injury?

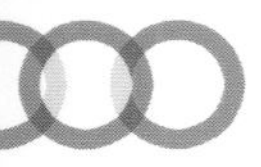

Answers

1. This patient is presenting with an atlanto-occipital dislocation. This is a rare and devastating injury, wherein there is disruption of ligaments connecting the base of the skull (i.e. occiput) from the C1 vertebral body (i.e. atlas). The most common mechanism is high-speed motor vehicle accidents and children are disproportionately affected due to the relatively larger size of their heads in relation to their bodies.

2. The injury has a very poor prognosis. The injury is fatal in 85% of patients, with 70% perishing at the scene. Low initial Glasgow Coma Scale score and a basion-dens interval of ≥16 mm is associated with worse outcomes.

Keywords: neurosurgery, neck injury, blunt trauma, do not miss, altered mental status, CT

Bibliography

Behar S. Cervical spine injury in infants and children. In *Tintinalli's Emergency Medicine: A Comprehensive Study Guide*, 8th ed., Tintinalli JE, Stapczynski J, Ma O, Yealy DM, Meckler GD, Cline DM, eds. New York: McGraw-Hill, 2016:chap. 139.

Cooper Z, Gross JA, Lacey JM, Traven N, Mirza SK, Arbabi S. Identifying survivors with traumatic craniocervical dissociation: A retrospective study. *J Surg Res* May 1, 2010;160(1):3–8.

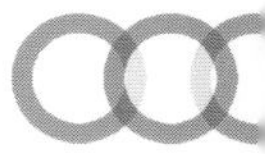

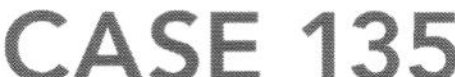

CASE 135

Timothy Ketterhagen

Questions

An 18-month-old boy presents to the emergency department with his parents with abdominal distention and constipation. Parents report that the patient's abdomen looks larger than it did a few weeks ago. The patient has also not been stooling as regularly as he had been in the past. He has only stooled once this week. The patient's appetite has also decreased recently, but the mother is unsure if he has lost weight. Prior to this the patient had been doing very well. The birth history is unremarkable. There is no prior medical or surgical history. His immunizations are up to date. No reported fevers, vomiting, diarrhea, cough, or rash.

Physical exam reveals an uncomfortable but non-toxic appearing boy. Vital signs are normal for age except for an elevated blood pressure (130/85). The abdomen is distended with hypoactive bowel sounds. A large mass is palpated in the left upper quadrant. The patient displays discomfort throughout the abdominal exam. Hepatomegaly is not appreciated. The GU (genitourinary) exam is unremarkable. The physical exam is otherwise unremarkable. Imaging of the patient is shown next.

135.1

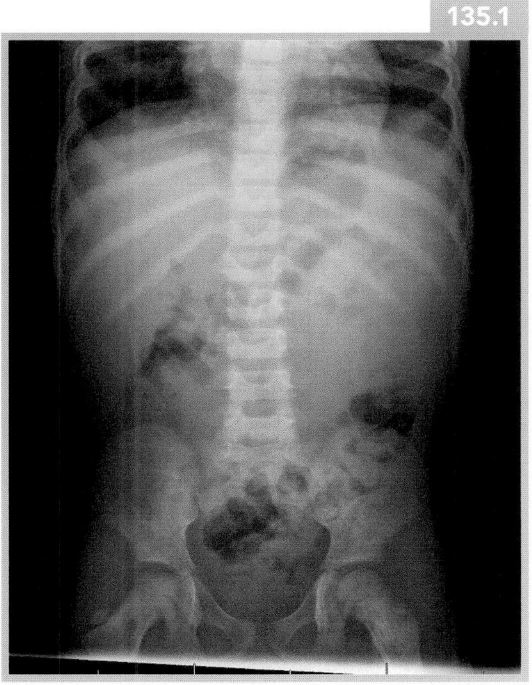

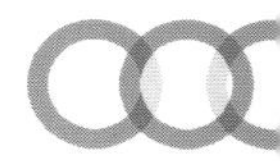

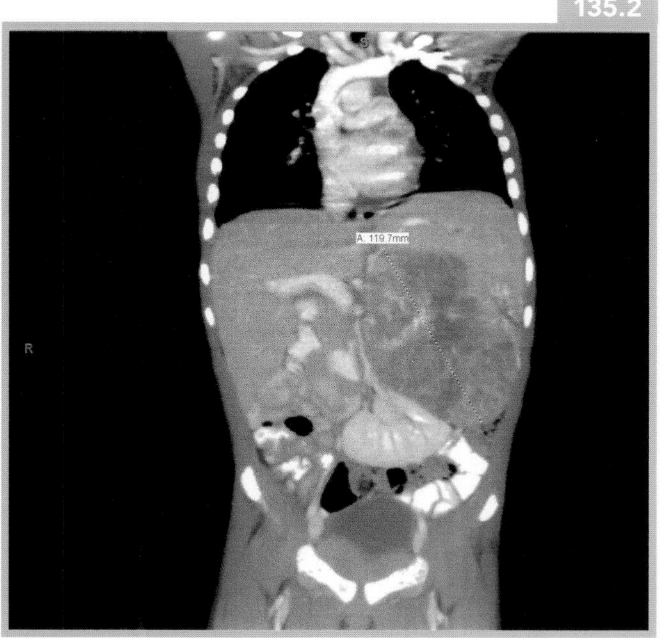

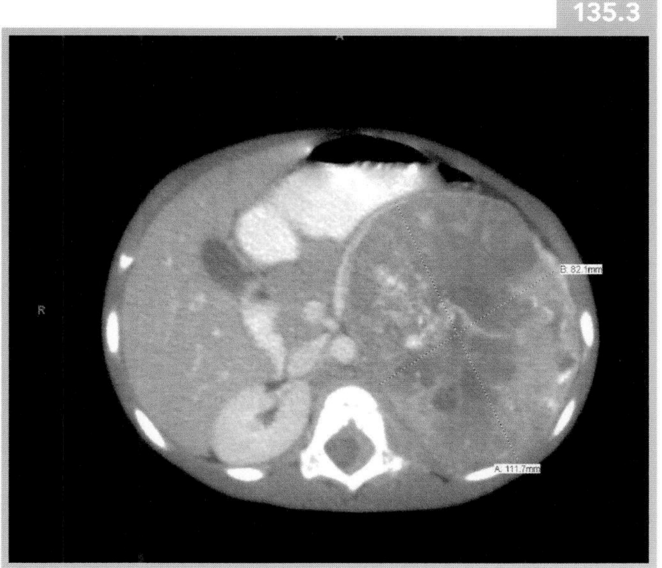

1. What is the diagnosis?
2. What syndromes are associated with this condition?
3. What diagnostic workup should be performed?

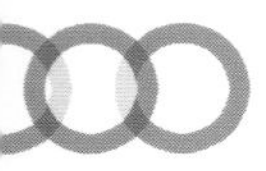

Answers

1. This patient has a diagnosis of neuroblastoma. Note the left upper quadrant mass and lytic lesions in the proximal femurs. Neuroblastoma arises from neural crest cells that exist in the adrenal medulla as well as the sympathetic chain. It is the most common extracranial solid tumor of childhood and usually occurs in the abdomen. Ninety percent of cases are diagnosed by the age of 5. Presentation is variable depending on the location of the tumor. Common presenting symptoms include abdominal pain, constipation, bone pain, bladder dysfunction, fever, weight loss, and fatigue.

2. Opsoclonus-myoclonus ataxia syndrome is seen in 2%–4% of patients with neuroblastoma. This is a paraneoplastic syndrome that consists of rapid eye movements, ataxia, and irregular muscle movements. Neuroblastoma is also associated with Turner syndrome, Beckwith-Wiedemann syndrome, Von Recklinghausen syndrome, Rubenstein-Taybi syndrome, and Hirschsprung disease.

3. Diagnostic testing includes CBC (complete blood count), lactate dehydrogenase, ferritin, urine catecholamines, electrolytes, and renal/hepatic function tests. If an abdominal mass is palpated, an ultrasound should be obtained with consideration of a pelvic CT or MRI. Treatment is based on tumor risk classification and consists of a combination of surgical resection, chemotherapy, and radiation. Prognosis is dependent on the patient age, stage, and biologic characteristics of the disease.

Keywords: oncology, neurology, abdominal pain, mass, CT

Bibliography

Fleisher GR, Ludwig S, eds. *Textbook of Pediatric Emergency Medicine*. 6th ed. Philadelphia: Lippincott Williams & Wilkins, 2010.

Hoffman RJ, Wang VJ, Scarfone R. *Fleisher & Ludwig's 5-Minute Pediatric Emergency Medicine Consult*. Philadelphia: Wolters Kluwer Health/Lippincott Williams & Wilkins, 2012.

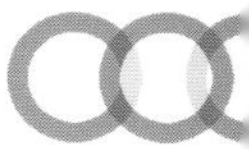

CASE 136

Leah Finkel

Question

A 15-year-old boy presents with right shoulder pain after colliding with another player during a football game.

The boy's physical exam is notable for pain at the medial aspect of the right clavicle with a palpable step off and mild shortness of breath. Range of motion of the shoulder is limited secondary to pain. The patient has strong pulses and a normal capillary refill of his right upper extremity. He is given a medication for pain control and a radiograph is ordered that shows no fracture (see images). The boy is discharged with a shoulder immobilizer, pain medications, and with follow-up to orthopedics where he is found to have a posterior sternoclavicular dislocation on ultrasound and confirmed with CT.

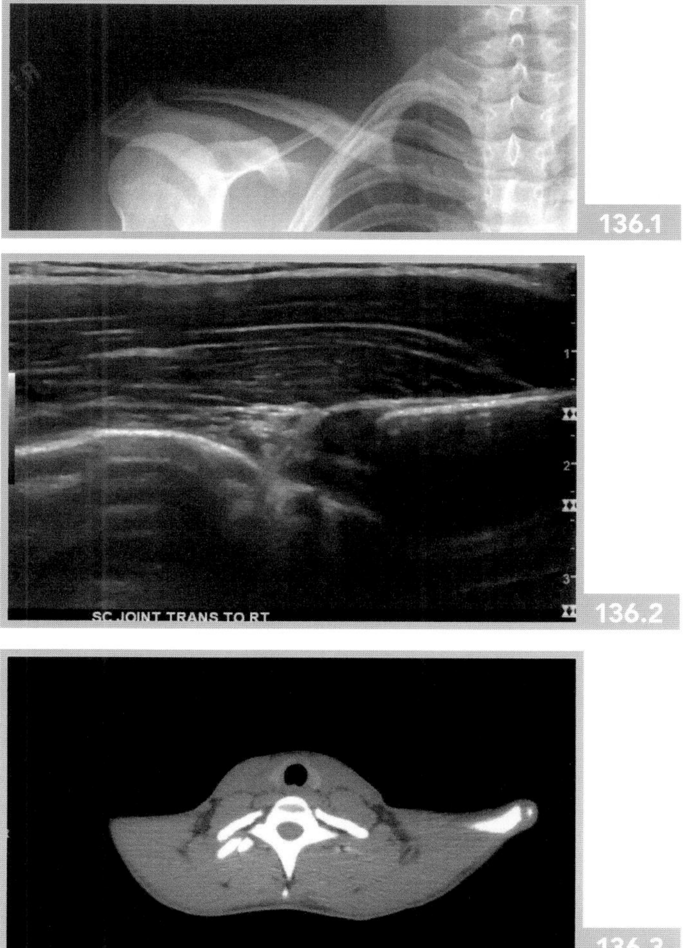

136.1

136.2

136.3

What types of sternoclavicular dislocations are there and which is most common? What type of imaging is most helpful for sternoclavicular dislocations?

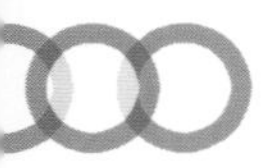

Answer

Traumatic and atraumatic dislocations can occur. Anterior dislocations are more common than posterior dislocations and often present with a deformity, a palpable bump. In contrast, posterior deformities are often associated with dyspnea, dysphagia, and increased work of breathing. Traumatic sternoclavicular dislocations are most commonly due to high impact injuries such as contact sports or motor vehicle collisions. Atraumatic subluxation typically occurs with overhead elevation of the arm. These dislocations are more common in patients with hypermobility syndromes (e.g. Ehlers-Danlos syndrome).

Radiographs may be helpful, but CT scan is the imaging of choice. Recommended views for radiograph are anteroposterior (AP) and serendipity views (angled 40 degrees cephalic). There may also be a utility for ultrasound in diagnosis.

Keywords: orthopedics, blunt trauma, extremity injury, ultrasound, CT

Bibliography

Bae DS. Traumatic sternoclavicular joint injuries. *J Pediatr Orthop* 2010;30:S63–8.

Tepolt F, Carry PM, Heyn PC, Miller NH. Posterior sternoclavicular joint injuries in the adolescent population: A meta-analysis. *Am J Sports Med* 2014;42.10:2517–24.

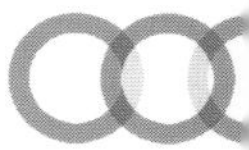

CASE 137

Timothy Ketterhagen

Questions

A 14-year-old boy presents to the emergency department with left leg pain. The patient was playing with his friends when he had a sudden onset of left leg pain after jumping from a ledge that was approximately 8 feet high. The patient noticed a deformity of his leg, just above his knee, and has not been able to ambulate since. The patient denies any head or neck trauma, and no loss of consciousness is reported. The patient denies any other injuries. The patient denies any numbness or tingling of his left lower extremity.

Physical exam reveals a healthy young main in a moderate amount of pain. The patient is minimally hypertensive and tachycardic, but vital signs are otherwise normal. Examination of the left lower extremity reveals swelling and deformity to the distal femur. The patient refuses to move his leg or ambulate due to pain. Severe pain is reported with any manipulation of the left lower extremity. There is also left knee swelling and tenderness with palpation of the superior and lateral aspect of the patella. There is no left tibial tenderness. Distal pulses are intact. Sensation is intact. Physical exam is otherwise unremarkable. The injury is shown next.

137.1

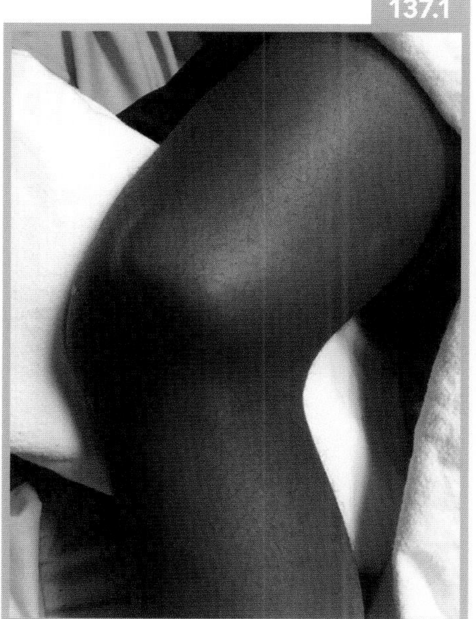

137.2

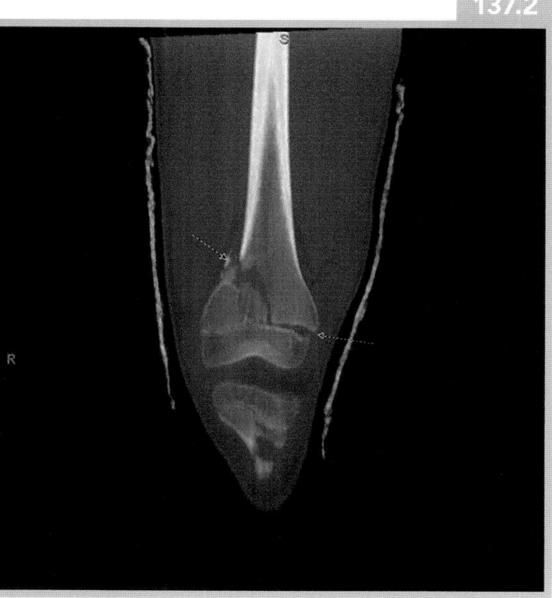

1. What are the different types of Salter-Harris fractures?
2. What is the Salter-Harris classification for this patient?

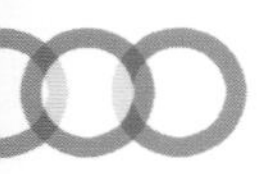

Answers

1. In children, fractures often occur at the physis. This is due to the fact that the growth plate is relatively weak when compared to the surrounding bone. The Salter-Harris classification is used to describe physeal fractures that may have prognostic and treatment implications.

   There are five types of Salter-Harris physeal fractures:

   Salter-Harris type I fracture—The fracture is through the physis. Separation of the metaphysis from the epiphysis.
   Salter-Harris type II fracture—The fracture is through the physis and the metaphysis. The epiphysis is spared.
   Salter-Harris type III fracture—The fracture is through the physis and the epiphysis. The metaphysis is spared.
   Salter-Harris type IV fracture—The fracture is through the epiphysis, physis, and the metaphysis.
   Salter-Harris type V fracture—The fracture is a compression fracture of the physis.

2. This patient has a Salter-Harris II femur fracture.

Keywords: orthopedics, extremity injury, blunt trauma, CT

Bibliography

Fleisher GR, Ludwig S, eds. *Textbook of Pediatric Emergency Medicine.* 6th ed. Philadelphia: Lippincott Williams & Wilkins, 2010.

Hoffman RJ, Wang VJ, Scarfone R. *Fleisher & Ludwig's 5-Minute Pediatric Emergency Medicine Consult.* Philadelphia: Wolters Kluwer Health/Lippincott Williams & Wilkins, 2012.

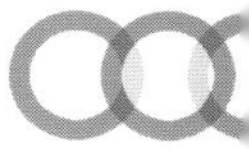

CASE 138

Veena Ramaiah

Question

A 7-year-old boy is brought in by his parents with concern for rectal bleeding. Both parents had gone to the store and left the child with relatives for about 4 hours. While they were away, a neighbor called the parents to say she called an ambulance after the child came to her apartment saying he was hurt. She saw blood on his shorts and underwear and thought there was bleeding from his rectum. He would not say how he got hurt. When questioned by the mother, the boy said he slipped and fell in the bathroom, but he would not give more details. He is otherwise healthy without any medical problems or surgical history. During a focused history, the mom states he is a developmentally normal child without any delays. His review of systems is negative for weight loss, fevers, chills, night sweats, rashes, or pallor.

On exam, he has moderate tachycardia but no tachypnea, fever, hypotension, hypertension, or hypoxia. He is quiet when left alone and lies on his side as a position of comfort. When asked to move around or lay on his back, he complains of pain in his rectal area. He has no pallor. His pulses are strong. His abdominal exam is positive for mild voluntary left lower quadrant (LLQ) guarding. All other quadrants are without pain, guarding, or rebound.

The physical exam is shown next.

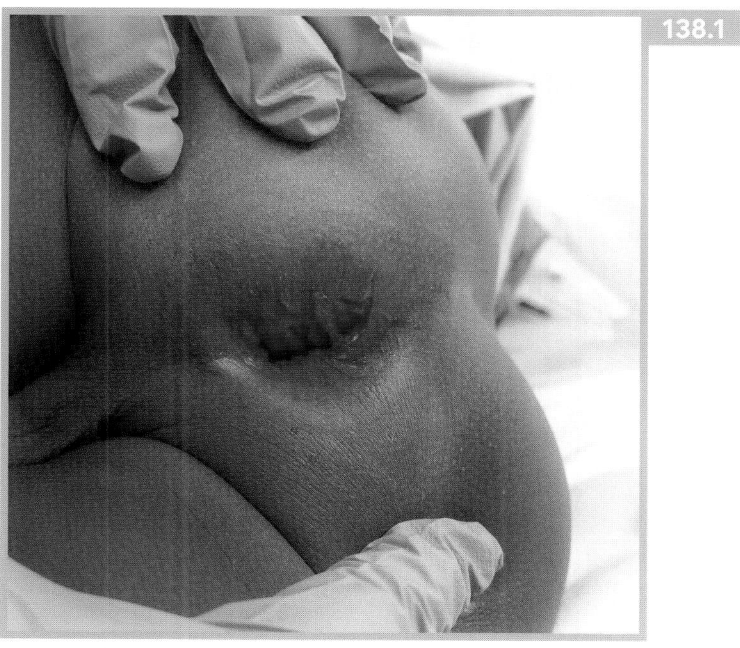
138.1

What is seen on exam? What is the first priority in his evaluation?

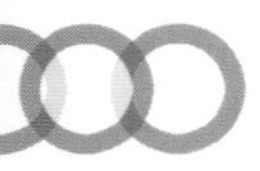

Answer

This patient has a rectal laceration. From the bedside exam, it is not clear how far it extends into the rectum. As with any trauma or medical evaluation, the first priority is the *ABCs*: attention to airway, breathing, and circulation.

In this patient, airway and breathing are stable. A rectal laceration raises concerns about circulation with concerns for hypovolemia, shock, peritonitis, and sepsis. Intravenous access is obtained and a normal saline bolus is infused. Laboratory studies are obtained to assess for anemia.

The physician and social worker asked the patient what had happened. He continued to repeat that he had fallen but without further details. Parents called the aunt who reported she went to the store leaving the patient in the care of his 19-year-old cousin. The cousin denied any trauma. Even without a disclosure, the injury met the criteria of a reasonable suspicion of abuse. The hospital staff made reports to police and child welfare services.

A surgical evaluation determined the need for operative intervention. A forensic evidence collection kit was sent to the operating room with the patient. Collection was obtained while the child was under anesthesia. Parents gave consent for evidence collection.

The rectal laceration was repaired and the patient was discharged home in 5 days. One week after the event, the patient underwent a forensic interview and gave a disclosure consistent with sexual assault by the cousin. He has had no contact with the cousin since the assault.

Discussion

Sexual assault is a highly traumatic and highly sensitive area of medicine. Child sexual abuse and assault rarely have physical evidence of trauma. The cases often rest on disclosures by children. An unusual traumatic injury with penetrating rectal trauma and lack of disclosure warrants investigation.

In this scenario, it was appropriate for the medical staff to ask the patient what happened. It is preferable to do this separate from caretakers, but only if the patient is willing to separate. Questions should always be non-leading and open-ended. This gives the opportunity for the patient to disclose if he or she wants to but does not introduce any suggestibility. Examples include "Can you tell me what happened? Can you tell me why you are here? Has anyone hurt you or made you uncomfortable?" These general questions are sufficient. One can then ask "Would you like to tell me more?" If there is a disclosure, the opportunity for disclosure to a trusted adult should be provided. The interview should be ended if the patient does not disclose anything with these general questions. Opportunities and resources for forensic interviews will vary in different regions.

The literature provides evidence that 90%–95% of exams in child sexual abuse/assault are normal, even when there is a history of penetrating trauma. Delayed disclosure is a common reason for this, which can be due to fear, shame, and lack of knowledge. An estimated up to 75% of perpetrators are known to the victim, contrary to popular belief, and 25%–50% of these are relatives.

In this scenario, it was also appropriate for medical staff to have a concern for sexual assault even without a disclosure. The majority of cases have no physical findings, although the presence of a finding is highly significant. Investigation is warranted if an accidental mechanism cannot be explained accurately, clearly, or reliably. The decision to collect forensic evidence is an

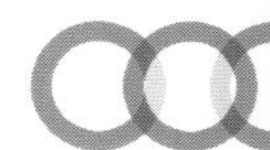

important consideration and is time-sensitive. The literature supports evidence collection out to 72 hours from an assault in pre-pubertal and pubertal children and out to 7 days in adolescents and adults.

Keywords: child abuse, abdominal pain

Bibliography

Adams JA, Kellogg ND, Farst KJ, Harper NS et al. Updated guidelines for the medical assessment and care of children who may have been sexually abused. *J Ped Adolesc Gynecol* 2016;29(2):81–7.

Fortin K, Jenny C. Sexual abuse. *Pediatr Rev* 2012;33(1):19–32.

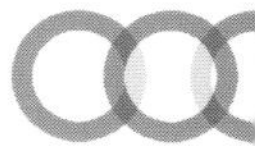

CASE 139

James Bistolarides

Questions

A father brings his 12-year-old boy to the emergency department after noticing a diffuse, pruritic rash that began on his trunk and has since spread "all over his body." The patient is generally comfortable with normal vital signs and otherwise the physical exam is unremarkable. The patient's father tells you that his son is otherwise healthy—except for an "infected lymph node" that his pediatrician has been treating with Bactrim (brand name for trimethoprim/sulfamethoxazole [TMP/SXT]) for the last week.

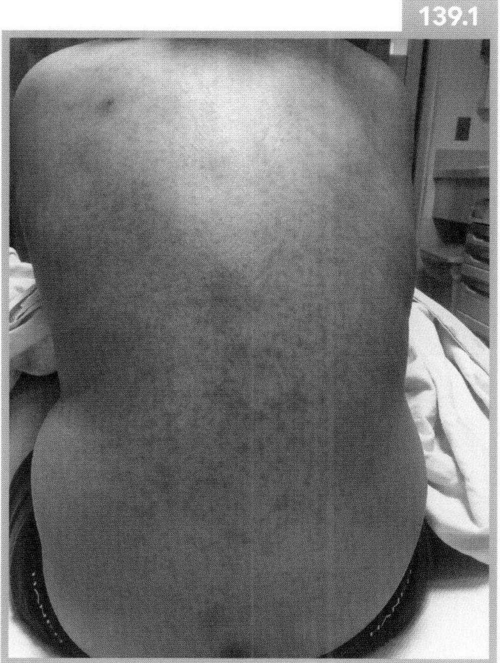

139.1

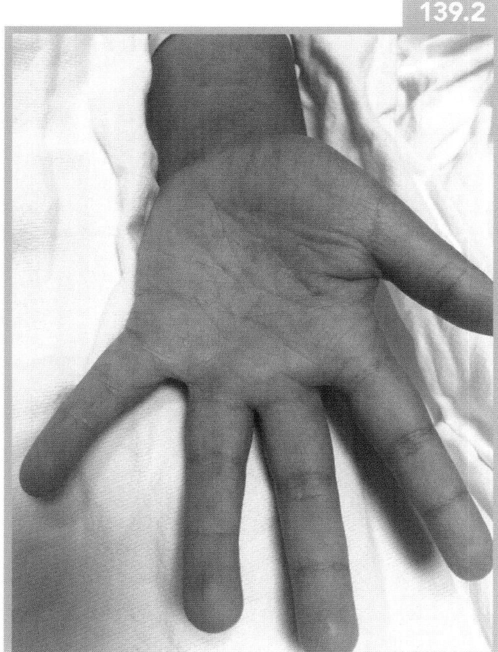

139.2

1. Describe the rash and provide a presumptive diagnosis.
2. What other aspects of the history and physical exam will help support your diagnosis and rule out others?
3. How would you treat and counsel this patient?

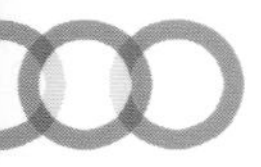

Answers

1. The rash can be best described as a combination of papules and macules, with occasional merging into patches or plaques. This presentation is most consistent with a drug eruption from exposure to TMP/SXT, also known as a morbilliform or exanthematous rash.

2. Medication history and timing is paramount to this diagnosis. The rash generally occurs within 5–14 days after exposure but can occur earlier if previously sensitized. On the other hand, a drug reaction with eosinophilia and systemic symptoms (DRESS) typically presents up to 2–6 weeks after exposure and is less likely to be due to TMP/SXT.

   The absence of viral symptoms, fever, or generalized lymphadenopathy makes an underlying viral exanthem less likely. Lack of severe or systemic symptoms (i.e. fever, mucosal involvement, edema, abdominal tenderness, arthralgia, skin blistering, or skin tenderness) help to reassure you that the rash is not a manifestation of DRESS, serum sickness, Stevens-Johnson syndrome (see Case 55 and Case 143), or toxic epidermal necrolysis.

3. A clinical diagnosis is appropriate in an otherwise well-appearing patient. This patient should be instructed to stop the offending agent, and should expect peeling and resolution of the rash within 7–14 days. You may prescribe topical corticosteroids, or simply recommend emollients and antihistamine for pruritus. If the patient has systemic symptoms or the diagnosis is unclear consider a laboratory workup.

Keywords: drug reactions, dermatology, mimickers

Bibliography

Farquharson NR, Coulson IH. Emergency dermatology: Drug eruptions. *Medicine* 2013;41(6):360–4.

Swanson L, Colven RM. Approach to the patient with a suspected cutaneous adverse drug reaction. *Med Clin North Am* 2015;99(6):1337–48.

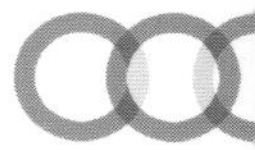

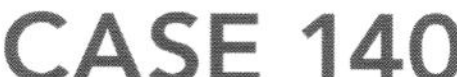

CASE 140

Veena Ramaiah

Questions

A 7-year-old male presents with a chief complaint of left hip pain and "walking funny," per the mother. Mom reports that he fell off his scooter last night and his left hip "twisted." He complained to her of left hip and anterior thigh pain. He was able to bear weight but is "walking funny" due to pain. The child says he had hip pain before the fall but cannot specify how long—maybe a few days prior. There is no prior history of trauma; however, he is a very active child. Of note, his pediatrician started him on cephalexin 5 days earlier for infected bug bites. These are improving. He had a tactile temperature yesterday.

Review of systems: No URI, weight loss, vomiting, abdominal pain, rash, or joint swelling.

He has no other medical problems, no allergies, and takes no medications except the cephalexin. His family history is non-contributory.

On exam, he is afebrile with normal vital signs. He is lying on his back with his leg flexed. There is mild pain if lying still. He has no pallor. Abdominal, back, and GU (genitourinary) exams are all normal. The neurologic exam is non-focal except his motor exam in his left leg is limited by pain. He is holding his left leg flexed 45 degrees and internally rotated. He has pain and decreased range of motion with extension and external rotation of his hip. He does not have pain with flexion, abduction, or internal rotation. There is no swelling or erythema anywhere on his left leg. His other extremities are normal except for some scabbed over pustules on his right knee. No signs of cellulitis or abscess.

1. What is in your differential diagnosis for a limp in a child this age?
2. How does the physical exam assist you?
3. What workup should be done?

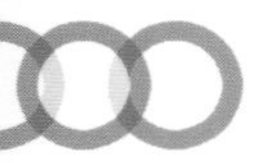

Answers

1. Trauma, infection, neoplasm, rheumatologic, neurologic, and congenital. Based on the history, trauma and infection are higher on your differential: fracture, SCFE (slipped capital femoral epiphysis), septic joint, osteomyelitis.
2. The position of comfort appears to be flexion with internal rotation. This is unusual for SCFE or septic joint. The absence of swelling and focal pain reduces the concern for a femur fracture. However, a femoral neck fracture can present without swelling. With femoral neck fractures, the hip is often held in external rotation and the leg may appear shortened. The position of comfort with flexion and internal rotation provides the clue that this may be a problem with the psoas muscle.
3. This patient underwent lab testing and x-rays. WBC 14.6, Hgb 12.5, Plt 423, ESR 50, CRP 8.6. Electrolytes were normal. Left hip and femur x-rays were normal. Left hip ultrasound showed normal hip joint space; however, there was a concern of possible fluid collection in the psoas muscle.

Abdominal CT showed the following.

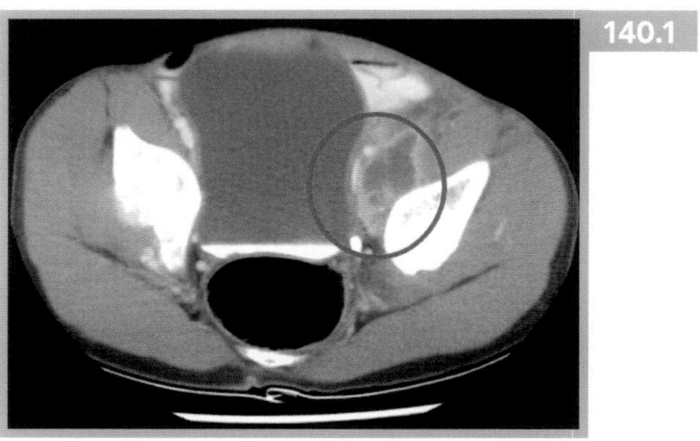

Diagnosis: Left Psoas Abscess

Psoas abscess is primarily seen in adults. Children often have no inciting event. The most common organism is *Staphylococcus aureus*. Other causes include gastrointestinal or urinary pathogens. Symptoms can be mild so diagnosis is often delayed. Median time to diagnosis has been reported as 22 days. The iliacus and psoas muscles are the main hip flexors and insert into the lesser trochanter.

Etiology is either primary or secondary. Primary is hematogenous or lymphatic seeding. Secondary abscess is due to direct spread from adjacent structures such as intra-abdominal infections, vertebral osteomyelitis, or retroperitoneal infections. Risk factors include diabetes, IV drug use, HIV, renal failure, immunosuppression, trauma, and hematoma formation. The most common disease associated with secondary abscess is Crohn's disease.

Clinical presentation can be mild and indolent with fever, lower abdominal/back/flank pain, or limp. There may be a flexion deformity of the hip and pain with extension of the leg or a positive psoas sign. This can also be seen with appendicitis. A mass may be palpable below the inguinal ligament if the abscess extends distally.

Treatment ranges from IV antibiotics alone to CT-guided drainage to surgical drainage.

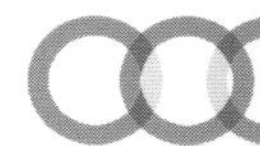

Keywords: orthopedics, limp, infectious diseases, CT

Bibliography

Shields D, Robinson P, Crowley TP. Iliopsoas abscess – A review and update on the literature. *Int J Surg* 2012;10(9):466–9.

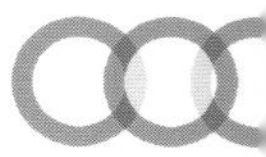

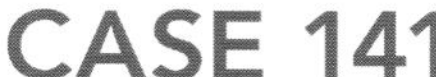

CASE 141

Michael Gottlieb

Questions

A 3-year-old girl presents to the emergency department with a rectal bulge. Her parents noticed a pink bulge in her rectal area when they were changing her diaper and brought her in for evaluation. The parents note that she has a history of frequent respiratory infections, but deny any known medical problems. The child was adopted and little is known about her medical history.

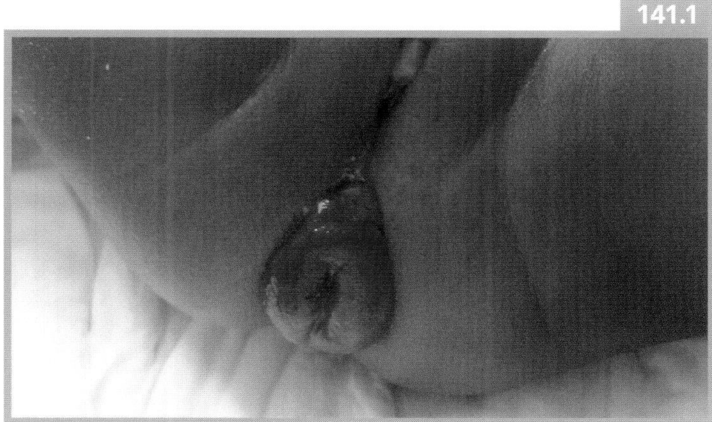

141.1

1. What is the medical problem demonstrated here?
2. What conditions are this associated with?

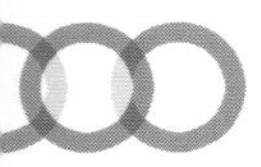

Answers

1. This patient is presenting with rectal prolapse. This is a condition where the layers of the rectal wall prolapse through the anal canal. It is important to reduce this to avoid mucosal breakdown. Reduction can be performed by applying gentle, steady pressure to the area until it re-enters the anal canal. This may be facilitated by applying granulated sugar to the area for 15 minutes to reduce the edema, allowing the prolapse to shrink in size. While adults frequently require surgery for this condition, children can often be managed conservatively by treating the underlying condition.

2. This occurs most commonly in children under the age of 4 and is associated with constipation, but may also be seen with cystic fibrosis. With increased screening for cystic fibrosis in newborns, this association is less commonly seen but can still be found in children who were born in countries without newborn screening.

Keywords: child abuse mimickers, procedures, mass

Bibliography

Cares K, El-Baba M. Rectal prolapse in children: Significance and management. *Curr Gastroenterol Rep* May 2016;18(5):22.

Fox A, Tietze PH, Ramakrishnan K. Anorectal conditions: Rectal prolapse. *FP Essent.* April 2014;419:28–34.

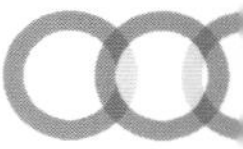

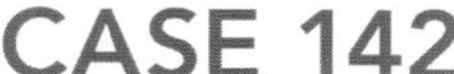

CASE 142

Emily Obringer

Questions

An 18-month-old boy presents with a 5-day history of progressive painful vesicular lesions over the tip of his finger. He is also noted to have an oral ulcer.

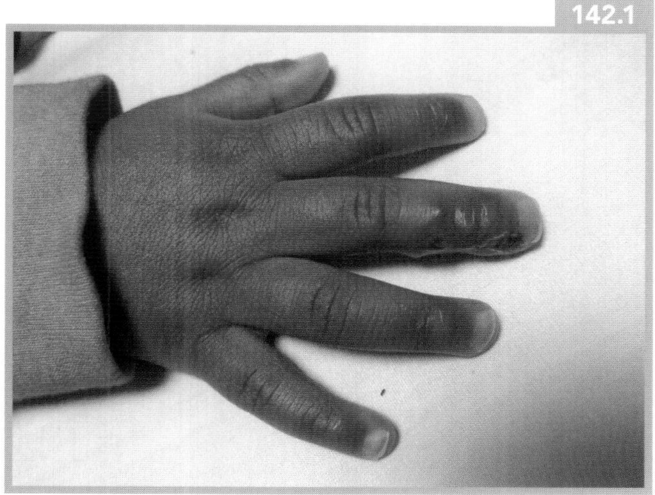

142.1

1. What is the etiology of this infection?
2. What is the primary treatment for this disease process?

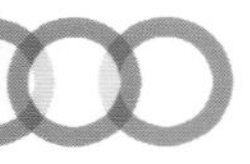

Answers

1. This patient has herpetic whitlow, a type of herpes simplex virus (HSV) infection that typically affects the thumb or fingers. The primary route of exposure is direct inoculation of the digits from herpes lesions or infected oral secretions (American Academy of Pediatrics, 2015). Thumb-sucking in toddlers with primary oral herpes infection may lead to autoinoculation. Medical and dental professionals may acquire infection through exposure to infected oral secretions when proper contact precautions (e.g. gloves) are not used. Most infections in children are caused by HSV-1, whereas persons in their 20s and 30s may be infected by HSV-2 through exposure to genital lesions (Szinnai et al., 2001).

2. Herpetic whitlow is a self-limited infection. Severe cases or those in immunocompromised hosts may be treated with oral or intravenous acyclovir. Incision and drainage are not recommended as this may cause the infection to spread.

Keywords: infectious diseases, skin and soft tissue infection, child abuse mimicker

References

American Academy of Pediatrics. Herpes simplex. In *Red Book: 2015 Report of the Committee on Infectious Diseases*, Kimberlin DW, Brady MT, Jackson MA, Long SS, eds. Elk Grove Village, IL: American Academy of Pediatrics, 2015:432–45.

Szinnai G, Schaad UB, Heininger U. Multiple herpetic whitlow lesions in a 4-year-old girl: Case report and review of the literature. *Eur J Pediatr* 2001;160(9):528–33.

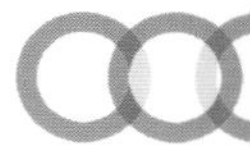

CASE 143

Diana Yan

Question

A 10-year-old male presents to the emergency room because of painful oral lesions. He has been complaining of myalgias, decreased energy, and upper respiratory symptoms for the last 3 days. The mouth lesions appeared this morning. The lesions have worsened throughout the day. He also has been having fevers for the last 2 days to a maximum of 101°F. He had normal oral intake until today due to pain but does have normal urine output. He has not had any diarrhea or vomiting. There are no other rashes on his body. No one else at school or home has a similar rash. There are no new contacts or exposures. He is otherwise healthy, but his mom does mention that he was treated with trimethoprim/sulfamethoxazole for a UTI 2 months ago.

Physical exam shows an alert and awake boy who is sitting on the pain in mild discomfort. He has no conjunctival injection and his tympanic membranes are normal. He has nasal congestion and is coughing on exam. He has multiple lesions on the lips and anterior oral cavity. There are perioral blisters and unroofed erythematous macules. There are multiple erythematous ulcers inside his mouth. One of the blisters sloughs off easily from pressure using a finger (+Nikolsky sign). He has slightly dry mucous membranes. No other rash is present on his skin. His lung, cardiovascular, and abdominal exams are within normal limits.

143.1

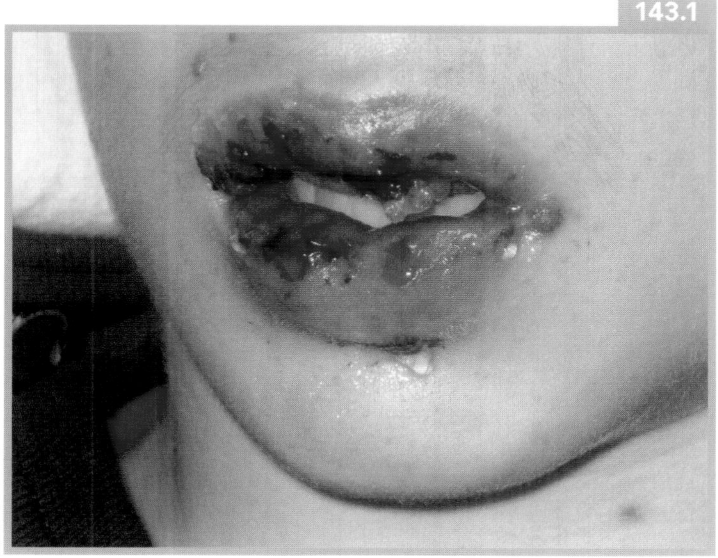

What is the diagnosis and what is the treatment?

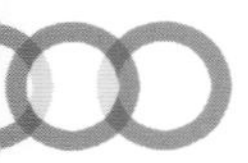

Answer

Stevens-Johnson syndrome (SJS). SJS and toxic epidermal necrolysis (TEN) are both severe mucocutaneous rashes associated with high mortality rates. They are differentiated by the amount of skin involved: SJS involves <10% of body surface area (BSA), whereas TEN involves >30% BSA with an overlap between the two processes from 10% to 30% BSA. The exact pathophysiology behind SJS and TEN is unknown, but it is thought that a drug, such as sulfa antibiotics, NSAIDs, or phenobarbital, or an infection, such as mycoplasma or herpes, causes a cell-mediated reaction against the keratinocytes of the skin, which causes detachment between the dermis and epidermis of the skin. Treatment includes discontinuing offending medications or treating the infection, aggressive supportive care with intravenous fluids, wound care, and pain medications, and possible transfer to a burn center. The larger the wound area, the more likely there will be fluid and protein loss with its associated electrolyte imbalances and potential progression to hypovolemic shock with organ dysfunction/failure. These patients can also easily become hypothermic and have superinfected wounds. *Staphylococcus aureus* and *Pseudomonas aeruginosa* are common bacteria that can infect these wounds and cause sepsis, the main cause of death in these patients. Sterile dressings and good wound care are essential. However, prophylactic antibiotics are not recommended. Other systems can also be affected such as the eyes (e.g. pain, photophobia, long-term vision loss), lungs (e.g. pneumonia, interstitial pneumonitis), and gastrointestinal (GI) tract (e.g. diarrhea, small bowel intussusception, stenosis). Subspecialty involvement is important depending on the systems involved. Recently, there have also been some small studies testing the efficacy of intravenous immunoglobulin (IVIG) and steroids. Results have been mixed, especially in children.

Keywords: drug reactions, dermatology, do not miss, fever

Bibliography

Alerhand S, Cassella C, Koyfman A. Stevens-Johnson syndrome and toxic epidermal necrolysis in the pediatric population a review. *Pediatr Emerg Care* 2016;32(7):472–8.

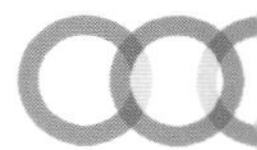

CASE 144

Michael Gottlieb

Questions

A 2-year-old boy presents with right foot pain. His mother thinks he may have stepped on a splinter in their new house. He has a small cut on the bottom of his foot with surrounding erythema and significant pain on palpation. A foot x-ray is obtained, which is unremarkable. An ultrasound is performed as demonstrated next.

144.1

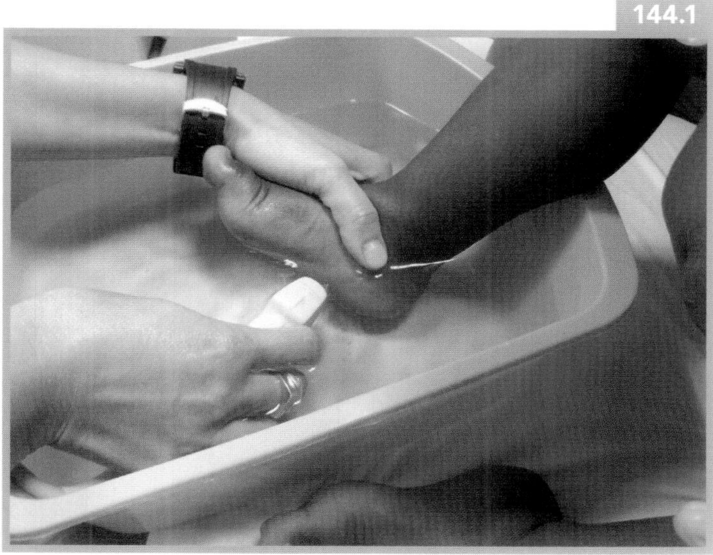

1. What is the value in ultrasound for identifying foreign bodies?
2. Why is a water bath utilized for this evaluation?

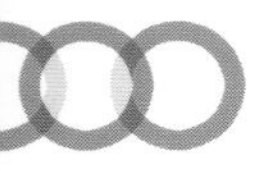

Answers

1. Ultrasound is both sensitive and specific for the identification of foreign bodies in soft tissue. While radiographs may identify larger, radiopaque foreign bodies, smaller objects and those that are radiolucent (e.g. wood [see Case 106], certain types of glass) can be missed by x-ray. Ultrasound can also be utilized for real-time guidance during foreign body removal.

2. The water bath allows the sonographer to visualize the superficial soft tissue without requiring direct contact with the area. Since the involved area is often painful for the patient, this allows one to perform the exam without applying additional pressure to the painful area. Additionally, ultrasound beams have poor image resolution in the very near field. The water bath allows for the image to be obtained at the point of the best image resolution, also referred to as the focal point.

Keywords: ultrasound, foreign body, skin and soft tissue infection, procedures

Bibliography

Chen KC, Lin AC, Chong CF, Wang TL. An overview of point-of-care ultrasound for soft tissue and musculoskeletal applications in the emergency department. *J Intensive Care* August 15, 2016;4:55.

Davis J, Czerniski B, Au A, Adhikari S, Farrell I, Fields JM. Diagnostic accuracy of ultrasonography in retained soft tissue foreign bodies: A systematic review and meta-analysis. *Acad Emerg Med.* July 2015;22(7):777–87.

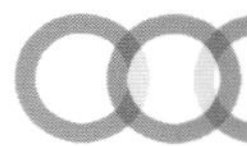

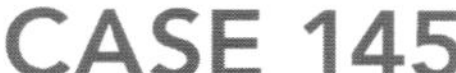

CASE 145

Michael Gottlieb

Questions

A 16-year-old girl presents to the emergency department with throat pain for the past 4 days. She reports worsening pain and difficulty swallowing. She also notes that her voice has sounded more muffled over the past day. She is afebrile with normal vital signs. Her throat exam is significant for swelling and uvular deviation to the right.

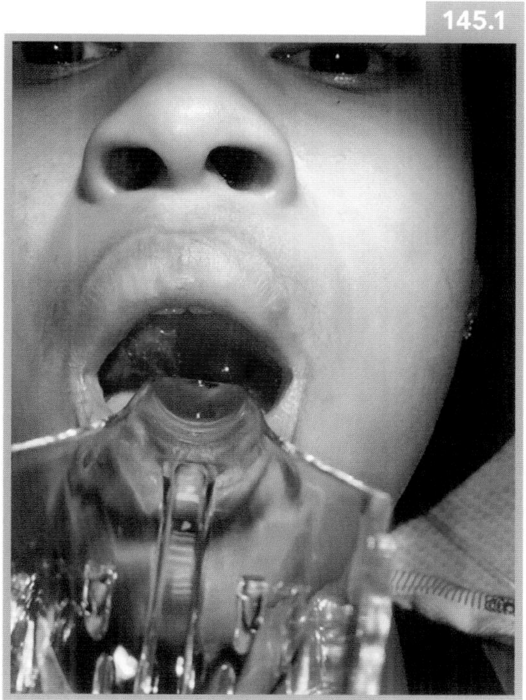

145.1

1. What is the diagnosis in this patient?
2. What is the treatment of this condition?

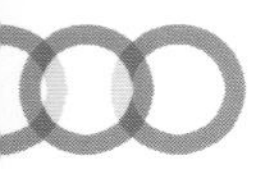

Answers

1. This patient is presenting with a peritonsillar abscess. This classically presents with unilateral peritonsillar swelling and deviation of the uvula away from the abscess. This can be differentiated from tonsillitis, which is not associated with swelling, and retropharyngeal abscess (see Case 174), which presents with neck pain and stiffness, as well as swelling in the posterior oropharynx.

2. The treatment of choice for peritonsillar abscesses is drainage. This may be performed either with a needle or scalpel based upon provider preference. Ultrasound may assist with identifying and performing real-time needle drainage. Steroids are commonly given to reduce inflammation along with empiric antibiotics covering oral flora.

Keywords: infectious diseases, head and neck/ENT, airway, procedures

Bibliography

Powell J, Wilson JA. An evidence-based review of peritonsillar abscess. *Clin Otolaryngol* April 2012;37(2):136–45.

Secko M, Sivitz A. Think ultrasound first for peritonsillar swelling. *Am J Emerg Med* April 2015;33(4):569–72.

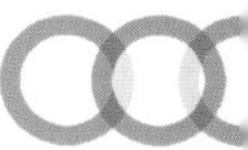

CASE 146

Michael Gottlieb

Questions

An 11-year-old girl presents to the emergency department with right arm pain after falling off her bike. She has pain and swelling to her arm with the skin deformity shown in the following. A radiograph is also obtained.

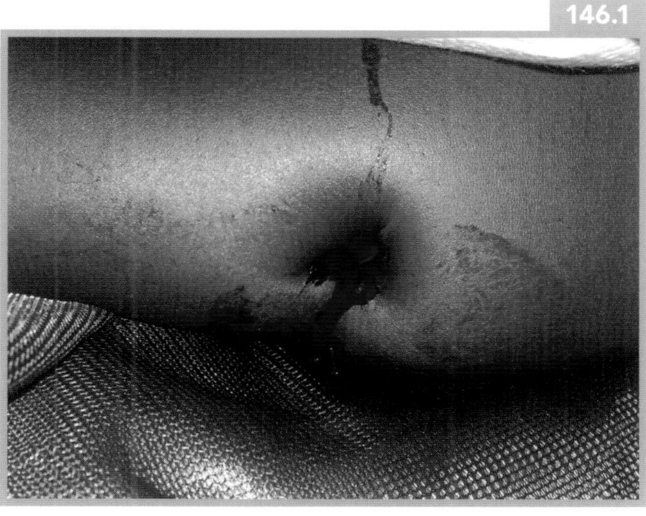

146.1

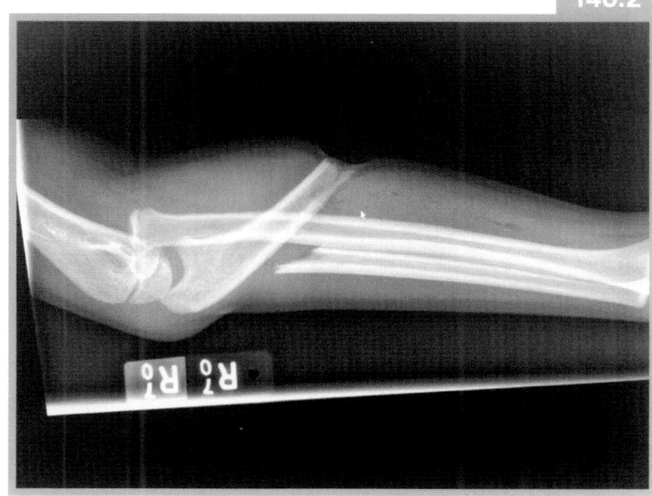

146.2

1. What type of fracture is demonstrated on the radiograph?
2. How does the open wound in the arm change the management of this patient?

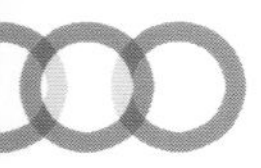

Answers

1. The radiograph demonstrates a Monteggia fracture, which is a combination of an ulnar fracture and radial head dislocation (see also Case 76). This is often confused with a Galeazzi fracture, which is a radial fracture with associated ulnar dislocation. Both fracture–dislocations may be treated conservatively with good outcomes but require reduction in the emergency department to reduce the risk of complications.
2. Whereas most fractures may be treated with closed reduction, an open fracture (i.e. a fracture with exposed bone) requires extensive irrigation, operative reduction, and empiric antibiotics to prevent infection. Orthopedic surgery should always be involved in the care of open fractures of long bones.

Keywords: orthopedics, penetrating trauma, extremity injury, pitfalls

Bibliography

Perron AD, Hersh RD, Brady WJ, Keats TE. Orthopedic pitfalls in the ED: Galeazzi and Monteggia fracture-dislocation. *Am J Emerg Med* May 2001;19(3):225–8.

Ring D. Monteggia fractures. *Orthop Clin North Am* January 2013;44(1):59–66.

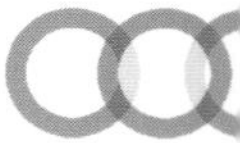

CASE 147

Leah Finkel

Question

An 18-month-old boy is brought in by his mom for increasing abdominal girth for the past month. There has been no emesis or diarrhea. The boy felt warm the day prior. He has been having normal intake with a normal number of wet and soiled diapers. On exam he is well-appearing but has a significant abdominal distension. A large abdominal mass is palpated. He does not appear jaundiced and appears well-hydrated.

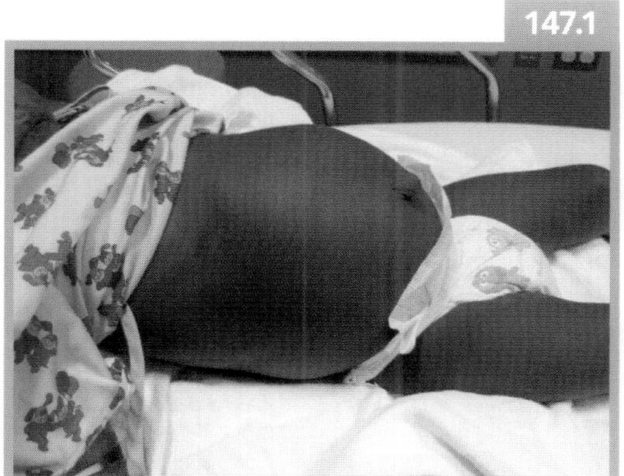
147.1

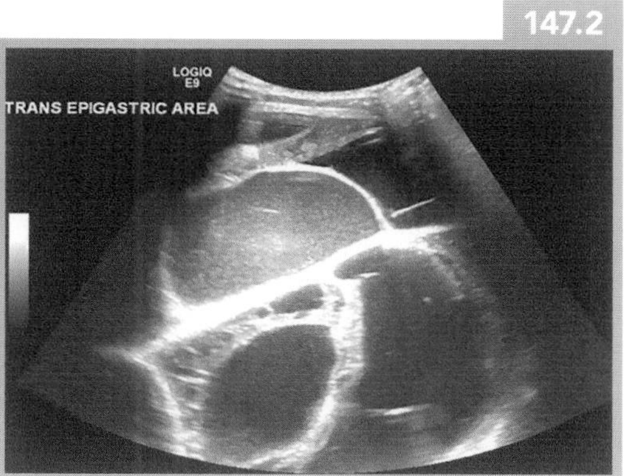

147.2

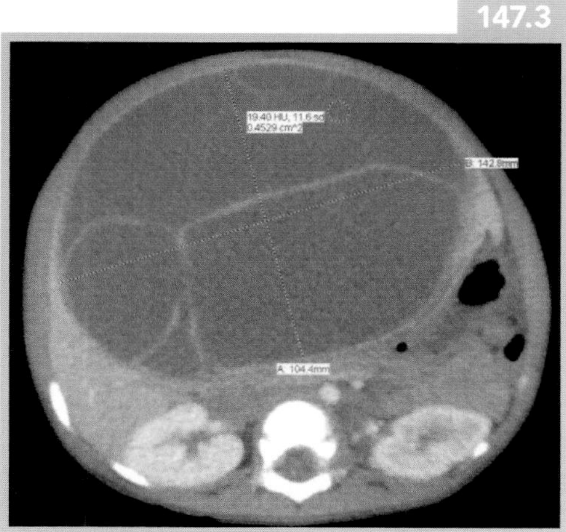

147.3

What imaging might be helpful to assess this abdominal mass? What does this patient have and what is seen on ultrasonography (US) and CT scans of this patient?

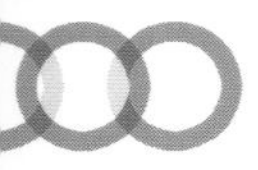

Answer

Both US and CT are helpful for confirming or excluding a "palpable" abdominal mass, with high sensitivity and specificity and can often identify the organ from which the mass is originating. US is frequently used as an initial diagnostic study in children (lower radiation and the smaller body habitus). Abdominal CT is the most sensitive imaging modality for detailed evaluation of solid organ pathology in the abdomen and may be helpful particularly when ultrasound imaging is inconclusive. The role of MRI in a palpable abdominal mass is unclear though it may be used to evaluate complex lesions not well characterized by US or CT. Plain radiographs have little utility in assessing a palpable mass.

This patient has a mesenchymal hamartoma, which is a rare, usually benign tumor of the liver that has occasional risk of malignancy. The patient is often asymptomatic but has rapid distension of the abdomen with a palpable mass. The US scan shows multiloculated fluid collections throughout the abdomen. The CT scan shows a large multiloculated cystic intra-abdominal mass with enhancing septa and mild splenomegaly.

Keywords: abdominal pain, mass, ultrasound, MRI, CT

Bibliography

American College of Radiology. ACR appropriateness criteria: Palpable abdominal mass. Available at https://acsearch.acr.org/docs/69473/Narrative/. Accessed May 25, 2017.

Gupta R, Parelkar S, Sanghvi B. Mesenchymal hamartoma of the liver. *Indian J Med Paediatr Oncol* October–December 2009;30(4):141–3.

Saeed O, Saxena R. Primary mesenchymal liver tumors of childhood. *Semin Diagn Pathol* March 2017;34(2):201–7.

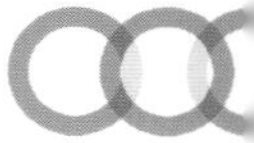

CASE 148

Timothy Ketterhagen

Question

A mother presents to the emergency department with her 14-month-old son because of bruising. The mother states that for the past several days she has noticed an increasing amount of bruising on her son. Initially the bruising was limited to the shins, but it has spread to the arms and face. The patient may have bumped his head a few times, but the mother denies any other traumatic events. The patient has otherwise been acting normally. No neurologic changes. No vomiting, diarrhea, weight loss, joint pain, or fever. The patient did have a URI a couple weeks ago, but symptoms have since resolved. The patient has not had any similar bruising in the past. No family history of any bleeding disorders. The patient is not on any medications. No recent immunizations.

Physical exam reveals a developmentally normal boy who is in no distress. Petechiae and various stages of ecchymosis are noted on the forehead, scalp, arms, and bilateral lower extremities. The skin is otherwise warm and well-perfused with no pallor or jaundice. There is no bleeding from the mouth or nose. Cardiac and pulmonary exams are unremarkable. Hepatosplenomegaly is not present. The patient is awake and alert, and there are no neurologic abnormalities. The physical exam is otherwise unremarkable.

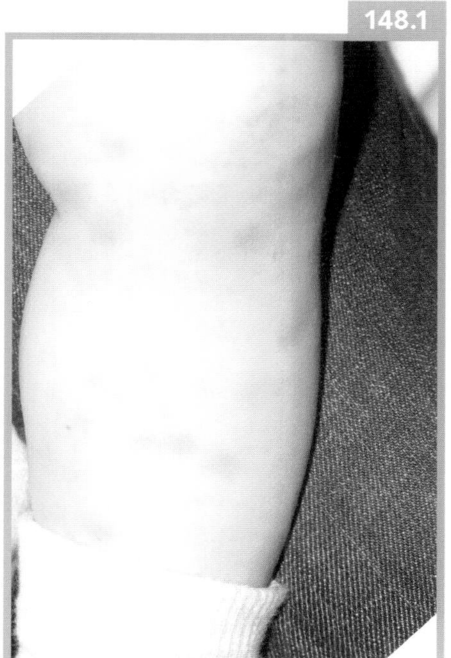

148.1

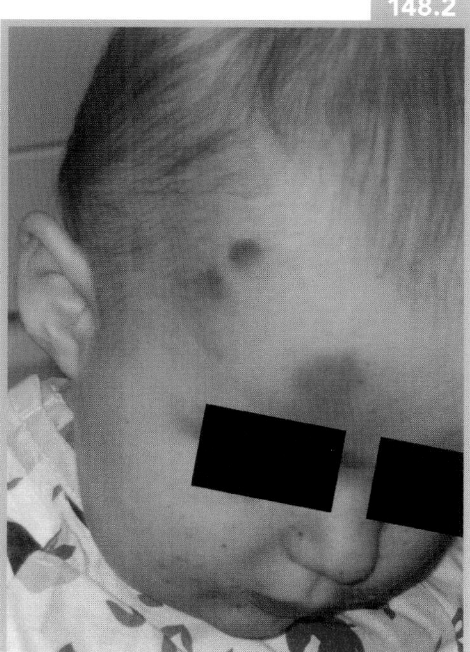

148.2

What is the diagnosis, cause, and treatment of this disorder?

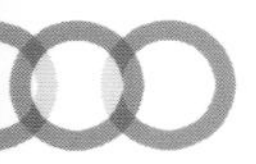

Answer

This patient has immune thrombocytopenic purpura (ITP). ITP is characterized by an isolated platelet count of less than 150 × 10^9/L, purpuric rash, and normal bone marrow (other cell lines are normal). This disorder is caused by the production of autoantibodies against platelet antigens. Platelet survival is significantly reduced. The initial presentation is typically an otherwise well child with acute onset of petechiae, purpura, and/or bruising. Mucosal bleeding may also be present. The majority of cases are preceded by a viral illness. ITP has also been found to follow administration of the MMR (measles-mumps-rubella) vaccine. Intracranial hemorrhage is a serious risk and should be considered when persistent headaches, neurologic changes, or platelet count $<20 \times 10^9$/L are present.

Constitutional symptoms, such as fever, weight loss, and fatigue, are rare in ITP. Family history is generally negative for bleeding disorders. Careful evaluation is required in order to rule out other causes of thrombocytopenia including medications, congenital platelet disorders, malignancy, and other inherited and acquired platelet disorders.

A CBC (complete blood count) is all that is required for diagnosis, but PT (prothrombin time), PTT (partial thromboplastin time), and type and screen are reasonable to obtain. Consultation with a hematologist is recommended in order to rule out other causes of thrombocytopenia. Treatment includes initial stabilization, IVIG (intravenous immunoglobulin), and corticosteroids. Hematology should be consulted prior to corticosteroid administration to help rule out leukemia. Anti-Rh (D) may also be used. Platelet transfusions alone are not useful due to the ongoing autoimmune platelet destruction. Most patients have a benign course and 60% of patients will have a normal platelet count within 3 months.

Keywords: hematology, dermatology, child abuse mimicker, do not miss

Bibliography

Hoffman RJ, Wang VJ, Scarfone R. *Fleisher & Ludwig's 5-Minute Pediatric Emergency Medicine Consult.* Philadelphia: Wolters Kluwer Health/Lippincott Williams & Wilkins, 2012.

McAninch S, Letbetter SA. Renal & genitourinary emergencies. In *Current Diagnosis & Treatment: Pediatric Emergency Medicine*, Stone CK, Humphries RL, Drigalla D, Stephan M, eds. New York: McGraw-Hill, 2015:chap. 38.

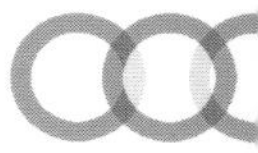

CASE 149

Diana Yan

Question

A 13-year-old female presents to the emergency room because of a painful bulge on her lower back. She has been complaining of pain in the sacral area for the last 3–4 days especially with sitting. The bulge has been there for 6 months but has not caused any issues. She has also been having a fever for the last 2 days with a maximum temperature of 101.3°F. There is no active drainage, no overlying redness, or changes in bowel pattern or urinary frequency. There is no pus or blood in urine or stool. She has had a normal appetite and oral intake. No history of trauma. She is otherwise healthy.

Physical exam shows an alert and awake teenage girl with a 3 cm × 3 cm lesion in the mid lower back that is fluctuant and indurated. There is no overlying redness or active drainage, but there is a small pit at the center of the mass. It is tender to palpation. There is a normal external and digital rectal exam. Her abdominal exam is normal. There are no other abscesses on exam.

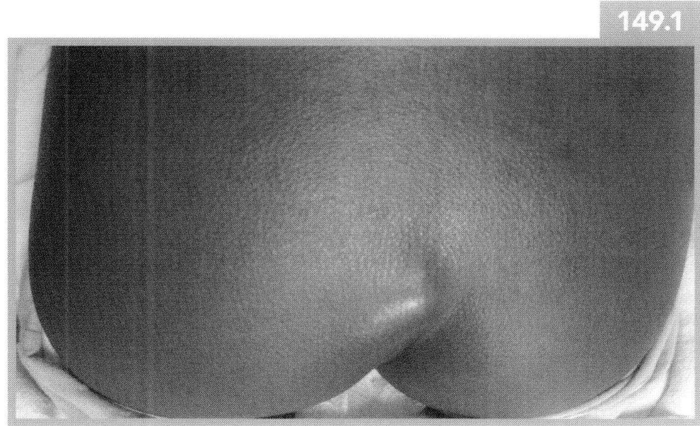

149.1

What is the mainstay of treatment for an infected pilonidal cyst abscess?

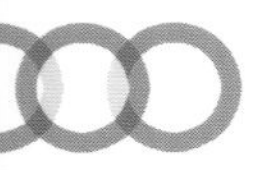

Answer

Surgery. Pilonidal cysts are caused by an inflammatory process in the gluteal region. They are most common in 15- to 20-year-old males with a deep natal or intergluteal cleft. Other risk factors include obesity, sedentary occupation (>6 hours a day sitting down), poor hygiene with <3 baths per week, and extensive body hair. These clefts can get infected due to trapping of perspiration and moisture in the deep pockets. An infected pilonidal cyst needs to be treated. They can cause systemic symptoms such as fever, chills, and pain. A sinus tract can also develop, and when present there can be intermittent discharge of pus or blood. Chronic pilonidal cysts can have multiple sinus tracts. During workup, physicians need to consider possible anal fistula development and perianal Crohn's disease. Management of these cysts involves antibiotics, pain control, surgery, and wound care. Antimicrobials should cover gram positive, gram negative, and anaerobic bacteria due to skin flora and close proximity to the anus. Hygiene is also very important in the treatment of these cysts. Baths need to be avoided while the wound heals and the use of handheld showerheads is recommended to be able to direct water to the site. Wounds must be cleaned after stooling and hair needs to be removed from wounds. Patients also need to be careful to avoid activities with excessive friction to the buttock such as cycling and driving/sitting for long periods.

Keywords: infectious diseases, mass, surgery, skin and soft tissue infection, congenital anomaly

Bibliography

Harris C, Sibbald RG, Mufti A, Somayaji R. Pilonidal sinus disease: 10 steps to optimize care. *Adv Skin Wound Care* 2016;29(10):469–78.

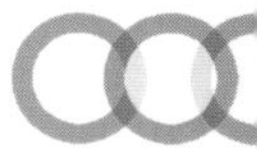

CASE 150

Diana Yan

Question

A 3-year-old female with a complex medical history presents to the emergency room because of a white object that her mom noticed in her vagina while changing her today. Mom states that there has not been any change in her urine or stool, and there is no blood. Mom believes that there may have been clear drainage from the object at one point but she is not sure. Mom states that she does not believe that the patient would or could put anything there. The patient has not had any fevers, increased fussiness, vomiting, or upper respiratory symptoms. She has been tolerating her G-tube feeds well and there is no change in her baseline mental status. The patient does have a past medical history of being born at 24-weeks gestational age, cerebral palsy, tracheostomy, G-tube–dependent feeds, and hydrocephalus status post ventriculoperitoneal (VP) shunt placement. The shunt has never been revised.

Physical exam shows a girl sitting up in her wheelchair, who, with tracheostomy in place, can breathe room air without a ventilator. She is at her baseline mental status: non-verbal but will grab at things occasionally. Her neurological, pulmonary, cardiovascular, and abdominal exams are at baseline. Her VP shunt is palpated along her scalp, along her neck, and her anterior chest wall. Her tracheostomy site and G-tube site are clean, dry, and intact. On genitourinary (GU) exam, she is Tanner I and a white tube is seen at the entrance of her vagina. It is immobile when you attempt to extract it gently. There is no active discharge. Her CT head shows stable hydrocephalus with VP shunt in place within the ventricle.

150.1

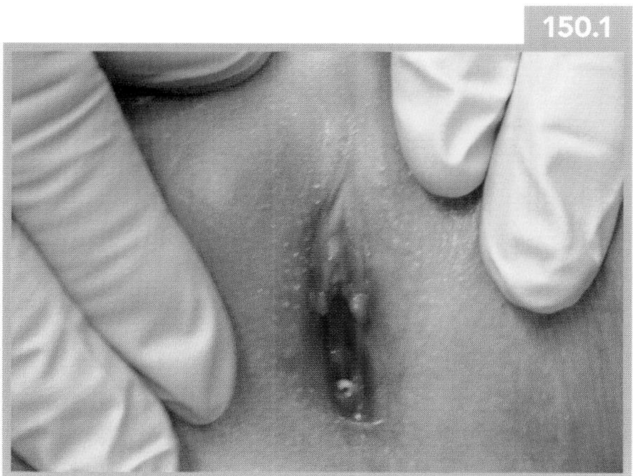

150.2

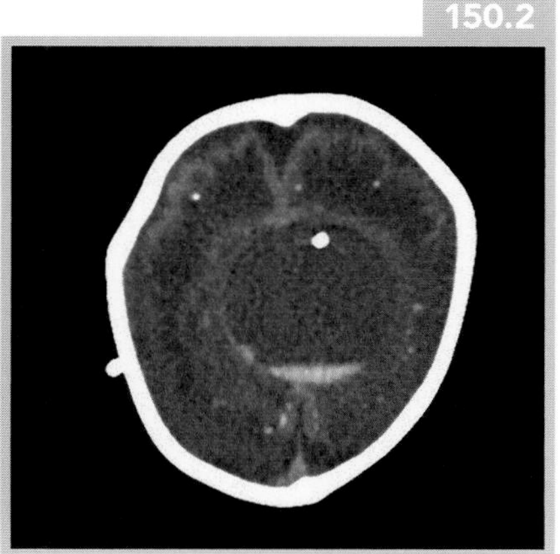

What are major complications of VP shunt erosion through the vagina?

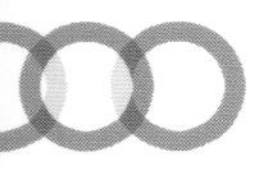

Answer

Worsening hydrocephalus and infection. The white tube in the picture is the patient's VP shunt. The risk of uterine erosion by the VP shunt is very rare. There are only four case reports of VP shunts perforating through the vagina in English literature. Other places that a VP shunt have migrated to are lateral ventricle, gastrointestinal tract, abdominal wall, bladder, and scrotum. The vagina, bladder, and scrotum are rarer, as that they are retroperitoneal organs. Most shunt malfunctions are due to mechanical obstruction and infection, and not migration or perforation of other visceral organs. Labs such as a CBC (complete blood count) with differential, C-reactive protein, and CSF (cerebrospinal fluid) studies (from tapping the VP shunt), and imaging such as a shunt series and CT are also important to the evaluation. Prophylactic antibiotics are started to prevent meningitis, as patients can also present with gram negative intracranial infections from ascending infection. Risk factors for vaginal erosion are thought to be weak vaginal muscles (such as in myelomeningocele), local inflammation from the hard VP plastic tubing, and a local allergic reaction to silicone that may lead to adherence of the shunt tubing to the Douglas pouch.

Keywords: neurosurgery, infectious diseases, gynecology, penetrating trauma, altered mental status, CT

Bibliography

Altas M, Tutanc M, Aras M, Altas ZG, Ariva V. Vaginal perforation caused by distal tip of ventriculoperitoneal shunt: Report of a rare complication. *Pak J Med Sci* 2012;28(3):550–1.

Pohlman GD, Wilcox DT, Hankinson TC. Erosive bladder perforation as a complication of ventriculoperitoneal shunt with extrusion from the urethral meatus: Case report and literature review. *Pediatr Neurosurg* 2011;47:223–6.

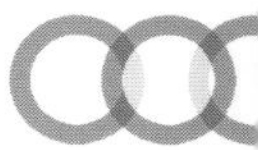

CASE 151

James Bistolarides

Questions

A 15-month-old male is brought to the emergency department by his mother for a "cold that just won't go away." When you ask her to elaborate she describes that her son has been having "belly pain and a poor appetite for the last few weeks." She decided to bring him in today since he's become progressively more "tired, sleepy, and is now making fewer wet diapers."

151.1

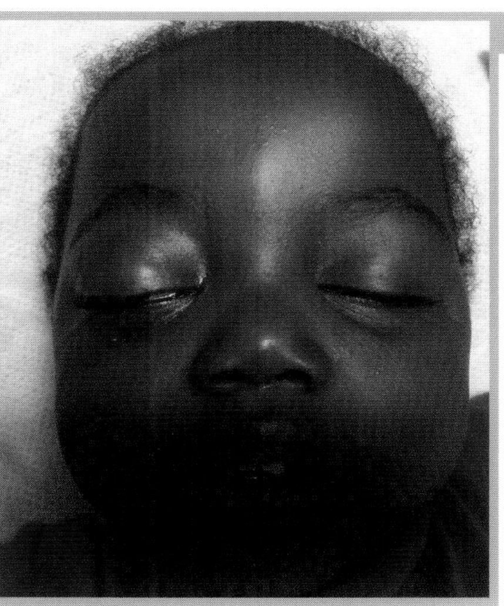

151.2

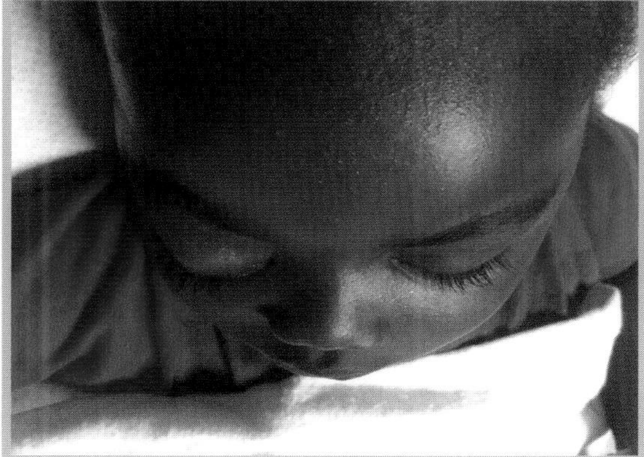

151.3

1. What do you notice on your initial visual inspection from the above images?
2. What is your initial assessment, and what would you do next?

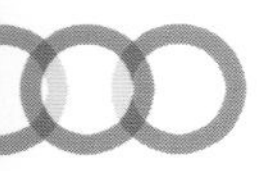

Answers

1. The patient has unilateral swelling and protrusion of the right eyelid while the eye is closed, along with right-sided periorbital ecchymosis. When the right eyelid is raised the patient has a clear anterior bulging—or proptosis—of the right eye.

2. This patient's history and physical exam have raised multiple red flags for neuroblastoma. Neuroblastoma presents at a median age of 18 months old, and is more common in both males and in African Americans. It rarely presents with ocular manifestations alone; typically it will manifest as a slow enlarging abdominal mass (see Case 135) with accompanying distension, fatigue, lethargy, fever, or dehydration. However, orbital metastatic neuroblastoma is considered one of the classic signs of neuroblastoma in children.

   Any child with proptosis and periorbital ecchymosis, Horner syndrome, or opsoclonus-myoclonus should undergo a thorough evaluation for neuroblastoma. Along with basic laboratory testing and rehydration this patient should have early consultation of a pediatric oncologist. Neuroblastoma is derived from primitive neuroectodermal cells; therefore it can arise wherever sympathetic nervous tissue is found. This child will need widespread imaging with either CT or MRI, and measurement of urine HMV (homovanillic acid) and VMA (vanillylmandelic acid).

Keywords: ophthalmology, oncology, do not miss

Bibliography

Alvi S, Karadaghy O, Manalang M, Weatherly R. Clinical manifestations of neuroblastoma with head and neck involvement in children. *Int J Pediatr Otolaryngol* 2017;97:157–62.

Musarella MA, Chan HS, DeBoer G, Gallie BL. Ocular involvement in neuroblastoma: Prognostic implications. *Ophthalmology* 1984;91(8):936–40.

Smith SJ, Diehl NN, Smith BD, Mohney BG. Incidence, ocular manifestations, and survival in children with neuroblastoma: A population-based study. *Am J Ophthalmol* 2010;149(4):677–82.

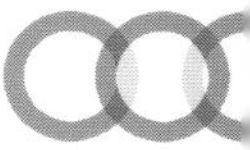

CASE 152

Michael Gottlieb

Questions

A 6-year-old boy presents with right thumb pain for 3 days. He denies any trauma and has no numbness or weakness. The swelling is most pronounced near the medial aspect of the nail bed. Both hands are shown next.

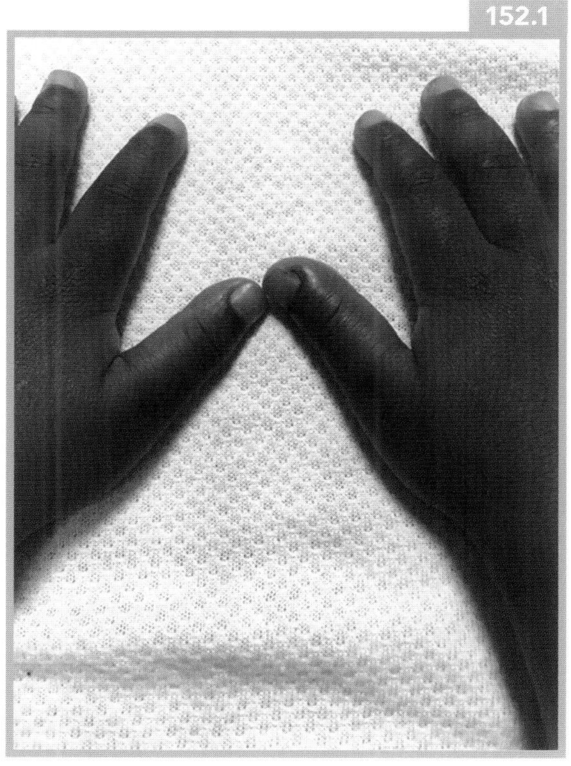

152.1

1. What is the diagnosis in this patient?
2. What is the treatment for this condition?

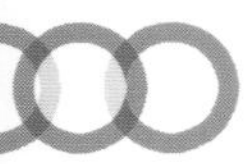

Answers

1. This patient has a paronychia. These are infections of the dorsal fingertip that track around and deep into the nail bed. Common causes include nail biting, hangnails, and artificial nails. Patients present with swelling and fluctuance surrounding the nail bed. If significant swelling is noted to the pulp of the finger, felon should also be suspected, as paronychia can be a precursor to the development of felons (see Case 153).
2. Early cases may be treated conservatively with antibiotics and warm soaks. However, when significant swelling is noted, incision and drainage is typically required. This involves sliding a #11 blade scalpel along the nail to elevate the eponychial fold, allowing for drainage of the abscess. Patients and parents should be provided information regarding the causes to avoid recurrences.

Keywords: skin and soft tissue infection, procedures

Bibliography

Franko OI, Abrams RA. Hand infections. *Orthop Clin North Am* October 2013;44(4):625–34.
Moran GJ, Talan DA. Hand infections. *Emerg Med Clin North Am* August 1993;11(3):601–19.

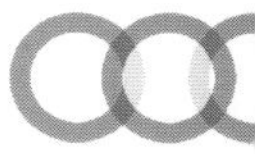

CASE 153

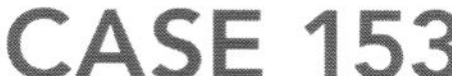

Michael Gottlieb

Questions

A 9-year-old girl presents with left index finger pain and swelling for 4 days. She had no trauma and denies numbness or weakness. On examination, her finger is tender, swollen, and erythematous.

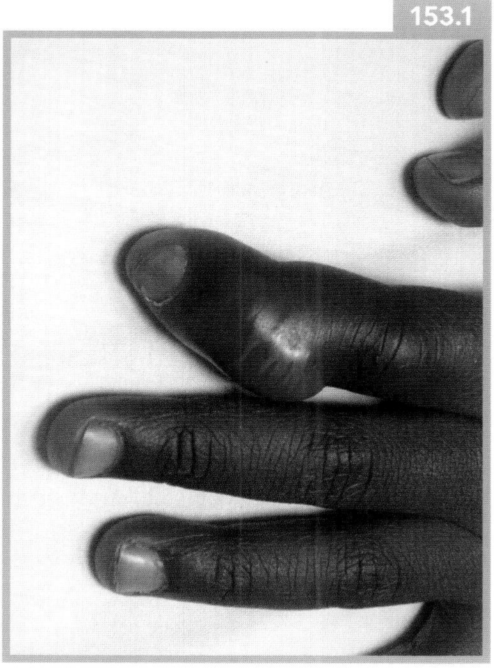

153.1

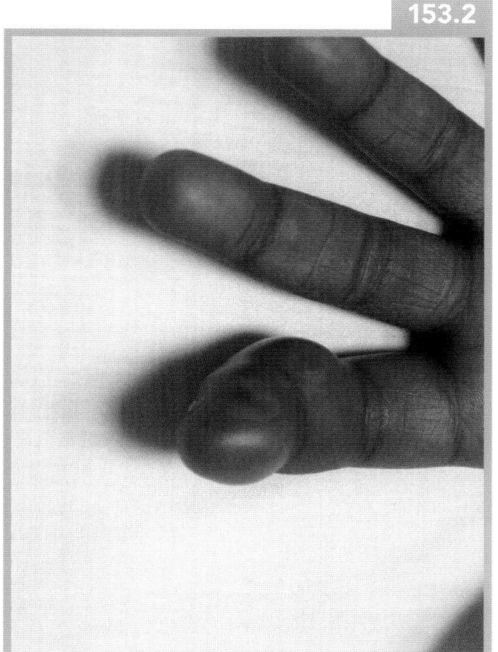

153.2

1. What is the diagnosis?
2. What is the treatment of this condition?

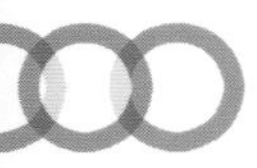

Answers

1. This patient is presenting with a felon. A felon is a closed infection of the pulp space of the finger. Typically, it begins as mild erythema and pain, progressing to swelling and fluctuance. This may be differentiated from a paronychia by noting that a felon is located on the palmar aspect, while a paronychia occurs on the dorsal aspect (see Case 152).
2. Early felons may be treated with elevation, oral antibiotics, and warm soaks. More significant felons require incision and drainage. Experts suggest making the incision over the area of greatest fluctuance. If there is no clear area of fluctuance, a mid-lateral incision is recommended. Dorsal and fish-mouth incisions are not recommended due to potential nerve injury and instability of the finger pulp space, respectively. Once the incision is made one needs to also break up the septa to decompress the infection.

Keywords: skin and soft tissue infection, procedures, pitfalls

Bibliography

Clark DC. Common acute hand infections. *Am Fam Physician* December 1, 2003;68(11):2167–76.
Franko OI, Abrams RA. Hand infections. *Orthop Clin North Am* October 2013;44(4):625–34.

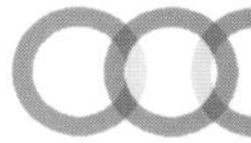

CASE 154

Diana Yan

Question

A 8-year-old male presents to the emergency room because of ingestion of a foreign body. He was with his 12-year-old cousin when the ingestion occurred. They were playing truth or dare in the living room and the 8 year old was dared to swallow an object. There was a small DVD remote cover nearby them and the patient swallowed it. Both the patient and the cousin state that no batteries were swallowed. The patient is currently complaining of sore throat, chest pain, and dysphagia. He is able to swallow his oral secretions and is not drooling. His voice is normal to his parents. There is no vomiting, abdominal pain, gagging, or choking. The event happened about 2 hours ago, as the children didn't tell their parents until about an hour ago. The patient is refusing any food or liquids. He is otherwise healthy without medical issues.

Physical exam shows an alert and awake but frightened boy sitting up in bed. He has some erythema in the posterior oropharynx without any visualized lacerations. There is no active bleeding in the posterior oropharynx. The patient states that he has chest pain but it is not reproducible on exam. His lungs and heart are normal on exam. The patient's abdominal exam is also benign. X-rays were obtained and are shown.

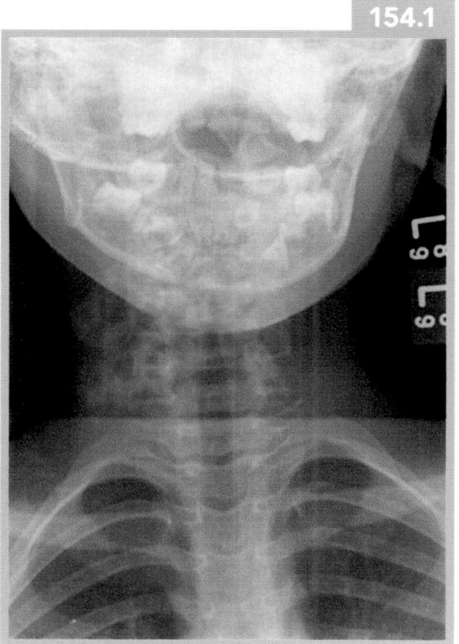

154.1

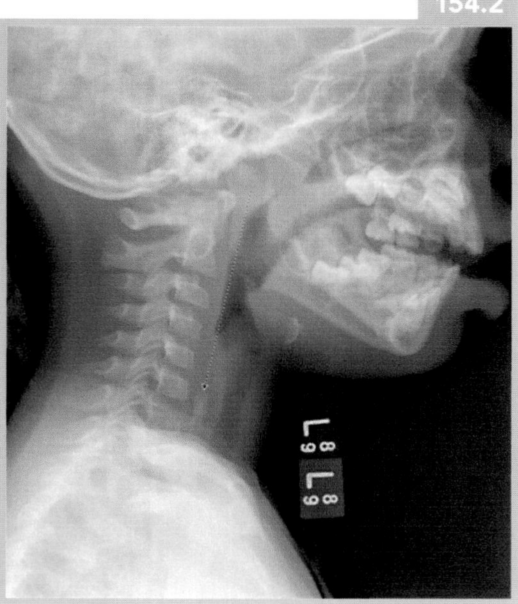

154.2

What are the most common sites for an ingested object to get caught?

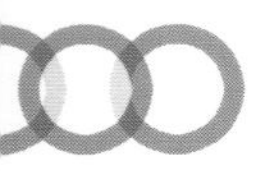

Answer

The most common sites for an ingested object to get trapped are (in descending order) upper esophagus, middle esophagus, lower esophagus, stomach, pharynx, and duodenum. However, up to 80% of ingested foreign bodies pass spontaneously and do not require intervention. These objects tend to be small and rounded. Commonly ingested objects include coins, button batteries (see Case 157), crayons, and toys such as beads and marbles. In our case, the object's exact size is unknown, but it is not rounded and is stuck in the mid-esophagus. An object such as this is unlikely to pass the pylorus as it is >6 cm in size and rectangular in shape and therefore requires endoscopic removal. If the object is less than 6 cm in size, then it will likely reach the stomach and be excreted in 4–6 days (see Case 78). X-rays are done to assess the size, location, shape, and number of foreign bodies. This modality is only useful if the foreign body is radiopaque. Other modalities used are ultrasound, which can detect radiolucent objects in the stomach, and CT scan, which is the most sensitive modality, as it can establish the diagnosis of a radiolucent foreign body, its exact location, and any associated complications. Complications of foreign bodies include impaction, obstruction, mucosal injury, and perforation. If the object is there chronically, it can lead to an abscess, peritonitis, or fistula formation.

Keywords: foreign body, airway, gastrointestinal, procedures

Bibliography

Bekkerman M, Sachdev AH, Andrade J, Twersky Y, Iqbal S. Endoscopic management of foreign bodies in the gastrointestinal tract: A review of the literature. *Gastroenterol Res Pract*. doi:10.1155/2016/8520767. Published online October 11, 2016.

Laya BF, Restrepo R, Lee EY. Practical imaging evaluation of foreign bodies in children: An update. *Radiol Clin North Am* 2017;55:845–67.

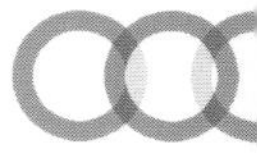

CASE 155

Veena Ramaiah

Question

A 2-year-old male presents to the emergency department (ED) with darkening of skin inside his diaper area. There is an irregular, patchy pattern of distribution on the buttocks and inguinal fold. Mom found him in the bathroom with a spilled bottle of bleach. She rushed him to the ED concerned he may have ingested some bleach. No lesions were seen in his mouth but lesions were found after undressing him in the ED. The mother did not notice them at home.

On exam, he is alert and well-appearing. There is no drooling or respiratory distress. He smells strongly of bleach including his diaper.

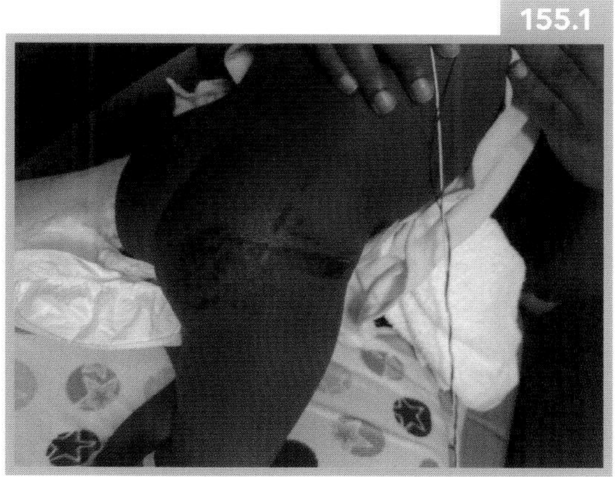

155.1

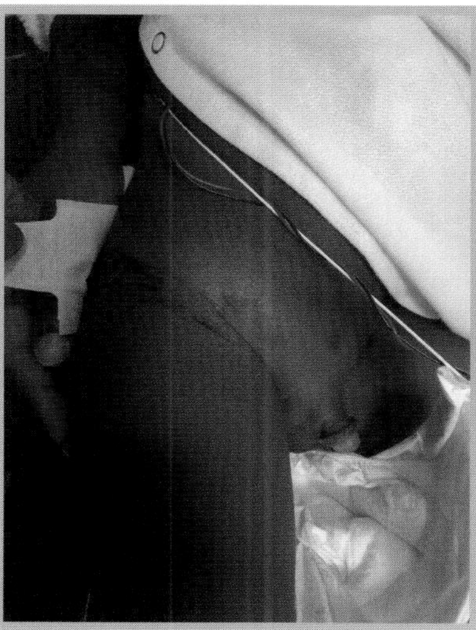

155.2

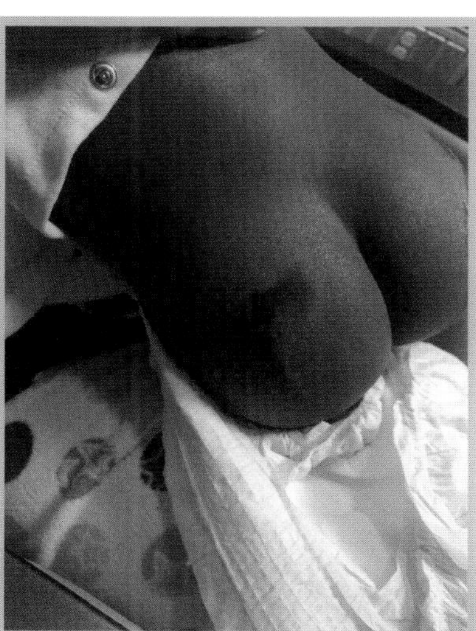

155.3

Do these lesions look like chemical burns? Could household bleach have caused these?

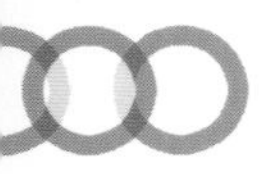

Answer

Yes, bleach can cause burns like this to the skin. This includes household bleach. The extent of burn is dependent on the concentration of the sodium hypochlorite combined with the time of exposure to the skin.

In this case, although the mom removed the child's clothing right away, the diaper was still on when he arrived to the ED and contained bleach. The diaper may have held the bleach to the skin in certain areas resulting in a superficial burn to the skin. This child was evaluated by endoscopy. There were no chemical burns to his gastrointestinal tract. He also was seen by the burn surgery team, and the burns were found to be superficial requiring no debridement or treatment other than topical emollients. There was concern for abuse or neglect because of the unusual appearance and pattern of the burns. However, these can occur from an accidental spill where the primary maltreatment concern is supervision of the child or safety of the environment.

Exposure to household bleach is not uncommon. According to Poison Control data in the United States for 2014, 48% of poison exposures are in children under 6 years of age totaling 1,031,927 (http://www.poison.org/poison-statistics-national). Out of these, 11% are due to exposure to household cleaning products. Household bleach is a type of household cleaning product that can cause chemical burns to the skin depending on how long the bleach was in contact with the skin.

A case series by Lang and Cox (2013) described chemical burns due to spilling of household bleach on the patients. One child's injury resulted in scarring to the burned areas. In two out of the three cases where the bleach specifics could be identified, the sodium hypochlorite concentration was between 5% and 10% resulting in a very basic pH.

Length of exposure of the substance on the skin can lead to more severe chemical burns. Removal of saturated clothing, including diapers, and aggressive irrigation of the skin is important in the management.

Keywords: child abuse, child abuse mimicker, dermatology, environmental

Bibliography

Lang C, Cox M. Pediatric cutaneous bleach burns. *Child Abuse Neglect* 2013;37:485.

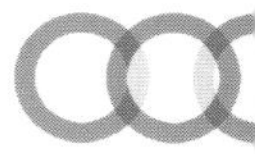

CASE 156

Nina Mbadiwe

Question

A 14-year-old male presents to the emergency department with right knee pain. He is a member of a tumbling team. He performed a front flip and heard a "pop" after he landed. He had severe pain in his right knee with subsequent swelling and was unable to ambulate. On exam he appears uncomfortable. He has limited range of motion of his right knee secondary to pain. There is swelling and tenderness to palpation at the knee joint. He is unable to ambulate. Radiographs of his knee show a tibial tubercle avulsion fracture.

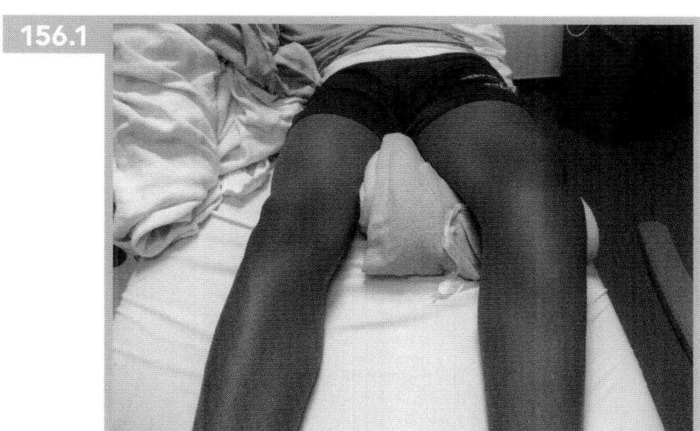

156.1

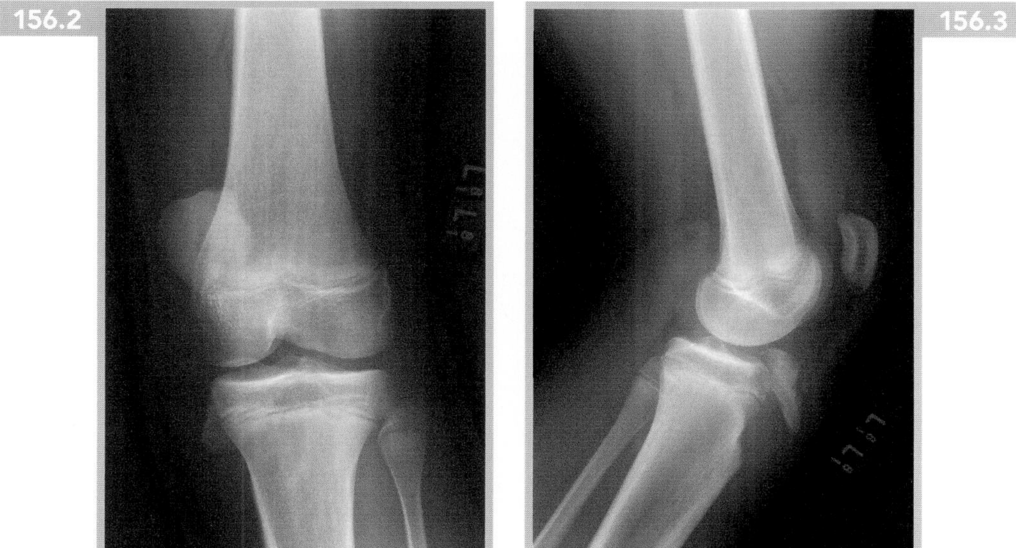

156.2 156.3

What are the three types of tibial tubercle avulsion fractures?

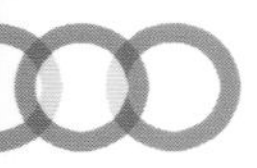

Answer

Tibial tubercle avulsion fractures are classified as follows: Type I, a small fragment of the distal tuberosity is avulsed and is displaced upward; type II, the anterior aspect of the tibial epiphysis is hinged upward without being completely fractured at its base; and type III, the entire tibial tuberosity is fractured at its base, with the line of fracture directed proximally and posteriorly into the articular surface (into the joint). Type III fractures carry the greatest risk for compartment syndrome.

Type I and II fractures are usually treated with immobilization. Displaced type II and type III injuries need reduction and fixation and require immediate orthopedic consultation.

Tibial tubercle avulsion fractures are most often seen in adolescent males (13–14 years of age) as a result of sports-related injuries. During strong contraction of the quadriceps against a fixed leg, force is exerted on the patellar tendon and its insertion site (the tibial tubercle), which may result in avulsion and displacement.

Keywords: orthopedics, blunt trauma, extremity injury

Bibliography

Skinner HB, McMahon PJ. *Current Diagnosis & Treatment in Orthopedics*. 5th ed. New York: McGraw-Hill Education, 2014.

Tintinalli JE. *Tintinalli's Emergency Medicine: A Comprehensive Study Guide*. 8th ed. New York: McGraw-Hill Education, 2016.

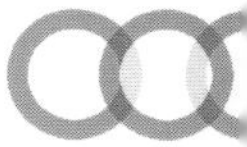

CASE 157

James Bistolarides

Question

An otherwise healthy 2-year-old boy is brought to the emergency department from a neighborhood birthday party when his mother noticed acute onset of coughing, drooling, and dysphagia after the children had emerged from playing in the basement. His mother suspects aspiration, but the episode was not witnessed by an adult. A chest x-ray is obtained.

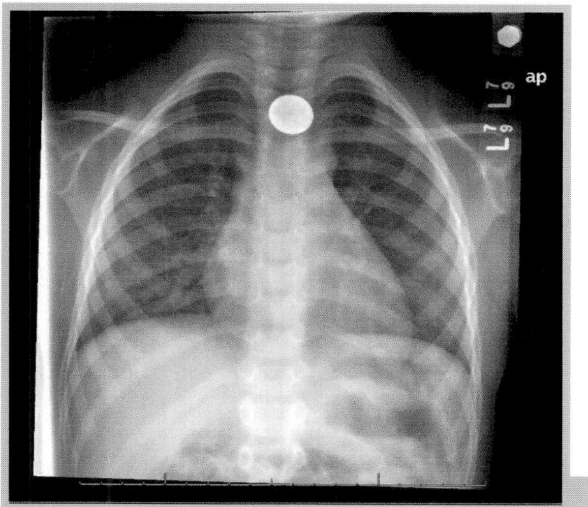

157.1

What do you see on the radiograph and how would you manage this scenario?

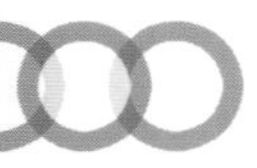

Answer

The radiograph show a cylindrical object in the upper chest, presumably in the esophagus. Round objects in the esophagus generally appear round on anterior view, whereas objects in in the trachea may be linear. A lateral view is generally recommended to confirm location. Similarly, including the abdomen in imaging is important based on the possibility that the object has passed beyond the pylorus—or that there are multiple ingestions.

A coin (Image 157.1) will appear as a flat disk with a uniform appearance and a sharp edge. A button battery (Image 157.2) can be distinguished based on a double-ring appearance in the coronal plane, as seen in this anterior film, and "step-off" appearance in the sagittal plane.

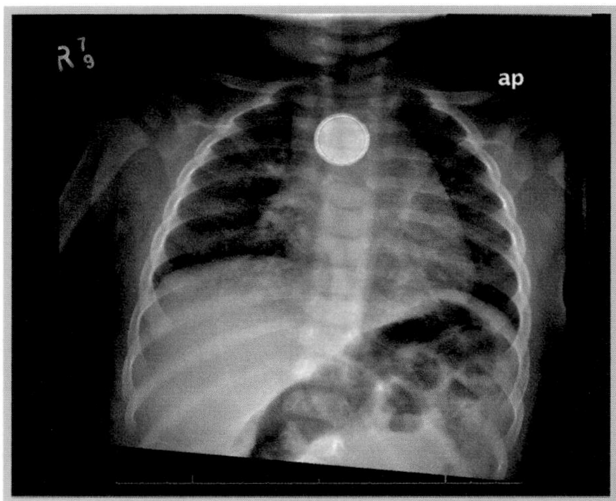

157.2

Button battery ingestion is a clinical emergency. Batteries greater than 20 mm in diameter are likely to lodge in the esophagus and cause damage within hours from direct pressure, as well as their chemical and electrical properties. Button batteries in the esophagus must be emergently removed to avoid complications (e.g. hemorrhage, strictures, fistulae, nerve damage). Batteries in the stomach are generally thought to be low risk and can be observed in an asymptomatic child, though evidence is emerging to advocate for removal. At minimum, a gastric battery larger than 20 mm in diameter should be re-evaluated by x-ray at 48 hours and removed if still in placed.

Coins in the esophagus should be removed urgently if the patient is symptomatic. If the patient is asymptomatic removal can be delayed up to 24 hours. Repeat x-ray should be obtained just before removal to ensure the coin has not passed. Coins in the stomach can be observed at home with return precautions and serial x-rays at 7–14 days if there has been no passage.

Keywords: foreign body, airway, pitfalls, gastrointestinal

Bibliography

Kramer RE, Lerner DG, Lin T, Manfredi M et al. Management of ingested foreign bodies in children: A clinical report of the NASPGHAN endoscopy committee. *J Pediatr Gastroenterol Nutr* 2015;60(3):562–74.

Pugmire BS, Lim R, Avery LL. Review of ingested and aspirated foreign bodies in children and their clinical significance for radiologists. *Radiographics* 2015;35(3):1528–38.

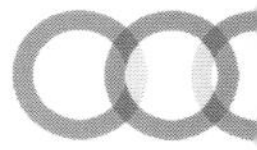

CASE 158

Nina Mbadiwe

Question

A 12-month-old girl presents to the emergency room with a chief complaint of coughing. The father states she has been coughing for the past month. The cough has worsened over the past 3 days with some grunting noted today. She occasionally has episodes of gagging with vomiting of partially digested food. She has no fevers, there is no drooling, and she has adequate weight gain. Her chest x-ray revealed an eroded coin in the proximal esophagus.

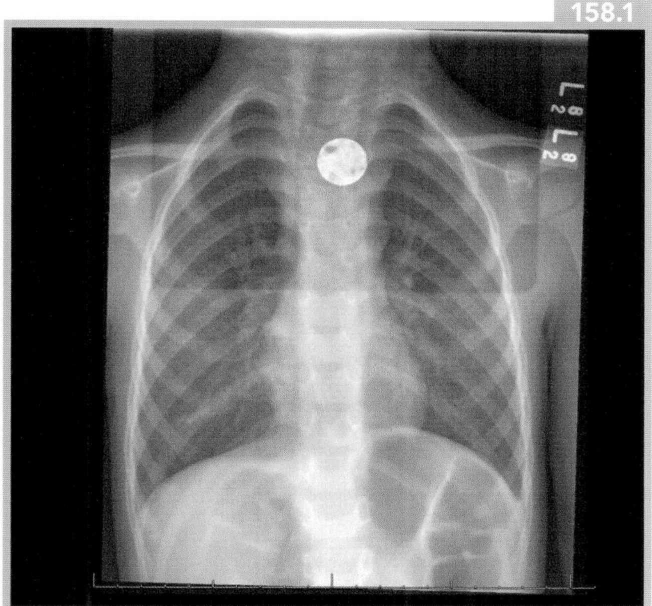

158.1

Asymptomatic patients with esophageal coins can have what types of complications?

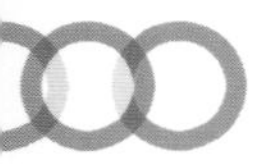

Answer

Long-standing esophageal foreign bodies can cause strictures, perforation, and/or erode the esophageal wall, which can create fistulas with the trachea and other nearby structures (e.g. esophageal-aortic fistulas).

Coins are the most common foreign body ingested by children. Patients with esophageal foreign bodies may be asymptomatic or present with refusal to eat, dysphagia, drooling, choking, wheezing, or stridor.

If a coin is visualized in the esophagus and the patient is asymptomatic, the patient can be observed for up to 24 hours from the time the coin was ingested. The coin should be removed if a patient is symptomatic or if a patient is asymptomatic and the coin does not pass spontaneously after 24 hours since this is the point at which complications can occur.

Keywords: gastrointestinal, foreign body, cough, vomiting, pitfalls

Bibliography

Waltzman M. Management of esophageal coins. *Pediatr Emer Care* 2006;22(5):367.

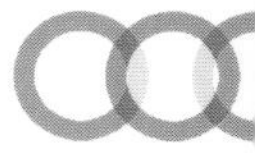

CASE 159

Diana Yan

Question

A 6-year-old male presents to the emergency room after ingesting a screw bit. The father was putting together furniture that they had brought into the living room, and the patient was playing nearby. The father had changed the screw bit of the power drill to a smaller sized bit. Later, the father noticed he was missing the screw bit. The patient told his father that he swallowed it while playing with it. He has some sore throat pain but does not have any globus sensation in his throat, chest pain, vomiting, or abdominal pain. The father thinks that the event happened 1 hour earlier. The patient has not eaten anything since the event. He is otherwise healthy without medical issues.

Physical exam shows an alert and awake boy who is watching TV in the room. He has some erythema in the posterior oropharynx but no lacerations, bleeding, or exudates. He has a soft, non-distended, non-tender, benign abdominal exam. External rectal exam is normal. An x-ray is obtained and shown next.

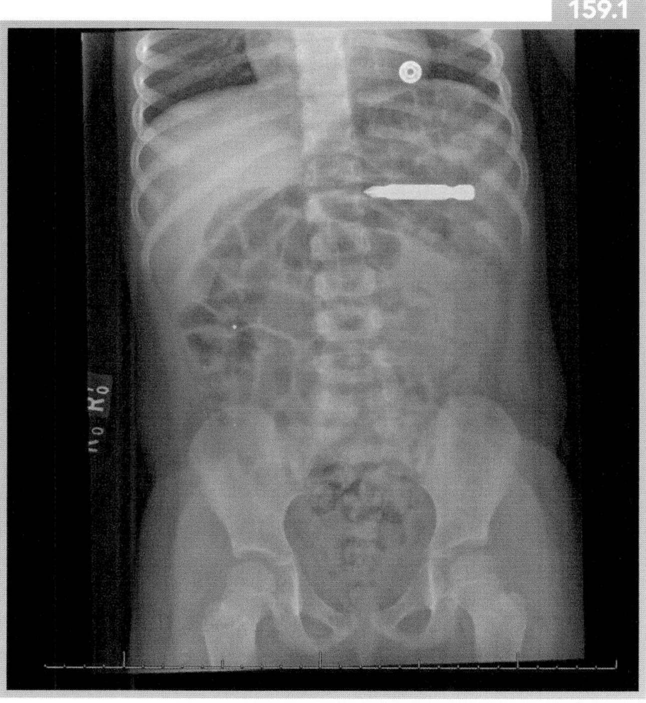

159.1

What signs/symptoms or exam findings would be worrisome in a patient who ingests a sharp object?

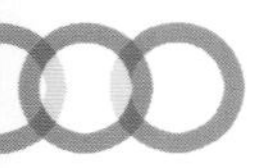

Answer

Abdominal tenderness, crepitus, guarding, or rebound, which would indicate signs of perforation. Intestinal perforation occurs in less than 1% of foreign body ingestions. Sharp objects need emergent endoscopic removal especially before they pass the stomach. This is because once they pass the stomach, there is an increased risk of perforation, especially at the ileocecal valve. Daily radiographs are needed to monitor progression if the initial management is to observe. Surgical intervention is necessary if there are symptoms of perforation or the object is not moving for >72 hours. Flexible endoscope removal tends to be very successful with a 95% success rate.

Animal bones such as fish bones are the most common sharp objects that cause perforation. Intestinal perforation can predispose a patient to hepatic abscess, sepsis, and retroperitoneal hematoma. Screws, in particular, can lodge into the appendix and cause appendicitis, appendiceal perforation, and appendiceal abscess due to its larger size. Other areas in which sharp objects can become trapped are the duodenal loop, the duodenojejunal junction, and terminal ileum, areas with acute angles or intestinal narrowing.

Keywords: foreign body, gastrointestinal, acute abdomen

Bibliography

Bekkerman M, Sachdev AH, Andrade J, Twersky Y, Iqbal S. Endoscopic management of foreign bodies in the gastrointestinal tract: A review of the literature. *Gastroenterol Res Pract.* Published online October 11, 2016. doi: 10.1155/2016/8520767.

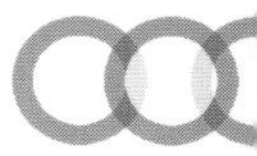

CASE 160

S. Margaret Paik

Question

A 14-month-old boy is brought into the emergency department (ED) by his grandmother with a history of decreased oral intake with some non-bilious, non-bloody vomiting for the past 3 days. There is no history of fever or diarrhea. The grandmother states he cries while feeding. There has also been a non-productive cough.

On physical examination, he is an alert, well-developed, and well-nourished boy. The heart rate is 120 beats per minute, with a respiratory rate of 28 with 98% oxygen saturation on room air. A chest radiograph is done.

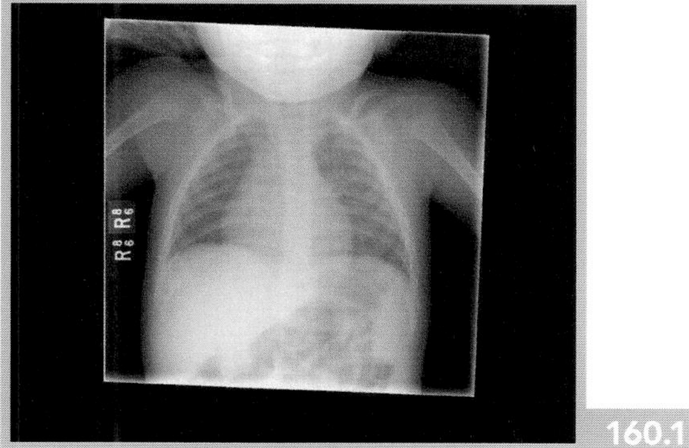

160.1

During the ED evaluation the child is noted to have episodes of gagging, coughing, and post-tussive emesis while drinking his milk. An esophagram contrast study is performed and a filling defect is identified. He is taken to the operating room and a sticker is removed from the esophagus.

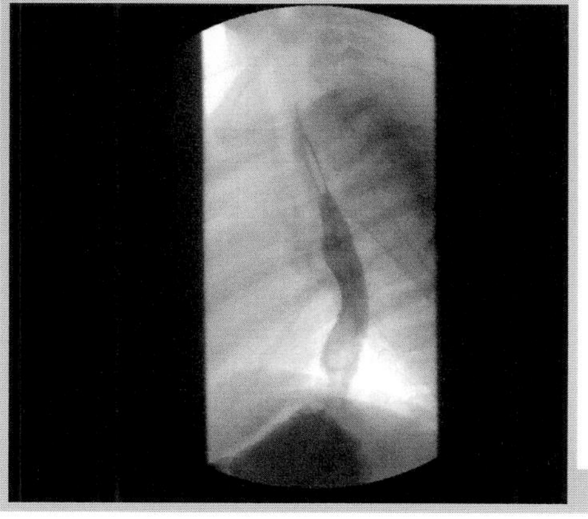

160.2

What are the most commonly ingested objects? Where are esophageal foreign bodies most likely to lodge?

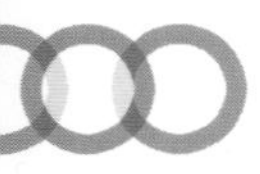

Answer

Coins are the most commonly ingested objects in the United States and Europe (Case 157). Coins are more likely to be retained at the level of the cricopharyngeus, the thoracic inlet, the aortic arch, and the lower esophageal sphincter. In Asia, fish bones cause a large portion of reported ingestions. Ingestions due to disk or button batteries and magnets have increased and can result in serious sequelae if not removed promptly. Food impaction is more likely to occur if there is underlying pathology.

Many cases of esophageal foreign body will present without a history of witnessed ingestion. Children can present with gastrointestinal (food refusal, gagging, vomiting, anorexia, dysphagia) and respiratory (cough, stridor, wheezing, apnea, pneumonia). Children may also present with chest or neck pain and nonspecific signs such as lethargy or irritability. Some children are asymptomatic at the time of presentation for a witnessed ingestion.

Keywords: gastrointestinal, foreign body, vomiting, cough

Bibliography

Macpherson RI, Hill JG, Othersen HB, Tagge EP, Smith CD. Esophageal foreign bodies in children: Diagnosis, treatment and complications. *Am J Roentgenol* 1996;166(4):919–24.

Waltzman ML. Management of esophageal coins. *Curr Opin Pediatr* October 2006;18(5):571–4.

Wyllie R. Foreign bodies in the gastrointestinal tract. *Curr Opin Pediatr* October 2006;18(5):563–4.

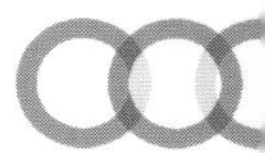

CASE 161

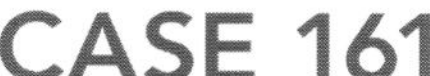

S. Margaret Paik

Question

A 21-month-old boy presents to the emergency department with one month of cough. Coughing occurs during the day and night, and is non-productive. The family reports occasional post-tussive emesis of food products, but otherwise he has been eating normally. They also report that the child is often found trying to put objects in his mouth. The family does not recall any episodes of choking or gagging. There is no history of fever, weight loss, or ill contacts. There is no significant past medical history and the family history is non-contributory.

Vital signs are unremarkable with respiratory rate of 26, pulse oximetry saturation of 98% on room air, and a temperature of 36.4°C. The child is alert and well-appearing. End-expiratory wheezing is auscultated in the right chest.

What types of imaging studies can be useful?

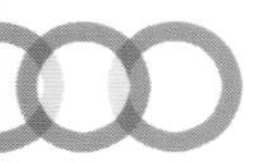

Answer

There is a strong concern for an inhaled foreign body because of the child's history and physical examination findings. Aspirated foreign bodies most frequently lodge in the right mainstem bronchus. The left mainstem bronchus, trachea, and larynx are additional sites. Posteroanterior and lateral chest radiographs are often obtained initially; non-radiopaque foreign bodies will not be seen on these studies. In these cases, films obtained during inspiration and expiration may demonstrate air trapping, but are difficult to obtain in young children. Bilateral decubitus chest radiographs can be used instead and may show segmental or lobar atelectasis or air trapping in a unilateral hyperlucent lung field. This is due to a "ball-valve" effect. Additional imaging modalities include fluoroscopy, computed tomography, and magnetic resonance imaging.

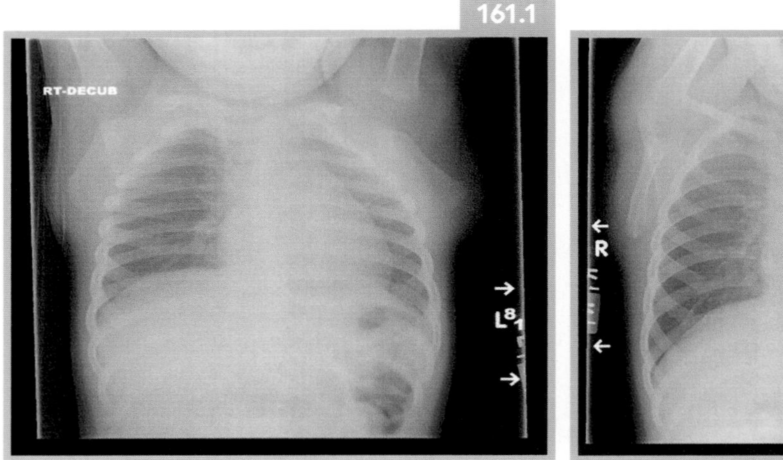

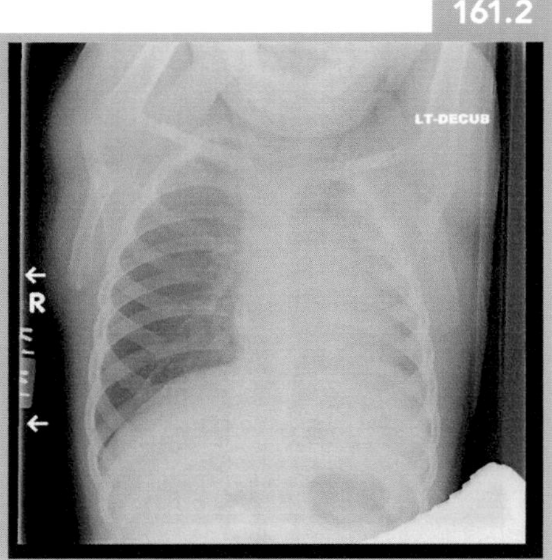

Keywords: pulmonary, cough, foreign body

Bibliography

Grassi R, Faggian A, Somma F, De Cecco CN, Laghi A, Caseiro-Alves F. Application of imaging guidelines in patients with foreign body ingestion or inhalation: Literature review. *Semin Ultrasound CT MRI* February 2015;36(1):48–56.

Lowe DA, Vasquez R, Maniaci V. Foreign body aspiration in children. *Clin Pediatr Emerg Med* September 2015;16(3):140–8.

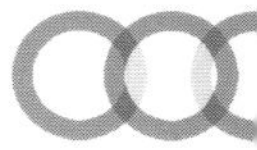

CASE 162

Barbara Pawel

Question

A 14-year-old boy presents to the emergency department after choking on a nail. He was helping his friend repair a fence and tripped over a board with a nail in his mouth. He had a brief episode of coughing shortly afterward which resolved. He denied any retrosternal chest pain, difficulty swallowing, abdominal pain, nausea, or vomiting. On exam he appeared comfortable with a respiratory rate of 16 and pulse oximetry of 98% on room air. There was focal wheezing in the right mid-lung without increased work of breathing, stridor, voice change, or drooling. Imaging for a possible foreign body was performed.

162.1

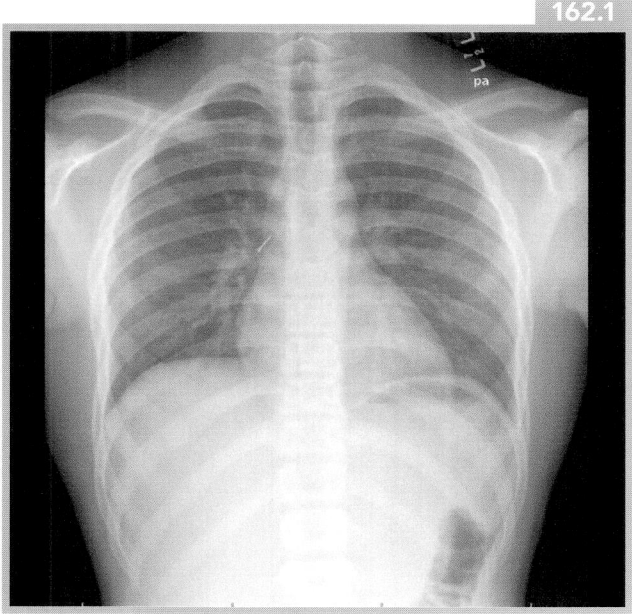

What is the preferred method for airway foreign body removal?

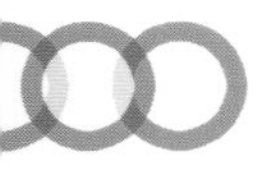

Answer

Rigid bronchoscopy is performed in the operating room and requires general anesthesia but has several advantages over flexible bronchoscopy for identification and removal of a foreign body (FB). The ability to control the airway and ventilate through the scope, availability of a variety of scope sizes and removal devices, larger working channels, excellent visualization, and improved suctioning make this a superior choice. It can be difficult to see small, thin, and radiolucent FBs on flexible bronchoscopy, especially in uncooperative patients, resulting in a delayed diagnosis. There is also a risk of dislodging the FB and further compromising the airway.

The diagnosis of an aspirated foreign body can be challenging. Only 57% of patients present with the classic triad of choking with cough, wheezing, and asymmetric breath sounds. FB aspiration symptoms also have significant overlap with common pediatric conditions (asthma, bronchiolitis, upper respiratory traction infection, pneumonia). The acute symptomatic episode may be followed by a symptom-free period and can be misinterpreted by parents as a sign of resolution. These factors often lead to a delayed diagnosis, increasing the risk of serious complications including recurrent atelectasis, pneumonia or bronchiectasis, prolonged hospitalization, and even death.

The degree of clinical suspicion will dictate the extent of the evaluation. Any stable symptomatic or asymptomatic patient with suspected FB aspiration should have a two-view chest radiograph with the awareness that plain radiographs have both low sensitivity and specificity. Moderate or high suspicion is suggested by (1) a witnessed aspiration regardless of symptoms, (2) a history of choking with symptoms and/or a suspicious radiograph, and (3) young children with suggestive respiratory symptoms without other explanations (see Case 161). These patients should have rigid bronchoscopy. Low-suspicion patients with no symptoms and a normal radiograph can be observed and re-evaluated in 2–3 days or sooner if they become symptomatic.

Keywords: pulmonary, foreign body, life-threatening, chest pain, penetrating trauma

Bibliography

Green, SS. Ingested and aspirated foreign bodies. *Peds Rev* 2015;36(10):430–6.

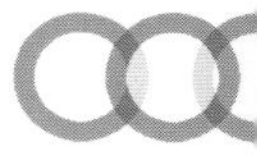

CASE 163

Diana Yan

Question

A 5-month-old female presents to the emergency room due to a large head size and vomiting. She was seen by her pediatrician a month ago when they noted the patient to have a slightly larger head. Her pediatrician instructed them to follow-up in a month as she was otherwise doing well and developmentally appropriate. Today, her mother brings her in with progressive vomiting. She states that the baby has been vomiting after some of her feeds for the last 2 weeks. She has been otherwise doing well. No fevers, seizures, abnormal movements, diarrhea, or upper respiratory symptoms. She has been meeting her developmental milestones and she is an otherwise healthy full-term baby without any prior medical issues.

Physical exam shows an alert and awake baby girl who will grab at things in front of her. She has a normal neurological exam and her pupils are equal and reactive. Her head circumference is 50 cm, which is >97 percentile. Her pediatrician sends her head circumference growth chart and you note that she has crossed 3 percentile lines over the last 2 months with the most dramatic increase over the last month. Neurosurgery comes to evaluate and a CT head is obtained.

163.1

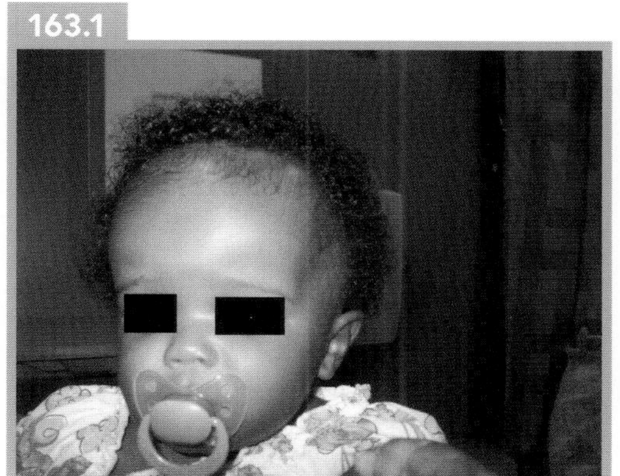

163.2

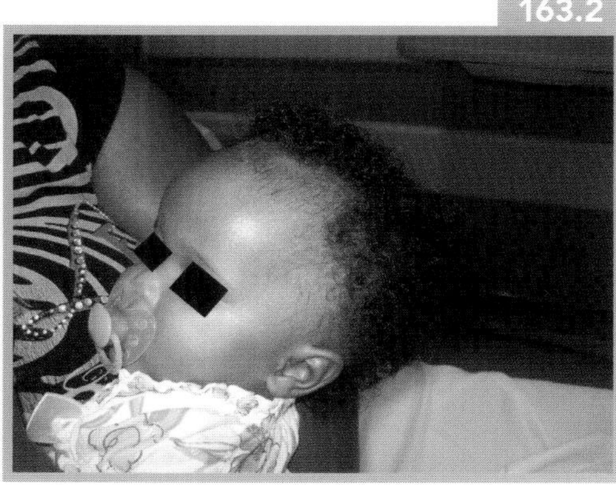

163.3

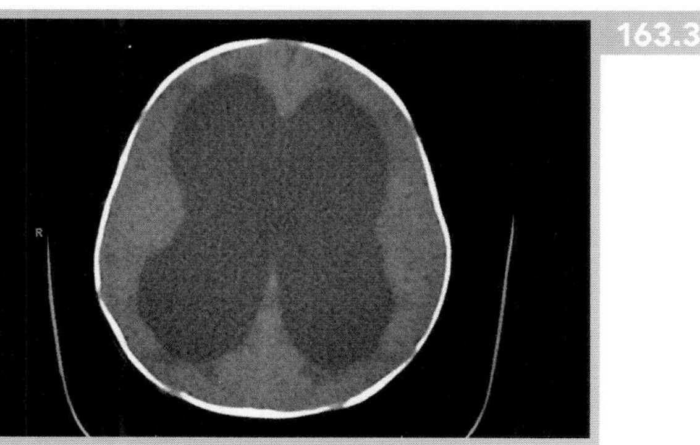

What is the treatment for this condition?

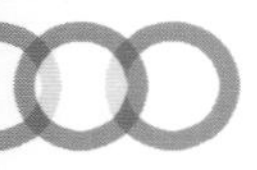

Answer

Placement of a ventriculoperitoneal (VP) shunt. This baby has hydrocephalus, which is an increase in volume of cerebrospinal fluid (CSF) in the ventricular system of the brain. In children whose sutures are still open, they can present with an increased head circumference. Hydrocephalus is caused by decreased normal CSF absorption, increased CSF production, abnormal flow of CSF, or another fluid (such as blood) occupying the ventricular space. With an increase in volume within the ventricular system comes increased intracranial pressure (ICP). As the ICP increases, brain structures become displaced (as shown in the CT head image).

There are many causes of hydrocephalus with the most frequent being intraventricular hemorrhage, aqueduct stenosis, meningitis, Arnold-Chiari malformation, Dandy-Walker syndrome, rachischisis from neural tube closure failure (such as myelomeningocele), and brain tumors. The etiology of this patient's hydrocephalus is still unknown. Surgical placement of a VP shunt is the mainstay of treatment, but in emergent cases, external ventricular drainage catheters can be placed. Other types of ventricular shunts are ventriculoatrial shunts, where the end of the shunt goes to the heart, and ventriculopleural shunts, where it ends in the pleural space. Infection and malfunction from mechanical issues such as kinking, fracture, or dislocation are the most common complications of VP shunt placement.

Keywords: neurosurgery, head and neck/ENT, CT

Bibliography

Wright Z, Larrew TW, Eskandari R. Pediatric hydrocephalus: Current state of diagnosis and treatment. *Pediatr Rev* 2016;37(11):478–90.

Zielińska D, Rajtar-Zembaty A, Starowicz-Filip A. Cognitive disorders in children's hydrocephalus. *Neurol Neurochir Pol* 2017;51:234–9.

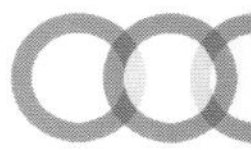

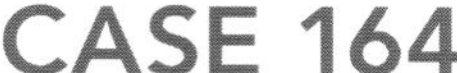

CASE 164

Nina Mbadiwe

Question

An 18-month-old boy is brought to the emergency room after his parents found him with a window cord wrapped around his neck. Currently, he is awake and alert with normal vital signs for age. His physical exam is unremarkable except for ligature marks on his neck.

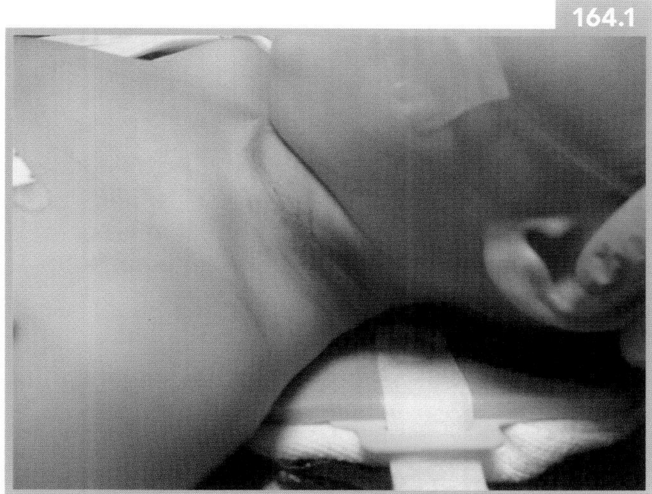

164.1

What are the findings seen in strangulation and hangings? What is the most common cause of death in window cord strangulation injuries?

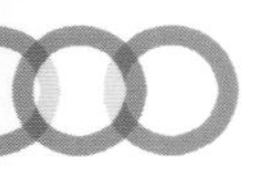

Answer

Strangulation in children is usually accidental but can also be a form of child abuse. Hanging, with strangulation and suspension of the neck, is classified as either complete with the entire body hanging off the ground or incomplete, with a portion of the body touching the ground and the weight not fully supported by the neck. Theories of the pathophysiology during strangulation and hanging include:

- Venous obstruction leading to hypoxia and loss of consciousness
- Arterial spasm caused by pressure on the carotid artery leading to decreased cerebral blood flow
- Vagal collapse due to the pressure on the carotid sinuses and increased parasympathetic tone

In all forms of strangulation, death is ultimately due to cerebral anoxia and ischemia with obstruction of cerebral venous return (vessel occlusion) rather than acute airway compromise.

Physical exam findings include abnormal vital signs, facial edema, petechiae, neck contusions and/or ligature marks around the neck, voice changes, difficulty swallowing, and respiratory symptoms.

Injury prevention is an important topic to address with parents and caregivers. Cribs, beds, furniture, and toys need to be placed away from windows. Window cords should be out of reach, either tying them up high or anchoring them to the wall. Cordless window coverings are the best option in children's bedrooms and play areas.

Keywords: blunt trauma, neck injury, airway

Bibliography

Muthukrishnan L, Raman R, Nagaraju K. An unusual cause of accidental hanging in a toddler. *Pediatr Emerg Care* 2012;28(9):924–5.

Sabo RA, Hanigan, WC, Flessner K, Rose J, Aaland M. Strangulation injuries in children. Part 1. Clinical analysis. *J Trauma* January 1996;40(1):68–72.

Tintinalli JE. *Tintinalli's Emergency Medicine: A Comprehensive Study Guide.* 8th ed. New York: McGraw-Hill Education, 2016.

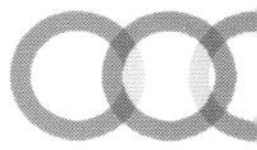

CASE 165

Nina Mbadiwe

Question

A 4-year-old boy presents to the emergency department with a right-sided scalp lesion for the past month. The boy has been scratching at the lesion. On physical exam there is a raised scaly circular scalp lesion with slightly irregular borders and some alopecia. There are also several non-tender mobile occipital nodes, all 0.5 cm or smaller.

165.1

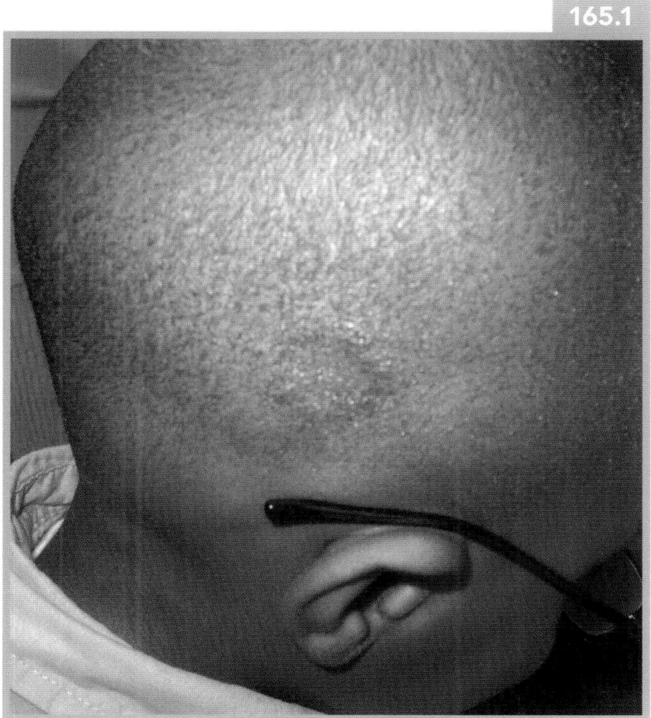

What is this condition? What are the treatment options for this condition? What are some associated findings?

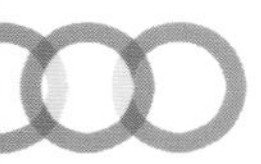

Answer

This is tinea capitis, which can occur at any age and is due to a fungal infection. The three main genera of fungi are Trichophyton, Microsporum, and Epidermophyton. Presenting symptoms can vary from minimal pruritus with little to no hair loss to purulent drainage, tenderness, and inflammatory kerion lesions. The kerion is a cell-mediated response to the fungal infection and is often misdiagnosed as an abscess. Additional findings include scaling, broken hair stubs with areas of alopecia ("black dot" sign), pustules, and lymphadenopathy.

165.2

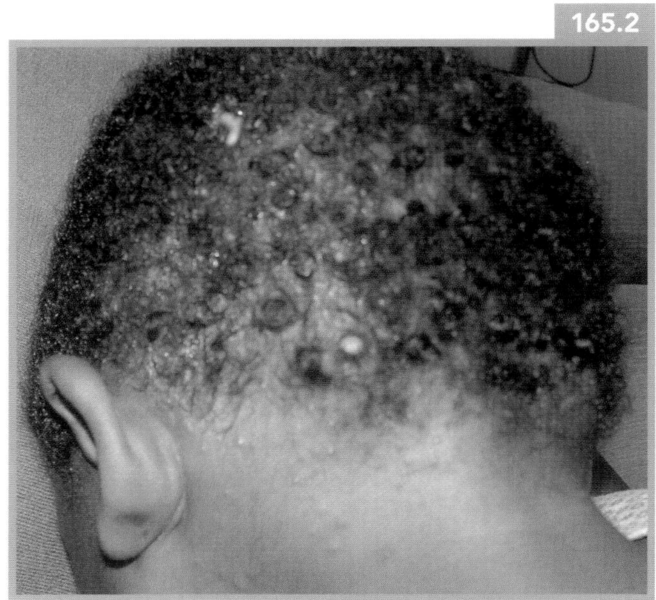

Infections involving hair-bearing skin usually necessitate oral antifungal treatment since dermatophytes penetrate the follicle and are out of reach of topically applied agents. Griseofulvin, terbinafine, itraconazole, or fluconazole are considered safe and effective in treating tinea capitis. Adjuvant therapy with selenium sulfide (1% and 2.5%), zinc pyrithione (1% and 2%), povidone iodine (2.5%), and ketoconazole (2%) are shampoo preparations that help eradicate dermatophytes from the scalps of children.

Keywords: dermatology, infection, infectious diseases

Bibliography

Ali S, Graham TAD, Forgie S. The assessment and management of tinea capitis in children. *Pediatr Emerg Care* September 2007;23(9):662–5.

Goldsmith LA. *Fitzpatrick's Dermatology in General Medicine*. 8th ed. New York: McGraw-Hill, 2012.

Kakourou T, Uksal U. Guidelines for the management of tinea capitis in children. *Pediatr Dermatol* 2010;27:226–8.

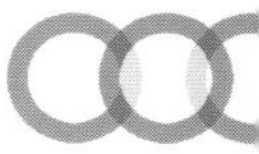

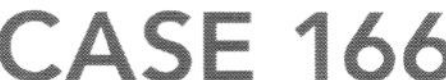

CASE 166

Catherine H. Chung

Question

A 15-year-old obese female with a presumptive diagnosis of cellulitis of her right knee by her pediatrician presents with more pain and swelling. She has been on cephalexin for 24 hours. She is mildly febrile and her knee exam reveals an indurated, warm, and mildly swollen area over a portion of her knee. She has some pain with flexion and extension of her knee. Due to her obesity, her knees are both large and difficult to assess for an effusion. She may have worsening cellulitis with or without possible joint involvement. You perform a bedside ultrasound of her knee.

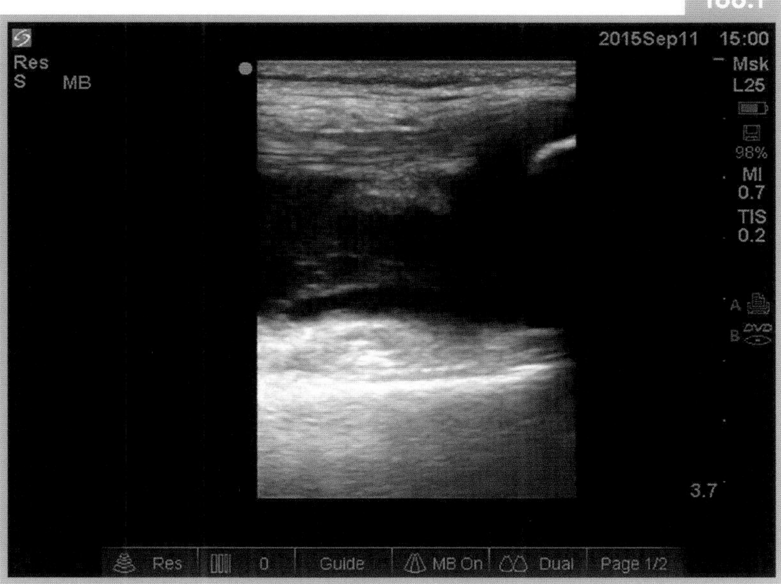

166.1

What does this ultrasound reveal?

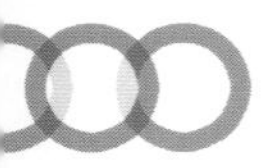

Answer

You visualize fluid in her knee joint with ultrasound. Effusions tend to be anechoic (i.e. black) if it is fresh blood or transudate. They may also be hyperechoic (i.e. gray or white) with or without a layer if it is congealed blood or purulent fluid. Ultrasound has been shown to be a simple and sensitive tool to evaluate for knee effusions. Bedside ultrasound helps augment your physical exam because effusions may be difficult to assess on exam or plain radiographs. Bedside ultrasound can also help guide arthrocentesis by finding the largest pocket of fluid or in settings of a failed arthrocentesis.

Keywords: ultrasound, procedures, extremity injury

Bibliography

Richardson ML, Selby B, Montana MA, Mack LA. Ultrasonography of the knee. *Radiol Clin North Am* 1988;26:63–75.

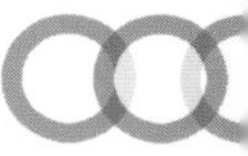

CASE 167

S. Margaret Paik

Question

A 10-week-old girl is brought in by her parents with a concern for a rash noted on the second day of life. The mother described the initial rash on a small portion of her arms and similar in appearance to blisters. The rash now appears to be red bumps and extends to the entire upper extremity including fingers and her legs. She is still feeding well and does not seem to be troubled by the rash. There is no fever.

The baby was born via normal spontaneous vaginal delivery, at term, without complications. The mother had prenatal care and denies any infections during her pregnancy. There is no other family member with skin disorders.

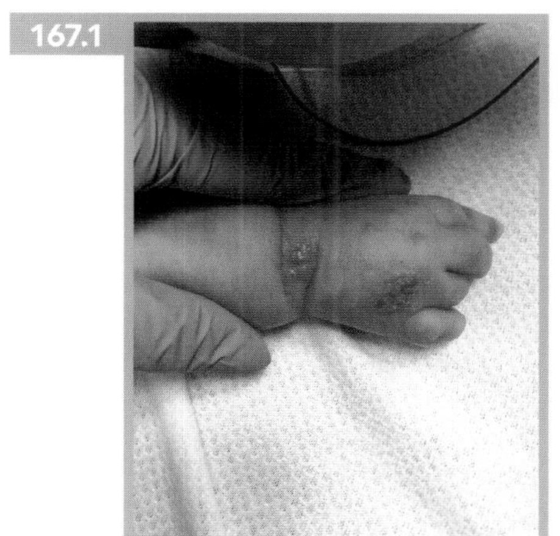

167.1

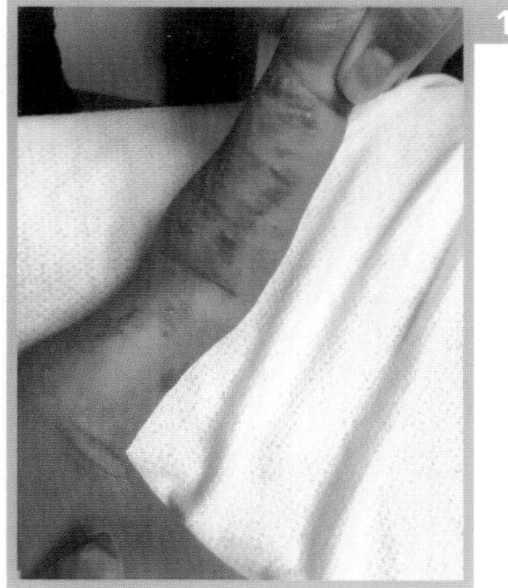

167.2

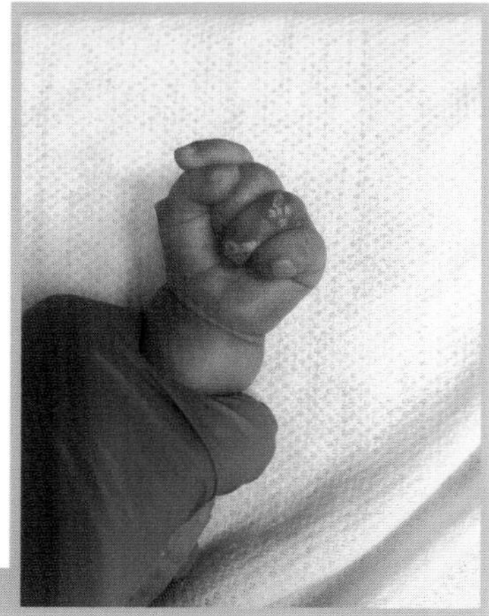

167.3

What is this condition? What are other organ systems that can be affected by this condition?

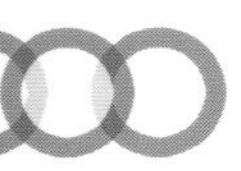

Answer

This is incontinentia pigmenti, also known as Bloch-Sulzberger syndrome. It is an X-linked dominant disease, usually fatal for males in utero. Four stages of cutaneous findings (some along Blaschko's lines) are described but not all stages are seen and there may be overlap. Bullous lesions are seen initially with vesicular linear patterned distributions and underlying erythema, and will occur for the first several months of life. The blisters can be mistaken for burns, and concern for child abuse may be considered. Linear wart-like verrucous plaques can be seen next, lasting from several months up to 2 years. The third stage is characterized by hyperpigmentation over the trunk and extremities with distinctive whorl and streak-like pattern, and can also be mistaken for bruising and child abuse. Hypopigmentation and overlying alopecia is seen in the final or atretic stage. This stage occurs in adulthood.

This is a multisystem disease that can lead to blindness from retinal ischemia and seizures, microcephaly, spastic paralysis, and mental retardation from central nervous system involvement. Some children may also have delayed dental eruption, impaction, and malformations of the crowns.

Keywords: dermatology, neonate, child abuse mimicker

Bibliography

Ciarallo L, Paller A. Two cases of incontinentia pigmenti simulating child abuse. *Pediatrics* October 1997;100(4):e6.

Landy SJ, Donnai D. Incontinentia pigmenti (Bloch-Sulzberger syndrome). *J Med Genet* 1993;30:53–9.

O'Doherty M, McCreery K, Green AJ, Tuwir I, Brosnahan D. Incontinentia pigmenti-ophthalmological observation of a series of cases and review of the literature. *Br J Ophthalmol* 2011;95:11–6.

Patel B, Butterfield R. Common skin and bleeding disorder that can potentially masquerade as child abuse. *Am J Med Genet* December 2015;169(4):328–36.

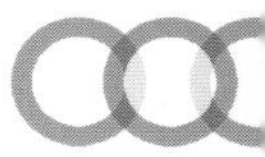

CASE 168

S. Margaret Paik

Question

A 15-year-old comes to the emergency department with swelling and drainage from her neck. There has been swelling on both sides of her lower neck for the past 3 months. She has had a poor appetite for one month and has been feeling warm for the past week. Her neck swelling has increased during the week and there was drainage from the left side of her neck today. She has not been living with her family and has been homeless, living in a shelter for the past year.

The vital signs are temperature 38.5°C, heart rate 98, respiratory rate 16, blood pressure 110/70. Her neck appears as shown.

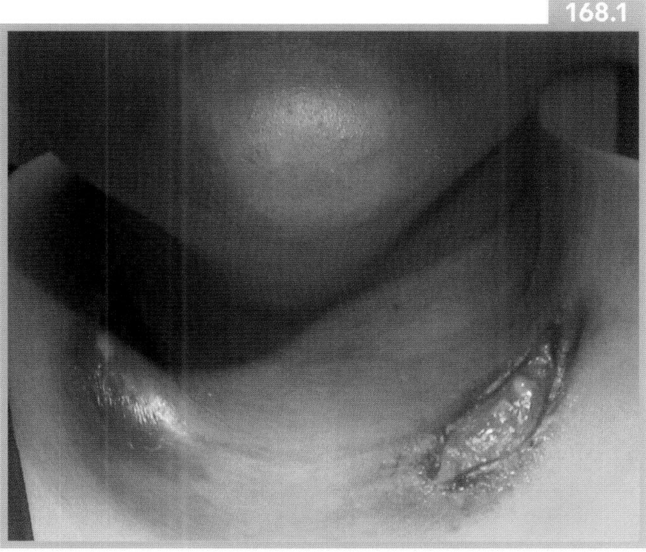

168.1

What is this condition and how should it managed? What additional studies should be done?

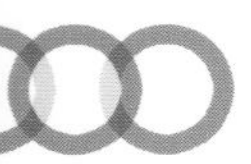

Answer

This case of lymphadenitis with ulceration has a differential diagnosis that includes malignancies (leukemia, lymphoma, neuroblastoma) and infectious causes. Infectious causes include viral (cytomegalovirus, Epstein-Barr virus), and bacterial (*Staphylococcus aureus*, *Mycoplasma pneumoniae*, group A streptococcus, anaerobes, cat scratch disease). Tuberculous as well as non-tuberculous or atypical mycobacteria are highly likely given the patient's presentation. Definitive diagnosis is made by histopathology (via excisional biopsy rather than incision and drainage or fine needle aspirate given the risk of forming a fistula) and acid-fast bacilli smear. Chest radiograph and neck imaging (ultrasound, CT, or MRI) is indicated to evaluate the extent of the disease. HIV testing is also indicated. Scrofula or king's evil are other terms used.

Keywords: infectious diseases, head and neck/ENT, skin and soft tissue infection, infectious

Bibliography

Danjani AS, Garcia RE, Wolinsky E. Etiology of cervical lymphadenitis in children. *N Engl J Med* 1963;268:1329–33.

Fontanilla J-M, Barnes A, Fordham von Reyn C. Current diagnosis and management of peripheral tuberculous lymphadenitis. *Clin Infect Dis* September 15, 2011;53(6):555–62.

Scobie WG. Acute suppurative adenitis in children: A review of 964 cases. *Scott Med J* 1969;14(10):352.

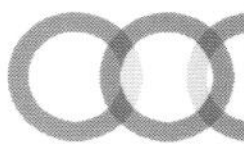

CASE 169

Nina Mbadiwe

Question

A 9-month-old boy presents to the emergency department with a rash on his trunk, extremities, and groin area. The rash has been present for 1 month. It is pruritic. He is otherwise well.

On exam there are multiple erythematous papules, excoriations, and eczematous lesions throughout the skin.

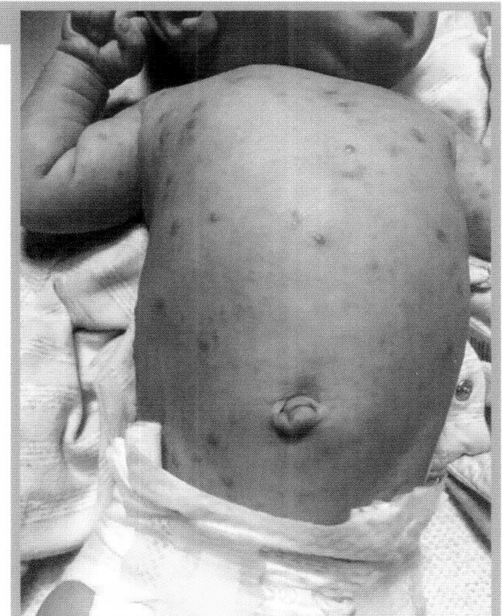

169.1

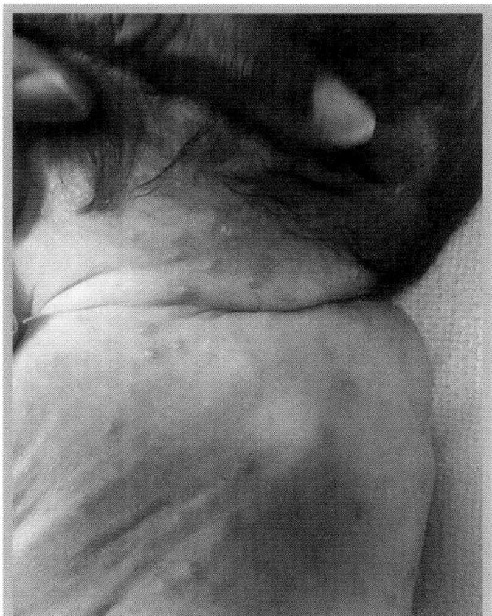

169.2

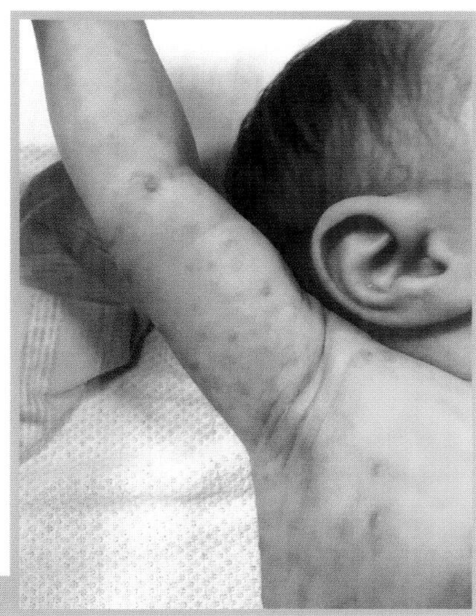

169.3

What is this condition and what is the best treatment?

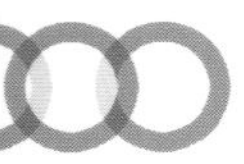

Answer

Scabies is worldwide and affects all ages, races, and socioeconomic levels. Close personal contact is the main route of transmission. It is caused by *Sarcoptes scabiei* var. *hominis*. The life cycle of mites is completed entirely on human skin. Some individuals remain asymptomatic despite being infested.

The diagnosis of scabies is suspected by pruritis associated with a characteristic distribution of lesions. On physical exam there are excoriations and eczematous dermatitis in the interdigital webs, volar aspects of the wrists, elbows, axillae, scrotum, penis, labia, and areolae. All skin surfaces are susceptible in infants. The pathognomonic lesion is a burrow: a thin, threadlike, linear structure.

The most common treatment is permethrin 5% cream, applied to the entire skin surface for 8 hours before rinsing. Treatment should be repeated 1 week after initial treatment to reduce the potential for reinfestation from fomites as well as to kill any nymphs that may have hatched after treatment. The rash and pruritis may persist for up to 4 weeks. Oral antihistamines (if appropriate for age) and emollients can be beneficial. All family members and close contacts should be treated simultaneously. All clothing, pillowcases, towels, and bedding should be washed in hot water and dried in high heat. Non-washables should be dry cleaned, ironed, put in the clothes dryer without washing, or stored in a sealed plastic bag in a warm area for 2 weeks. Carpets, floors, and furniture should be carefully vacuumed.

Keywords: dermatology, infestation, infection, rash

Bibliography

Goldsmith LA, Katz SI, Gilchrest BS, Paller AS, Leffell DJ, Wolff K. *Fitzpatrick's Dermatology in General Medicine*. 8th ed. New York: McGraw-Hill, 2012.

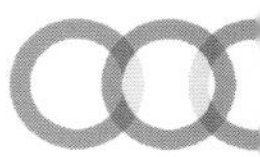

CASE 170

Barbara Pawel

Question

A 3-year-old boy presents to the emergency department with a history of fever for 2 days, knee pain, and a limp. On exam he is non-toxic appearing and there is point tenderness over the distal femur with minimal erythema, edema, and decreased range of motion. The patient has an antalgic gait. All other joints appear normal with full range of motion. There is no history of trauma or recent illness. He is fully immunized.

170.1

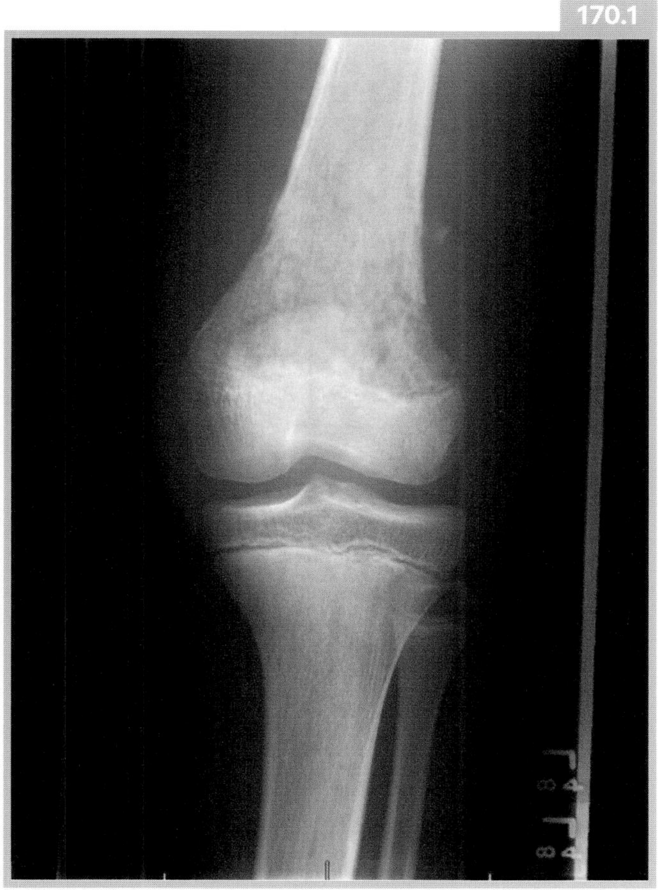

What would your initial workup be for this patient?

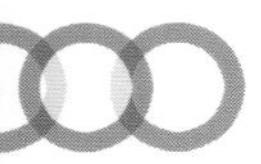

Answer

This patient has a history and exam that may indicate a musculoskeletal infection and should have laboratory investigations including a complete blood count with differential, erythrocyte sedimentation rate, C-reactive protein levels, and a blood culture. Synovial fluid should be obtained if there is a concern for septic arthritis. Lyme titers should be drawn if the patient has been in an area that is endemic for Lyme disease. Imaging with plain radiographs can be supplemented with ultrasound or MRI.

Acute hematogenous osteomyelitis develops when blood-borne bacteria seed the trabecular network of the bone, most commonly near the hip or knee. Bacterial cytotoxins and proteolytic enzymes cause tissue invasion and destruction. Osteomyelitis near the joint capsule can progress to secondary septic arthritis. Early recognition and use of appropriate antibiotics can reduce short term (sepsis) and long-term (growth disturbance, permanent joint destruction) sequelae.

Staphylococcus aureus is the most common causative organism. There has been up to a tenfold increase in methicillin-resistant *S. aureus* (MRSA) as the causative agent in musculoskeletal infections in children. Patients with MRSA have more extensive local soft tissue destruction, more rapid spread of infection, increased length of hospital stay, and often need repeated surgical interventions. They are also at high risk for serious complications, including persistent bacteremia, deep vein thrombosis (DVT), septic pulmonary emboli, and pathologic fractures.

The differentiation between methicillin-sensitive *S. aureus* (MSSA) and MRSA infections pre-culture can be difficult. A clinical predictive algorithm created to allow providers to predict the presence of MRSA has not been reproducible across varied patient populations. Molecular methods for rapid identification of MRSA are emerging but are not yet widely available. Awareness of epidemiological trends of MRSA within a local community can help guide initial treatment options.

Keywords: infectious diseases, orthopedics, limp, do not miss

Bibliography

Ratnayake K, Davis AJ, Brown L, Young TP. Pediatric acute osteomyelitis in the postvaccine, methicillin-resistant *Staphylococcus aureus* era. *AJEM* 2015;33:1420–4.

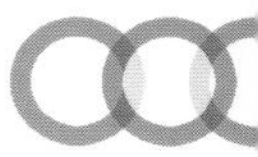

CASE 171

S. Margaret Paik

Question

A 5-month-old boy was brought for evaluation of bruises in his lower gums. The child has a past medical history of hemophilia (factor VIII deficiency). He has been doing well without any issues related to his hemophilia. The child drinks formula from a bottle and was started on rice cereal last month. The parents have noticed he has been chewing on the nipple of the bottle more.

The child is alert and smiling. There is no active bleeding from his mouth. There is ecchymoses of the lower gum.

171.1

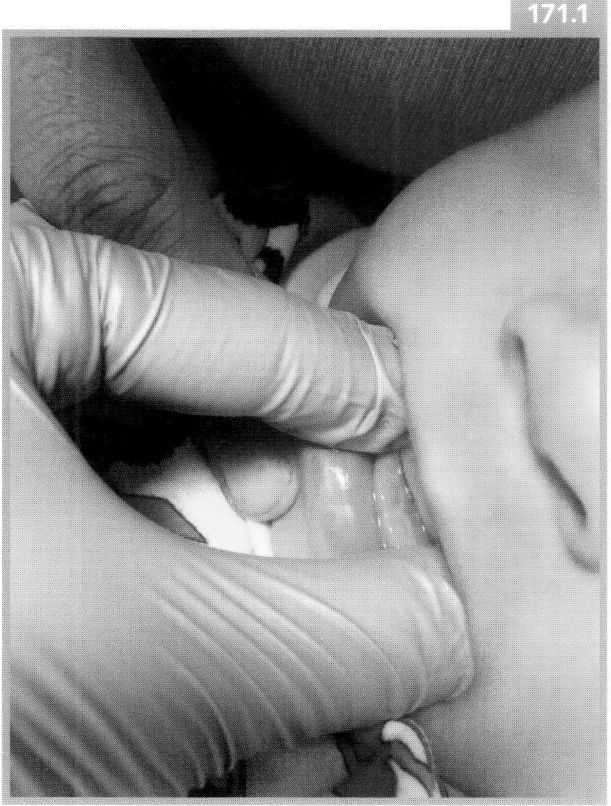

What is the most likely cause of this condition?

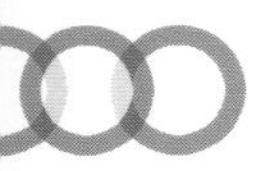

Answer

Ecchymoses outlines the erupting deciduous teeth as a result of bleeding due to hemophilia. Hemophilia A (factor VIII deficiency) is an X-linked recessive disorder and is more common than hemophilia B or Christmas disease (factor IX deficiency). Severity of hemophilia is classified based on percentage of the factor level.

- Severe: Factor level less than 1% normal
- Moderate: Factor level 1%–5% of normal
- Mild: Factor level more than 5%–40% of normal

Clinical manifestations will vary based on the severity and can range from intracranial hemorrhage in the newborn, epistaxis, easy bruising intramuscular hematomas, and gastrointestinal bleeding. Hemarthrosis is a hallmark presentation. Administration of factor is based on the severity and location of the bleeding.

Keywords: dental, hematology/oncology, dental injury

Bibliography

Shastry SP, Kaul R, Baroudi K, Umar D. Hemophilia A: Dental considerations and management. *J Int Soc Prev Community Dent* December 2014;4(Suppl 3):S147–52.

Smith, JA. Hemophilia: What the oral and maxillofacial surgeon needs to know. *Oral Maxillofacial Surg Clin N Am* 2016;28:481–9.

Srivastava A, Brewer AK, Mauser-Bunschoten EP, Key NS et al. Guidelines for the management of hemophilia. *Haemophilia* January 2013;19:e1–47.

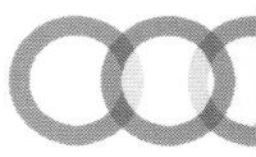

CASE 172

S. Margaret Paik

Question

A 10-year-old boy is brought with a concern for peeling of skin on his hands. He had complained of a sore throat and rash several days ago, but both symptoms have resolved. He is eating normally. His family feels he is improved but became concerned when they noticed skin peeling from his palms.

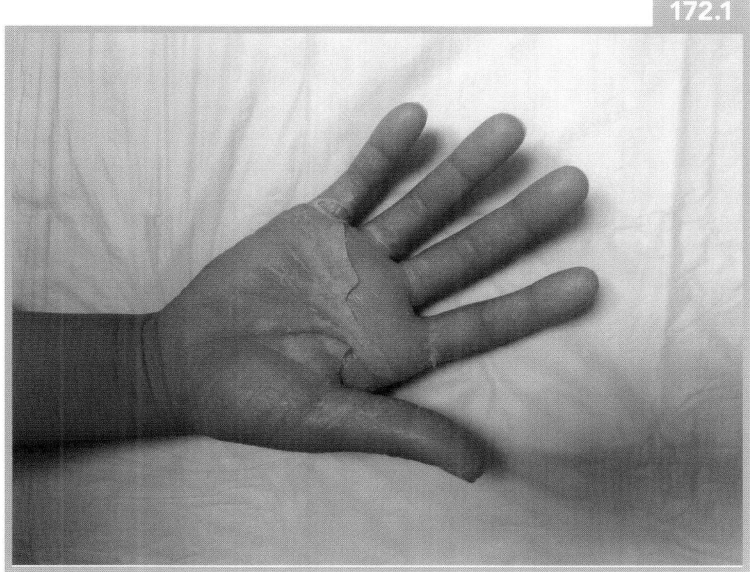

172.1

What is the most likely diagnosis? What additional studies can be done to confirm the diagnosis?

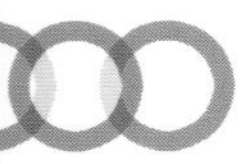

Answer

The history of sore throat and rash which preceded the peeling from the palms is consistent with a recent streptococcal infection (see Case 23). Several rapid antigen detection tests with varying sensitivities and specificities are commercially available. Throat culture can also be obtained. One or both of these tests may be negative due to the time course of the infection. Rising antistreptococcal antibody titers, antistreptolysin O (ASO), and antideoxyribonuclease B (DNase B) are reliable methods to detect a recent streptococcal infection. The ASO will rise after 1 week and reach a maximum level in 3 to 6 weeks. DNase B titers can appear at 2 weeks after infections and reach maximum titers levels in 6 to 8 weeks. Similar skin findings are seen after viral infections as well, most classically after coxsackie infection (hand-foot-mouth disease).

Keywords: dermatology, infectious diseases, benign

Bibliography

Block SL. Streptococcal pharyngitis: Guidelines, treatment issues, and sequelae. *Pediatr Ann* January 2014;43:1.

Schermer K, Gwynn L. Peeling rash in a 4-year-old boy. *Contemp Pediatr* 2016;33(9):41–8.

Spellerberg B, Brandt C. Laboratory diagnosis of *Streptococcus pyogenes* (group A streptococci). In *Streptococcus pyogenes: Basic Biology to Clinical Manifestations*, Ferretti JJ, Stevens DL, Fischetti VA, eds. Oklahoma City, OK: University of Oklahoma Health Sciences Center, February 10, 2016. Available from https://www.ncbi.nlm.nih.gov/books/NBK343617/.

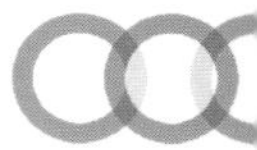

CASE 173

S. Margaret Paik

Question

The parents of an 8-year-old boy are concerned about swelling to both sides of his neck. They initially noticed the swelling one month ago and they have increased in size. They noted drainage today. He has been acting well and eating normally. There is no fever, change in voice, or drooling. The parents do not recall a history of fall or trauma to the neck.

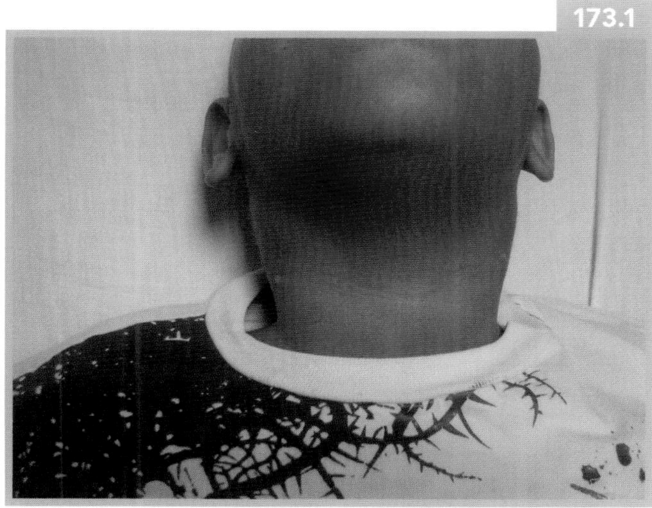

173.1

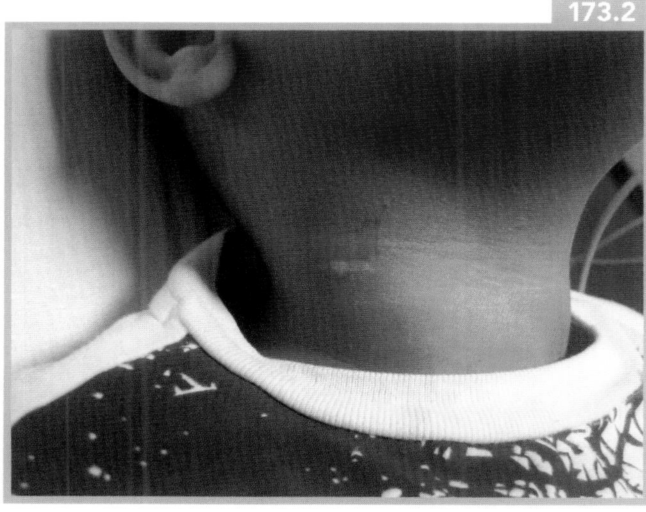

173.2

What is this and what is the best management for this?

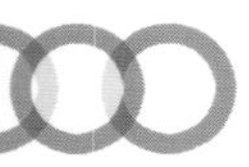

Answer

This is a branchial cleft cyst. Branchial cleft anomalies may present as a cyst, sinus, fistula, or cartilaginous remnant. The majority are cystic structures arising from the region of the second branchial arch. Most present in the first or second decade of life but some are noted at birth. A branchial cleft cyst is usually located superior to the clavicle, along the anterior border of the sternocleidomastoid muscle and presents as a painless, mobile, fluctuant mass. The differential diagnosis includes cervical lymphadenopathy, dermoid cyst, and cystic hygroma fibrous dysplasia of the sternocleidomastoid muscle. A thyroglossal duct cyst will present in the midline or paramidline at or below the level of the hyoid bone.

Patients should be referred for complete surgical excision. Incision and drainage or aspiration is associated with recurrence, wound infection, and hemorrhage.

Keywords: head and neck/ENT, congenital anomaly, skin and soft tissue infection

Bibliography

Gaddikeri S, Vattoth S, Gaddikeri RS, Stuart R, Harrison K, Young D, Bhargava P. Congenital cystic neck masses: Embryology and imaging appearances, with clinicopathologcial correlation. *Curr Probl Diagn Radiolo* 2014;43:55–67.

Leung AKC. Branchial cleft cyst. In *Encyclopedia of Molecular Mechanisms of Disease*, Lang F, ed. Berlin: Springer-Verlag, 2009, 244–5.

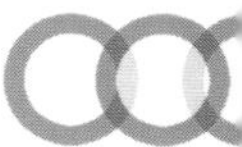

CASE 174

S. Margaret Paik

Questions

A 3-year-old girl, with a history of drooling and lethargy for the past day, is urgently brought to the emergency department by her mother. The mother notes a decrease in her daughter's oral intake for the past 2 days. She has had a runny nose and nonproductive cough for the past week. There was a temperature measured to 39.2°C today. The mother also noticed some swelling to the left side of her daughter's neck. The immunizations are up to date and she attends a day care facility.

On physical examination the child has a heart rate of 148, a respiratory rate of 30, oxygen saturation of 97% on room air, and a temperature of 39.6°C. The child is sleepy but able to be aroused. Her voice sounds hoarse when she cries. She is drooling clear oral secretions. There is swelling and tenderness to the left side of her neck with some mild overlying erythema. She cries when her head is moved to the left. Her lungs are clear to auscultation.

A peripheral IV is placed and she receives a normal saline fluid bolus of 20 mL/kg. The lateral neck radiograph and neck CT are obtained.

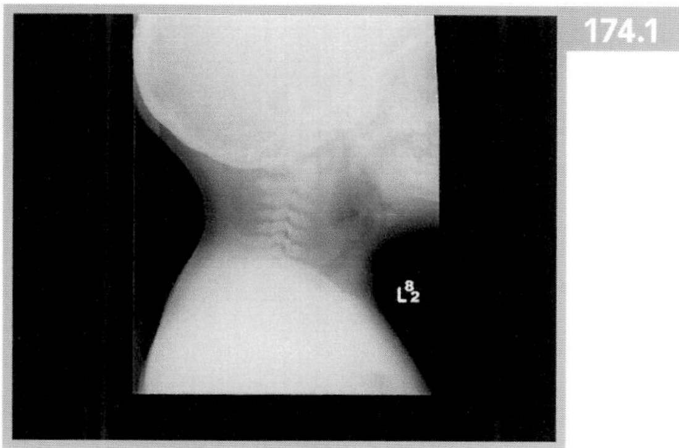

174.1

1. What is seen in the lateral neck radiograph and what are the potential pitfalls in interpretation? What is seen in the CT scan of the neck?
2. What organisms are seen in a retropharyngeal abscess?
3. What are the complications associated with a retropharyngeal abscess?

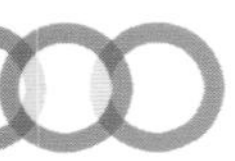

Answers

1. The prevertebral soft tissue space is widened. Thickening of the prevertebral soft tissue space greater than 7 mm at the level of the second cervical vertebrae and/or greater than 14 mm at the level of the sixth cervical vertebrae is abnormal. A lateral neck radiograph has a high false-positive rate due to positioning, swallowing, and respiratory effort. Computed tomography with intravenous contrast of the neck is done. The key image demonstrates an abscess in the retropharyngeal space. A retropharyngeal abscess is a suppurative deep neck infection occurring in the potential space between the posterior pharyngeal wall and prevertebral fascia, from the base of the skull to the posterior mediastinum.

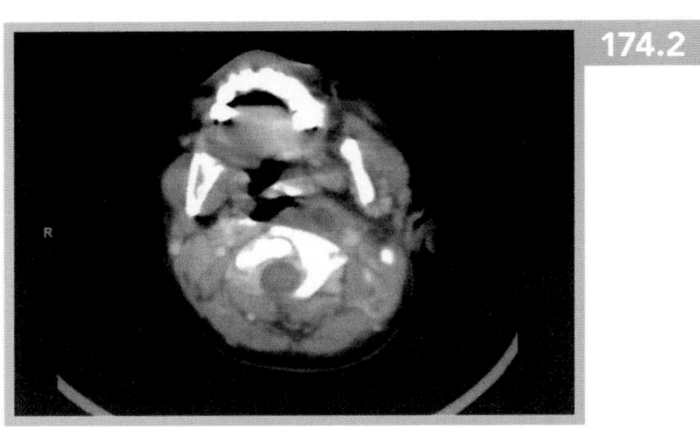

174.2

2. Causative organisms include group A beta-hemolytic *Streptococci*, *Staphylococcus aureus*, *Moraxella*, *Haemophilus*, polymicrobial, and mixed oropharyngeal flora including anaerobes.
3. Complications include airway compromise, especially with children <1 year of age. A definitive airway, when necessary, must be established cautiously and carefully to avoid rupture of the abscess. Mediastinitis is more common in younger children and in those with methicillin-resistant *S. aureus* with a mortality rate from 16.5% to 50%. Lemierre syndrome with thrombosis of the ipsilateral internal jugular vein is a rare complication but is increasing in incidence.

Keywords: head and neck/ENT, infectious diseases, airway, do not miss, CT

Bibliography

Bochner RE, Gangarm M, Belamarich PF. A clinical approach to tonsillitis, tonsillar hypertrophy, and peritonsillar and retropharyngeal abscesses. *Pediatr Rev* February 2017;38(2):81–92.

Jenkins IA, Saunders M. Infections of the airway. *Paediatr Anaesth* July 2009;19(Suppl 1):118–30.

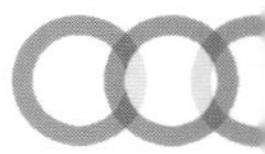

CASE 175

S. Margaret Paik

Question

A 5-year-old girl is brought to the emergency department with a complaint of bilateral lower leg pain for the past 2 days. There is a history of intermittent fever 1 week ago for 4 days, maximum temperature to 38.9°C. She had rhinorrhea, cough, and vomiting for 4 days at the start of her illness but these symptoms have resolved. The leg pain has increased in severity. Last night she refused to walk without assistance, prompting the visit to the emergency department.

The temperature is 37.6°C with a heart rate of 110 beats/minute and respiratory rate of 26 breaths/minute. The examination is remarkable for tenderness of both lower extremities, maximum at the calves. Motor strength is 4/5 bilaterally. The deep tendon reflexes are normal. She will only walk with assistance and is unable to flatten either foot as she bears weight on her feet.

175.1

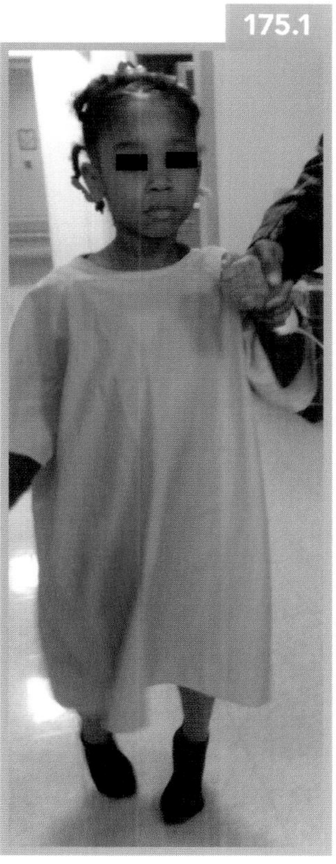

175.2

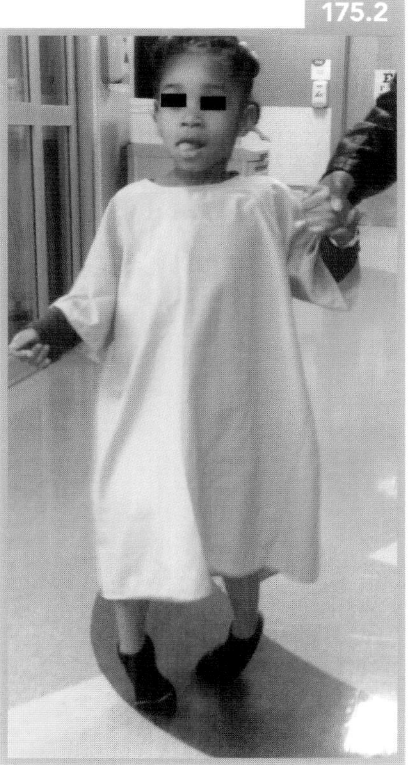

What laboratory test would be useful in making a diagnosis on this child? What conditions are associated with this condition?

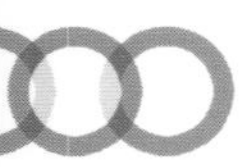

Answer

The serum creatine phosphokinase (CK) was elevated at 3310 U/L and physical findings indicate a diagnosis of myopathy. Additional laboratory studies demonstrated an elevated aspartate aminotransferase (AST) at 127 U/L. The white blood cell count was 6.6 K/uL with an unremarkable differential. The erythrocyte sedimentation rate and C-reactive protein were not elevated. The urine analysis had <3 red blood cells per high-power field. The respiratory viral panel was positive for influenza B, consistent with a diagnosis of viral myositis.

Influenza infections typically begin with systemic symptoms of fever, chills, headache, myalgia, and anorexia. Complications associated with influenza include pulmonary (pneumonia, croup, bronchiolitis), apnea in young infants, and myocarditis. Children may also have gastrointestinal complaints of abdominal pain, vomiting, and diarrhea. Myositis can present with sudden onset calf pain, associated with inability or difficulty in walking. It is more commonly associated with influenza B than with influenza A. This usually presents after the prodromal symptoms and differs from the diffuse myalgia that is usually seen during the initial onset of influenza. Boys are more frequently affected. Serum CK levels are markedly elevated. Myositis is generally self-limited and usually lasts less than a week. Rhabdomyolysis with myoglobinuria (see Case 194) and acute renal failure is uncommon.

Keywords: infectious diseases, neurology, limp

Bibliography

Dietzman DE, Schaller JG, Ray G, Reed ME. Acute myositis associated with influenza B infection. *Pediatrics* February 1976;57(2):255–8.

Hu J-J, Kao C-L, Lee P-I, Chen C-M, Lee C-Y, Lu C-Y, Huang L-M. Clinical features of influenza A and B in children and association with myositis. *J Microbiol Immunol Infect* 2004;37:95–8.

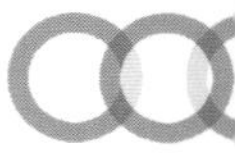

CASE 176

S. Margaret Paik

Question

An 18-month-old girl is brought in for yellow hands and feet. The parents believe they have seen the yellow discoloration for the past 2–3 months. There is no history of fever, vomiting, or weight loss. Her stool has been brown and formed. She is healthy otherwise and does not take any medications or nutritional supplements. Her immunizations are up to date.

Her vital signs are within normal limits. She is alert and very active. The physical exam is unremarkable except for an orange-yellow discoloration to her palms and soles. The sclerae are white in color. No hepatosplenomegaly is appreciated.

176.1

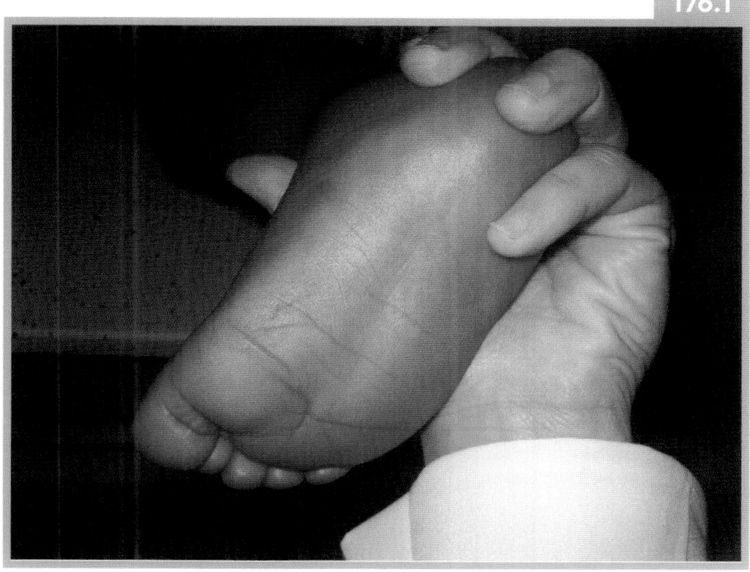

What is the differential diagnosis for this?

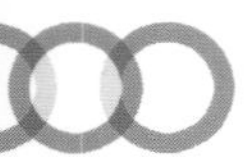

Answer

Jaundice is a consideration; however, the lack of icteric sclera makes this less likely. During the more detailed dietary history, the parents comment that their daughter is a very selective eater and will only take pureed carrots and sweet potatoes. She eats these several times a day, making carotenemia the most likely diagnosis. Carotene is found in pigmented fruits and vegetables. Carrots, squash, sweet potatoes, and pumpkin have a large amount of carotene. Serum carotene levels can be obtained to confirm the diagnosis, but in the setting of a suggestive dietary history, is not required. Elevated carotene levels can be associated with other conditions such as diabetes mellitus, hypothyroidism, and liver disease but is uncommon. Treatment is the reduction of carotene-rich foods.

Keywords: dermatology, benign, mimickers

Bibliography

Karthik SV, Campbell-Davidson D, Isherwood D. Carotenemia in infancy and its association with prevalent feeding practices. *Pediatric Dermatol* 2006;23:571–3.

Leung, AKC. Benign carotenemia in children. *Can Fam Physician* January 1989;35:81–3.

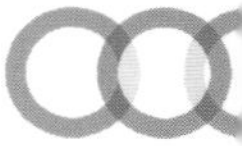

CASE 177

S. Margaret Paik

Question

A 4-month-old girl is brought by her parents with a concern for fever for 2 days. There was a temperature of 39.3°C today. She is taking a normal amount of formula from her bottle. The mother notes some loose stools without blood for one day. Bladder catheterization is ordered to evaluate for a urinary tract infection. The nurse is having difficulty in obtaining a specimen and asks you to examine the child.

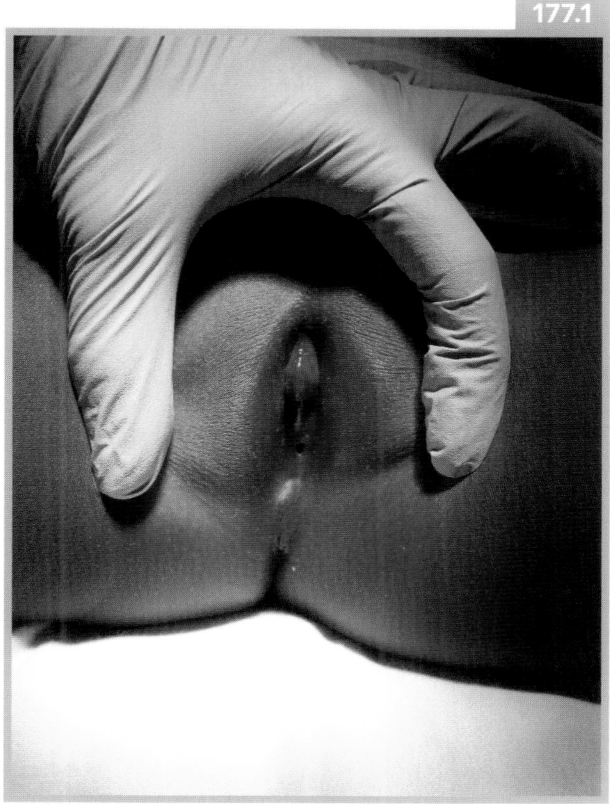

177.1

What is seen on visualization of the genital urinary and how should this be treated?

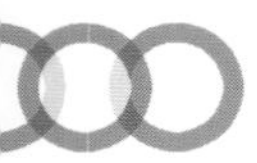

Answer

This child has labial adhesions (also called labial fusion, labial agglutination, and synechia vulvae). The cause is not known but may be associated with the low estrogen levels in pre-pubertal girls. Labial adhesions may be noted during a routine genital examination. Fusion can occur at the midline or below the labia minora. Presenting complaints include dysuria, recurrent urinary tract infections, vaginal pain, or discharge. Poor hygiene, candida vulvovaginitis, frequent diaper dermatitis, and genital trauma can lead to adhesions. Patients can also be asymptomatic. Topical estrogen cream is a conservative approach for symptomatic patients. Topical steroid cream can also be used. Manual or surgical separation of adhesions is indicated for patients with severe urinary flow obstruction and should be performed by an experienced physician.

Keywords: child abuse mimicker, gynecology, fever

Bibliography

Bacon JL, Romano ME, Quint EH. Clinical recommendation: Labial adhesions. *J Pediatr Adolesc Gynecol* October 2015;28(5):405–9.

Soyer T. Topical estrogen therapy in labial adhesions in children: Therapeutic or prophylactic? *J Pediatr Adolesc Gynecol* August 2007;20(4):241–4.

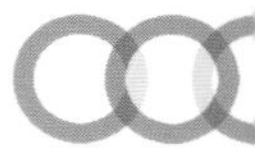

CASE 178

S. Margaret Paik

Questions

A 12-year-old boy is brought in after a fishhook was accidentally embedded into his scalp during a family fishing trip. There was some minor bleeding initially. There was no loss of consciousness and he has been acting normally.

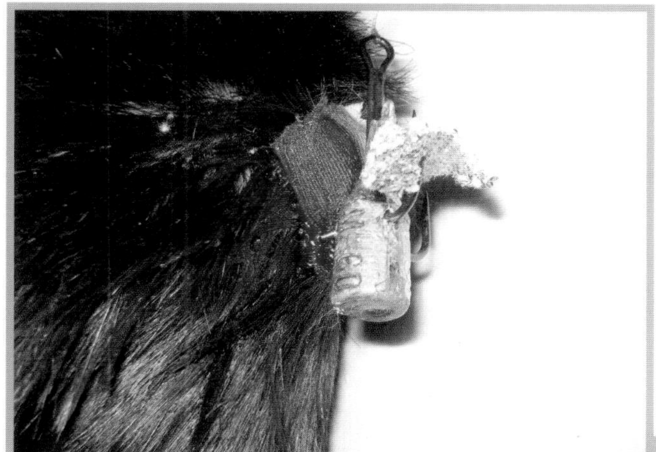

178.1

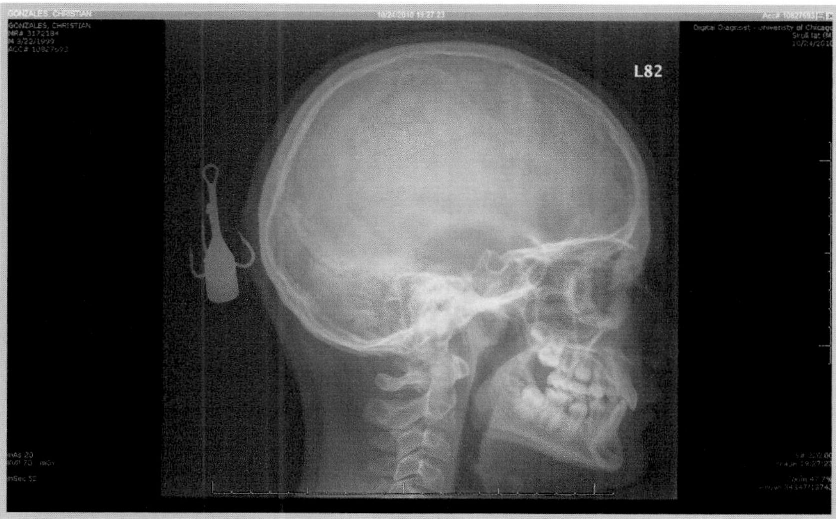

178.2

1. What additional information will aid in the management and removal?
2. What are methods for removal of a fishhook? What are the complications associated with removal?

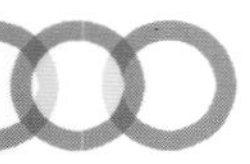

Answers

1. A radiograph of the skull can approximate the depth of the embedded hook and consider evaluate for bony penetration. The skull radiograph shows the fishhook in the soft tissue of the scalp.

2. Four primary methods for removal are (1) retrograde, (2) string-yank, (3) needle cover, (4) advance-and-cut (see Case 43). The method selected is based on anatomic location and the type of fishhook. The retrograde and string-yank method are less invasive than the needle cover and advance-and-cut methods, resulting in less tissue trauma. Post-removal wound care includes exploration for additional foreign bodies (e.g. grass, bait) and tetanus administration if indicated. Studies do not support the use of prophylactic antibiotics. Prophylactic antibiotics may be considered in immunosuppressed patients, those with poor wound healing (e.g. diabetes mellitus), and deeper wounds involving the tendon, cartilage, or bone.

Keywords: penetrating trauma, head injury, procedures, foreign body

Bibliography

Dose C, Cooper WL, Ediger WM, Magen NA, Mildbrand CS, Schulte CD. Fishhook injuries: A prospective evaluation. *Am J Emerg Med* September 1991;9(5):413–5.

Gammons M, Jackson E. Fishhook removal. *Am Fam Physician* June 2001;63(11):2231–6.

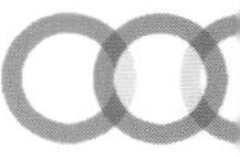

CASE 179

Barbara Pawel

Question

A 4-year-old girl presented to the emergency department with difficulty sleeping and restlessness for 2 weeks. The mother has notes that she is rubbing her buttocks.

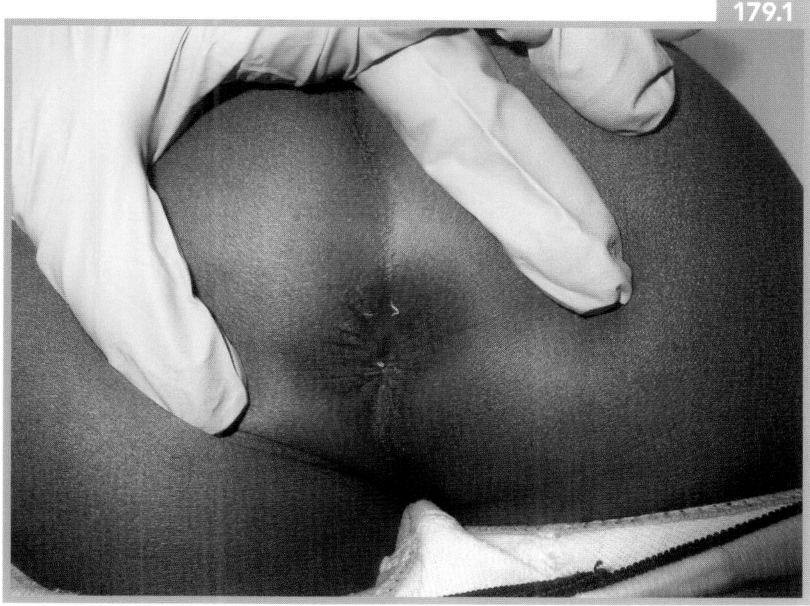

179.1

What gynecologic complications can be associated with the extraintestinal migration of adult pinworms?

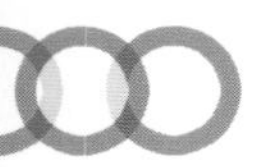

Answer

Vulvovaginitis with increased incidence of UTI (urinary tract infection), salpingitis, oophoritis, and peritoneal inflammation have been described in association with pinworm infestations.

Pinworm infestation (*Enterobius vermicularis*) is the most common helminth infection in the United States. Humans are the only natural host. Infections are common in pre-school and school-age children, their caretakers, and in institutionalized patients. Autoinfection occurs after scratching (fecal-oral route). Eggs beneath fingernails contaminate food, clothing, linens, and carpeting facilitating spread among household members. Adult worms lay eggs on perianal skin at night causing inflammation. Infections can be asymptomatic but a common complaint is anal itching causing difficulty sleeping and restlessness. A high worm burden can cause abdominal pain, nausea, and vomiting. Pinworms should be part of the differential for vulvovaginitis in prepubescent females. Adult pinworms have been found in surgically removed inflamed appendices but causality has not been proven. The diagnosis can be confirmed by an adhesive pad or tape pressed to the perianal area at night or in the early morning pre-bathing. Eggs and adult worms (8–13 mm) can be seen. These are generally not passed in the stool. Pinworms can be treated with antihelminthics such as mebendazole or albendazole: Two doses given 2 weeks apart. Reinfection is common and can be reduced by treating the entire household, washing all clothes and bed linens, good hand hygiene, daily bathing, and frequent nail clipping.

Keywords: infectious diseases, gynecology, child abuse mimicker, infestation

Bibliography

Rajpal TM, Mottaghi TM, Keith L, Patel A. A prepubertal girl with persistent vaginal pruritus. *Pediatr Ann* 2014;43(7):262–4.

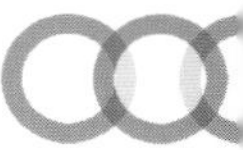

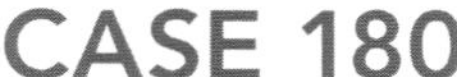

CASE 180

Barbara Pawel

Question

A 2-year-old boy presents to the emergency department with red swollen lips, a perioral rash, and drooling after drinking callus remover. The active ingredients were available on the product container. The pH was tested in the emergency department and was 12.

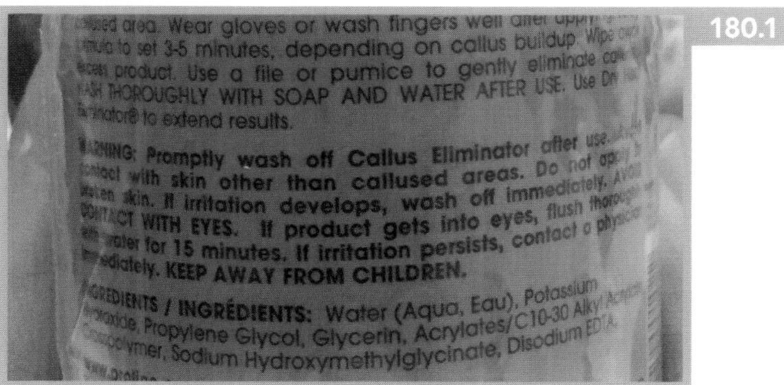

180.1

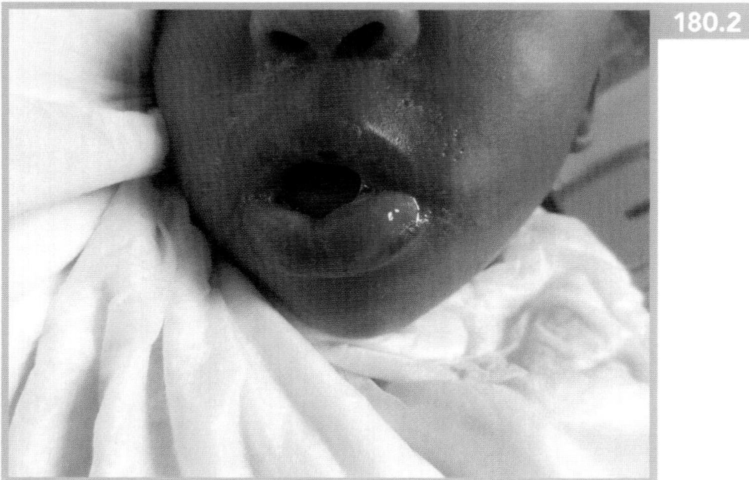

180.2

What common modalities of treatment for ingestions are not recommended in this patient?

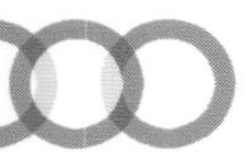

Answer

- Ipecac is contraindicated in caustic ingestions due to the potential for re-exposure of the esophageal mucosa leading to further injury.
- Oral dilution/neutralizing agents may also result in vomiting and re-exposure to the caustic agent.
- Blind nasogastric tube insertion carries a high risk of esophageal perforation. An nasogastric tube may be placed during endoscopy for circumferential burns to act as a stent.
- Corticosteroids have not been proven to prevent strictures but can be considered if there are symptoms of airway involvement (uncommon).
- Broad-spectrum antibiotics have been used if steroids are administered, in patients with deep ulcerations and necrosis on endoscopy or if there are signs and/or symptoms of infection. There have been no prospective studies on the use of antibiotics post caustic ingestion and are not routinely recommended.

Most caustic ingestions in children occur in the 12 to 48 months age group, are accidental, and involve alkali agents such as household cleaners, especially if not in the original container (commonly a water or soda bottle). Alkali substances are usually odorless and tasteless allowing for ingestion of large volumes. Even small volumes with a pH above 11 can cause severe burns. Strong alkali agents cause liquefactive necrosis most typically involving the esophagus. Acids have a bitter taste but more rapid transit. Lesser volumes may be ingested but more gastric injuries occur.

Endoscopy should be done within 12–24 hours if there is a history of significant ingestion with symptoms (drooling, dysphagia, feeding refusal, abdominal pain, vomiting) or if there are oral burns. Patients with a questionable history of ingestion, who are asymptomatic and without oral burns should have an oral challenge of fluids and a period of observation. Minor oral burns in children tolerating oral fluids may not need further therapy. Greater than 50% of ingestions in teenagers/adults are part of a suicide attempt. These ingestions involve larger volumes that are more rapidly swallowed, sparing the oropharynx. Endoscopy should be strongly considered even if the patient is asymptomatic.

Long-term complications include esophageal strictures, perforation, abnormal motility, gastric, or intestinal injury. There is an increased risk of esophageal carcinoma developing 1–3 decades post ingestion.

Keywords: head and neck/ENT, oropharyngeal injury, toxicology, gastrointestinal

Bibliography

Kurowski JA, Kay M. Caustic ingestions and foreign bodies ingestions in pediatric patients. *Pediatr Clin N Am* 2017;64(3):507–24.

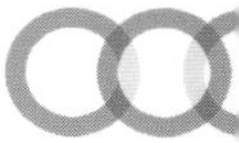

CASE 181

S. Margaret Paik

Questions

A grandmother brings her 3-year-old grandson to the emergency department for a rash she has noted for 2 weeks. She initially noticed a few lesions on his right upper arm, now spreading to his chest and back. He has been well otherwise without fever.

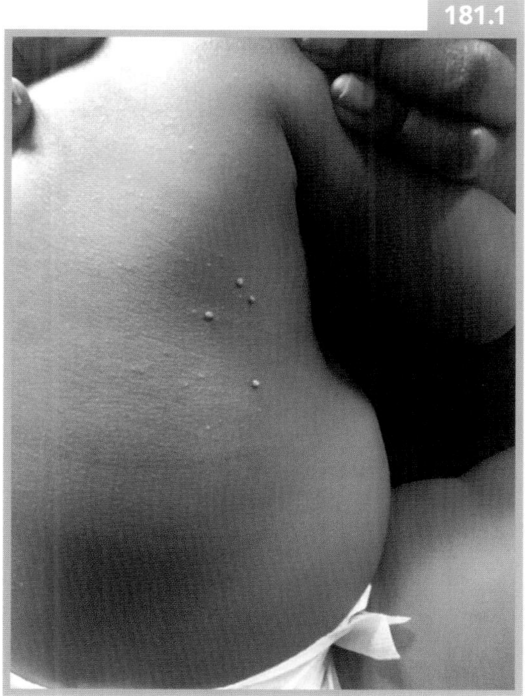

181.1

1. What is cause of these lesions?
2. What are the treatment options?

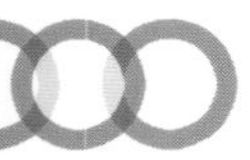

Answers

1. This is *Molluscum contagiosum* caused by a poxvirus and presents with discrete, dome-shaped, flesh-colored papules. Some papules can have central umbilication. The papules average 3–5 mm in diameter. The condition is commonly seen in childhood; it can also be seen in adolescents and adults. The infection is localized to the skin in immunocompetent individuals. *Molluscum contagiosum* is generally self-limited with an average duration of 2 months for a single lesion. Scratching and trauma can cause autoinoculation increasing the duration of symptoms for 8–12 months or longer.

2. Therapy options include physical (curettage, cryotherapy, pulsed dye laser), destructive chemical agents (phenol), non-destructive chemical agents (cantharidin 0.9%, podophyllotoxin 0.3%–0.5% cream, salicylic acid gel 12%, benzoyl peroxide 10% cream, retinoic acid 0.5% cream, potassium hydroxide solution 5%–10%), and immune modulators (imiquimod 5% cream, cimetidine). No single therapy has been shown to be more effective than the others. Some patients will choose supportive therapy given the potential complications of pain, scarring, hyperpigmentation, and hypopigmentation as a result of the therapy options.

Keywords: dermatology, rash, skin and soft tissue infection

Bibliography

Chen X, Anstey AV, Bugert JJ. *Molluscum contagiosum* virus infection. *Lancet Infect Dis* 2013;13(10):877–88.

Dohil MA, Lin P, Lee J, Lucky AW, Paller AS, Eichenfield LF. The epidemiology of *Molluscum contagiosum* in children. *J Am Acad Dermatol* January 2006;54(1):47–54.

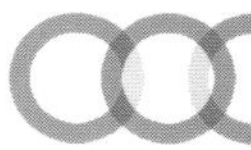

CASE 182

Barbara Pawel

Questions

An 11-month-old infant presents to the emergency department with the chief complaint: "cries when mother picks him up." No fever or other symptoms were reported. A chest x ray demonstrates a healing rib fracture of the left 10th rib.

182.1

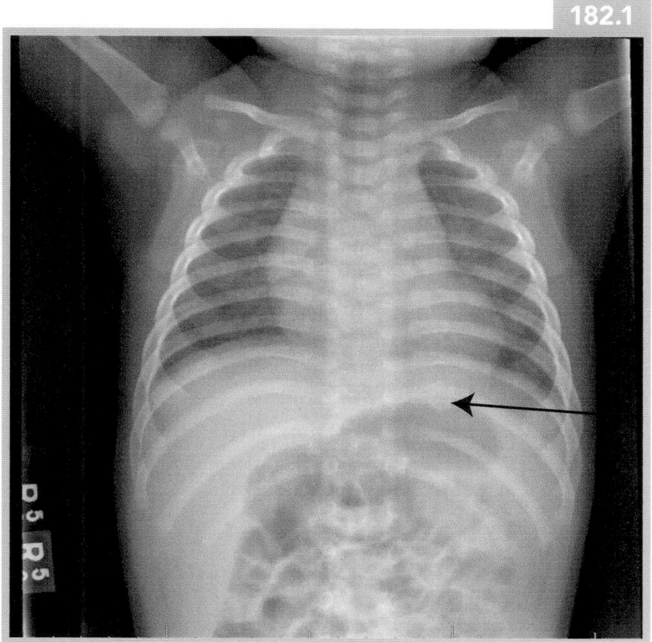

1. List some findings in the history and physical examination of a child with a rib fracture that would concern you for non-accidental trauma (NAT).
2. Which rib fracture patterns are more concerning for additional injuries?

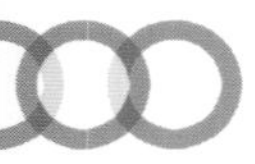

Answers

1.
- Rib fractures in infants (extremely uncommon)
- Rib fractures without a history of significant trauma (ribs pliable)
- Non-displaced multiple sequential rib fractures (finger placement)
- Multiple fractures in various stages of healing
- Different co-existing injuries
- Inconsistent/variations in history for developmental age, injury severity, or pattern

2.
- Fracture of ribs 9–12 (right: liver injury, left: spleen injury)
- Fracture of ribs 1, 2, or 3 (mediastinal/aortic injury)
- Consider additional imaging (CT chest or abdomen) and labs (liver function tests, lipase, urine analysis) if concerned for internal injuries

Most rib fractures are caused by direct blunt trauma to the chest wall. A single blow can cause multiple fractures at the site of impact or at the posterolateral bend (weakest area of rib). Rib fractures can present with focal tenderness exacerbated by breathing and movement. Non-displaced fractures and fractures at the costochondral margins are often missed on chest radiographs. Oblique views or a bone scan can identify missed fractures. Rib fractures become most apparent during callus formation (at 10–14 days after injury). The chest radiograph may show pneumothorax and/or hemothorax. When fracture is the only concern for NAT consider consulting subspecialists to help rule out metabolic or genetic disorders such as rickets or osteogenesis imperfecta. These entities are rare and do not exclude co-existing NAT.

Keywords: child abuse, blunt trauma, do not miss

Bibliography

Kellogg ND, Committee on Child Abuse and Neglect. Evaluation of suspected child physical abuse. *Pediatrics* 2007;119(6):1232–41.

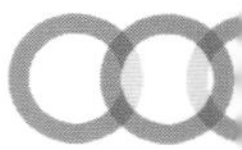

CASE 183

S. Margaret Paik

Question

A 3-year-old is brought into the emergency department after falling onto his right shoulder on the playground. He did not hit his head and he is acting normally. His only complaint is right shoulder pain.

He is alert and cooperative with normal vital signs. He cries when his right upper chest wall is palpated. There is tenderness and swelling along the right clavicle. The overlying skin is intact. He is able to move his right hand and fingers normally with a strong grip strength of his fingers but refuses to lift his right upper extremity above his head.

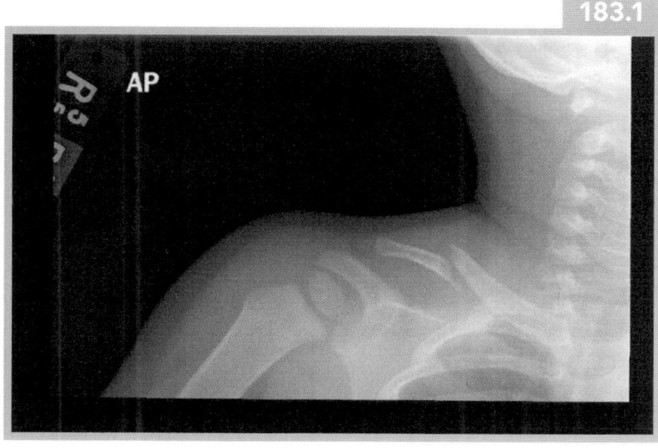

183.1

What is the most likely diagnosis? What are the treatment options?

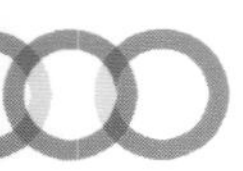

Answer

This is a closed midshaft clavicle fracture. Clavicle fractures are divided into three groups: proximal, middle, and distal third of the clavicle. Fractures of the middle third are the most frequent with either an oblique or transverse fracture line. Shortening, displacement, and comminution are common. The usual mechanism of injury is either a fall onto an outstretched hand or a fall onto the shoulder. Stabilization of the airway with appropriate management of any hemodynamic instability is paramount if there has been any compromise as a result of injury. Emergent specialist consultation is required for displaced fractures with tenting of the overlying skin, open fractures, and those with neurovascular compromise. Non-operative therapy with either a sling or figure-of-eight device is used for comfort and is the treatment of choice in children and adolescents. There is a very low incidence of complications because of bone remodeling in children and adolescents.

Fractures distal to the coracoclavicular ligament can result in nonunion. Fractures of the proximal end of the clavicle are usually not displaced and nonunion is rare.

Keywords: orthopedics, blunt trauma, chest pain

Bibliography

Allman FL Jr. Fractures and ligamentous injuries of the clavicle and its articulation. *J Bone Joint Surg Am* 1967;49(4):774–84.

van de Meijden OA, Gaskill TR, Millett PJ. Treatment of clavicle fractures: Current concepts review. *J Shoulder Elbow Surg* 2012;21(3):423–9.

Zlowodzki M, Zelle BA, Cole PA, Jeray K, Mckee MD. Treatment of acute midshaft clavicle fractures: Systematic review of 2144 fractures: On behalf of the evidence-based orthopaedic trauma working group. *J Orthop Trauma*, August 2005;19(7):504–7.

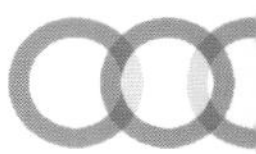

CASE 184

Nina Mbadiwe

Question

An 18-month-old girl presents to the emergency department for a limp which has been present for the past day. There is no history of fevers or URI (upper respiratory infection) symptoms. The parents deny any trauma or falls. She has been crying on and off for the past day but otherwise is eating and drinking normally. She has no other symptoms. On physical exam, she is able to bear weight on both of her legs but appears uncomfortable when doing so. There is no erythema, swelling, or warmth of the joints and she has full range of motion of both lower extremities without discomfort. A radiograph of her lower leg shows a fracture.

184.1

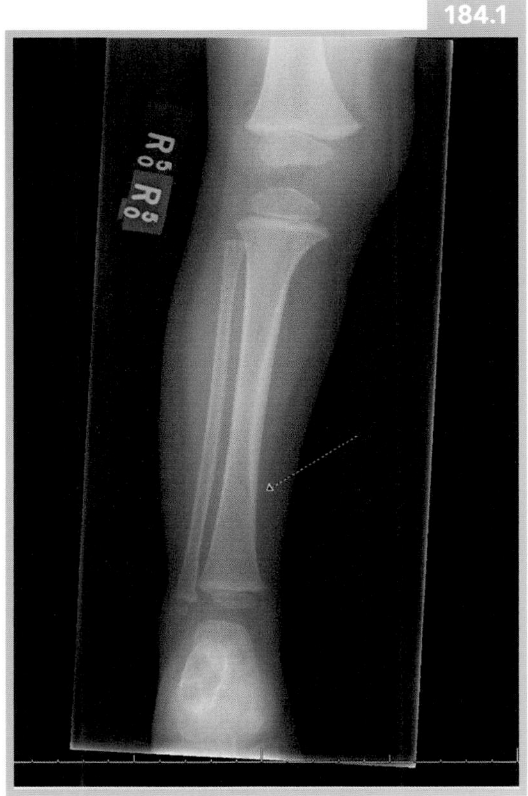

What type of fracture is this? What is the most common mechanism for this type of injury?

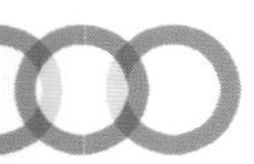

Answer

This is a toddler's fracture, one of the most common fractures in children younger than 4 years old. In most cases, the fracture is located in the distal two-thirds of the tibia. Typically, it has a non-displaced and spiral pattern. It is usually caused by low energy trauma with a rotation component as when a child twists the leg during a fall. This commonly occurs when the child is first learning to walk and run. On physical examination, localized tenderness with minimal swelling or bruising is common. Patients also refuse to walk or bear weight and may regress to crawling.

Treatment is placement in a long leg cast with non-weight-bearing for 3–4 weeks.

Keywords: orthopedics, extremity injury, limp

Bibliography

Miller D, Rosenwasser K, Hsu A, Franzone J. Toddler's fracture. In *Orthopedic Emergencies*, Makhni MC, Makhni EC, Swart EF, Day CS, eds. Cham, Switzerland: Springer, 2017:493–6.

Schuh AM, Whitlock KB, Klein EJ. Management of toddler's fractures in the pediatric emergency department. *Pediatr Emerg Care* July 2016;32(7):452–4.

Zitelli BJ, Davis HW. *Atlas of Pediatric Physical Diagnosis*. 5th ed. Philadelphia: Mosby/Elsevier, 2007.

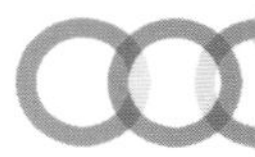

CASE 185

Barbara Pawel

Question

A previously healthy 3-year-old male presents to the emergency department with progressive shortness of breath, cough, and ankle swelling. He was diagnosed by his primary medical doctor 1 week ago with an upper respiratory infection and was started on antibiotics after an urgent care visit 3 days ago. A chest radiograph shows an enlarged cardiothymic silhouette with pulmonary congestion. The ECG is shown.

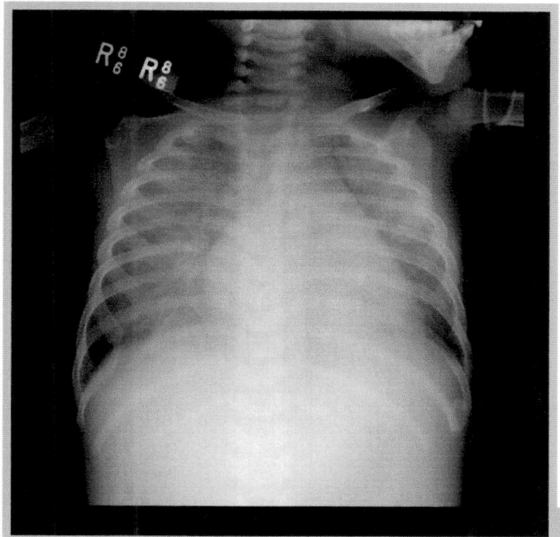

185.1

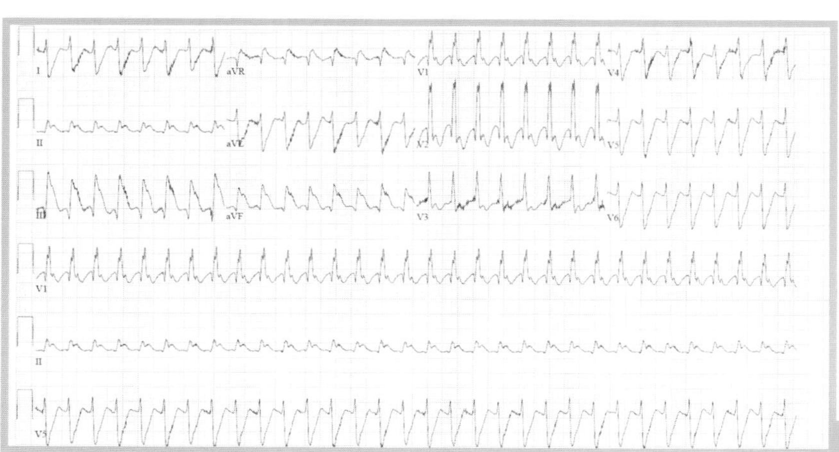

185.2

What is the most common cause of myocarditis in pediatric patients?

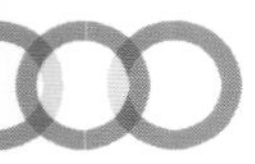

Answer

Viral infections such as enterovirus (coxsackie group B), adenovirus, parvovirus B19, EBV, HHV6, influenza, and others.

Myocarditis is inflammation of the heart muscle with myocyte damage causing myocardial dysfunction and subsequent heart failure. Presentation varies from subclinical cases to sudden cardiac death. A mild prodrome (nonspecific upper respiratory infection or gastrointestinal symptoms) precedes cardiovascular symptoms by 7–14 days (congestive heart failure, palpitations, syncope). Tachypnea, grunting, increased work of breathing, and tachycardia are common. Variability in presentation and nonspecific labs make initial diagnosis difficult. Less invasive tests are preferred over biopsy due to procedural risks. Inflammatory markers are nonspecific. Cardiac enzymes (troponin T $\geq$ 0.01 ng/mL: Sn 100%, Sp 85%) are the most useful studies in the initial workup. Sinus tachycardia on ECG is common. Dysrhythmias (SVT and VT—as shown in this case), conduction abnormalities (heart block), and pseudo-infarct patterns have also been described. The chest radiograph is abnormal in 90% (cardiomegaly and pulmonary edema). Echocardiograph (ECHO) is abnormal in 98% (wall motion or valvular abnormalities). Neither ECHO, ECG, nor chest radiograph are specific for myocarditis but are helpful to rule out pneumonia, pulmonary embolism, structural abnormalities, and acute coronary syndrome. Cardiac MRI is more sensitive and specific than echocardiogram. Initial management is based on severity and includes supportive therapy and cardiovascular stabilization (monitoring, antiarrhythmics, vasodilators, inotropes, and diuretics). In fulminant disease, mechanical support (ECMO, VAD) acts as a bridge before transplant.

Keywords: cardiology, infectious diseases, ECG, chest pain

Bibliography

Pettit MA, Koyfman A, Foran M. Myocarditis. *Pediatr Emerg Care* 2014;30(11):832–6.

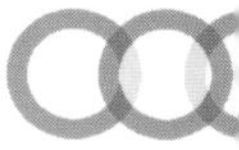

CASE 186

S. Margaret Paik

Question

An 11-year-old girl with sickle cell disease (SCD) hemoglobin SS is brought in by her mother with a complaint of nonproductive cough and fever to 38.7°C for one day. She is complaining of chest pain that is made worse with coughing and deep inspiration. She has a history of vaso-occlusive pain crisis starting at 18 months of age, typically presenting with upper and lower extremity pain. She has not had other complications associated with sickle cell disease. She has never received transfusion of any blood products.

She is quiet but alert with a respiratory rate of 34 breaths/minute, heart rate 122 beats/minute, blood pressure 112/80, temperature 39.0°C, oxygen saturation on room air 89%. The lung sounds are diminished bilaterally with crackles in both lower lung fields. She is given supplemental oxygen. Intravenous access is established, blood for laboratory studies and cultures is drawn, and a dose of parenteral antibiotics is started. The chest radiograph is shown.

186.1

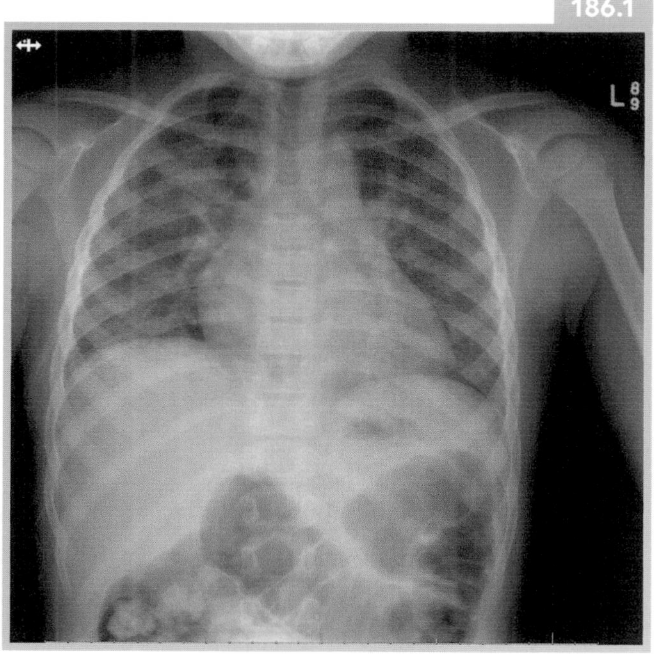

What is the likely diagnosis in this patient? What complications are related to this condition?

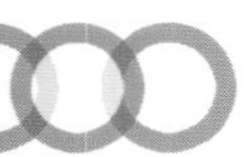

Answer

The chest radiograph demonstrates hazy opacities in the upper lung fields. The history of fever, tachypnea, hypoxia, and new pulmonary infiltrate on the chest radiograph is consistent with acute chest syndrome (ACS) in this patient with SCD. The syndrome of ACS includes both infectious and non-infectious causes. ACS has a disease spectrum ranging from mild pneumonia to respiratory distress syndrome and multi-organ failure. ACS is one of the more common reasons for hospitalization and is a leading cause of morbidity and mortality. Patients may present initially with vaso-occlusive pain crisis without signs and symptoms of ACS until 24–72 hours later. The most common presenting symptoms are cough, pleuritic chest pain, and shortness of breath. Younger children may present with fever, cough, and wheezing. Clinical signs can precede radiographic findings. Other considerations and complications include evaluation for pulmonary embolism, fluid overload/overhydration, respiratory depression due to opiate use, and hypoventilation secondary to pain.

The patient was admitted to the hospital. Several hours later she became more short of breath with tachypnea and an increased need for supplemental oxygen. A second chest radiograph shows increased opacifications.

186.2

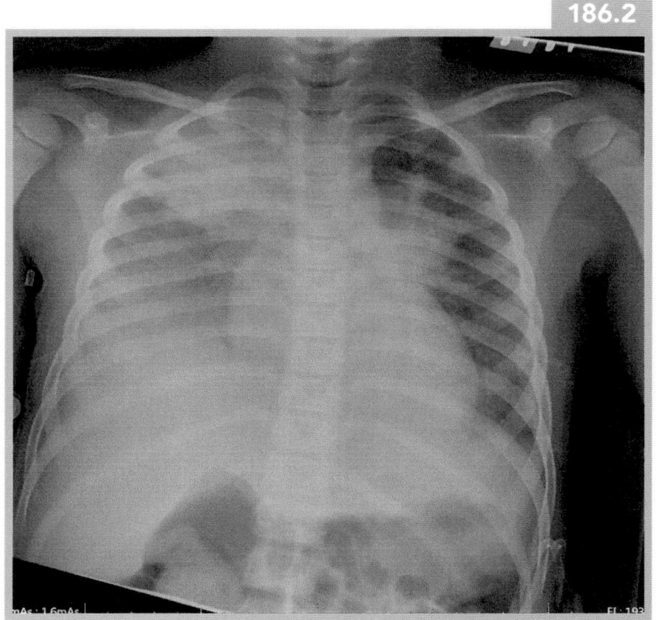

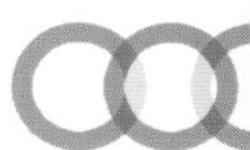

She was transferred to the intensive care unit. Her respiratory status continued to deteriorate, necessitating intubation, mechanical ventilation, and an exchange transfusion.

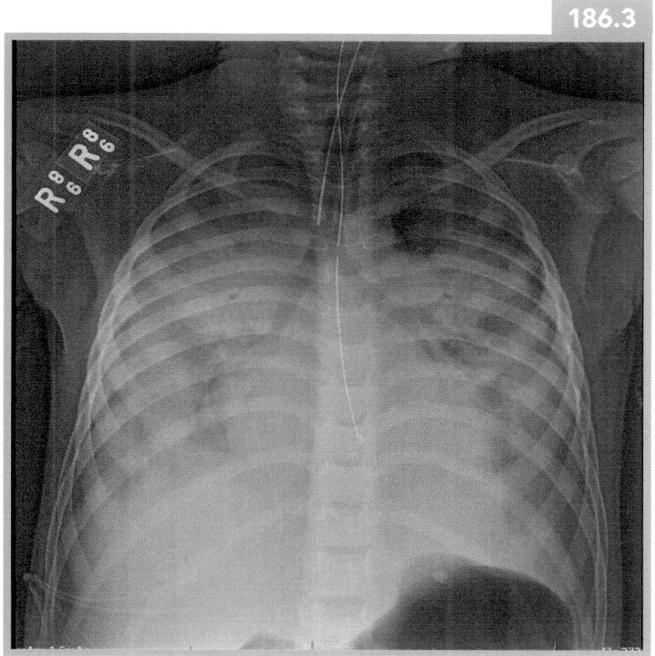

186.3

Keywords: hematology/oncology, pulmonary, chest pain, respiratory distress, do not miss

Bibliography

Castro O, Brambilla DJ, Thorington B, Reindorf CA, Scott RB, Gillette P, Vera JC, Levy PS. The acute chest syndrome in sickle cell disease: Incidence and risk factors. The Cooperative Study of Sickle Cell Disease. *Blood* 1994;84(2):643–9.

Howard J, Hart N, Roberts-Harewood M, Cummins M, Awogbade M, Davis B on behalf of the BCSH Committee. Guidelines on the management of acute chest syndrome sickle cell disease. *Br J Haematol* 2015;169:492–505.

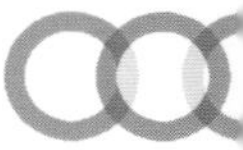

CASE 187

S. Margaret Paik

Question

The parents of a 2-week-old baby boy come to the emergency department after they had seen clear drainage and a red knot on his umbilicus today after the umbilical cord fell off. The baby is a term infant, delivered by normal spontaneous vaginal delivery. The mother received prenatal care and did not have any infections during her pregnancy. The baby has been nursing normally. There is no history of fever.

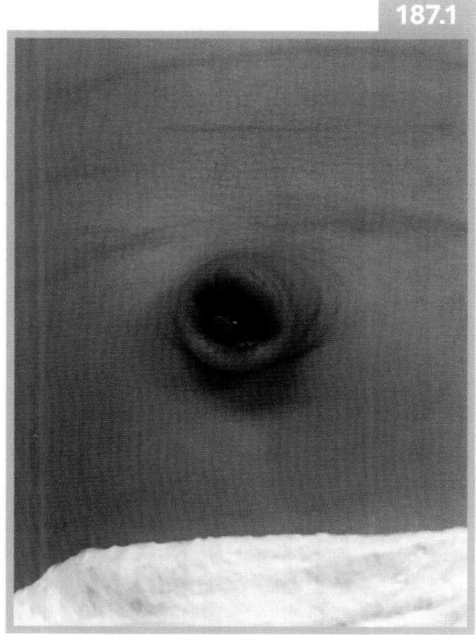

187.1

What does this baby have? What are the treatment options and complications associated with this condition?

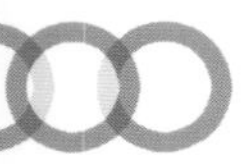

Answer

This baby has an umbilical granuloma. Incomplete epithelialization after separation of the umbilical cord can lead to reddish granulation tissue and is not infected as seen in omphalitis (see Case 195). Overgrowth of this granulation tissue can result in the formation of an umbilical granuloma. The lesion may be friable, moist with drainage, and can measure from 3 to 10 mm. Application of silver nitrate (75%) sticks to the umbilical granuloma produces a chemical cautery and must be done cautiously. Burns to the surrounding skin have been reported. Patients usually require several applications. Excision and application of absorbable hemostatic material is another treatment option.

Keywords: neonate, dermatology, benign

Bibliography

Chamberlain JM, Gorman RL, Young GM. Silver nitrate burns following treatment for umbilical granuloma. *Pediatr Emerg Care* 1992;8(1):29–30.

Nagar H. Umbilical granuloma: A new approach to an old problem. *Pediatr Surg Int* September 2001;17(7): 513–4.

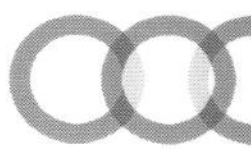

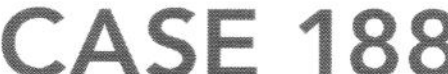

CASE 188

S. Margaret Paik

Question

A 13-year-old boy is brought in by a school coach after he complained of sudden onset of left hip pain during soccer (football) practice. There was acute onset of pain after he had kicked the ball with his left foot. There is increased pain at his left hip with internal rotation of his left leg in extension. He is unable to bear weight.

188.1

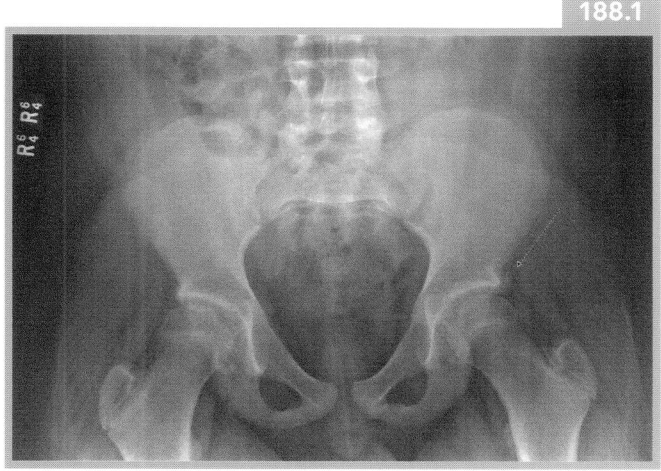

What does the radiograph of his pelvis and left hip show?

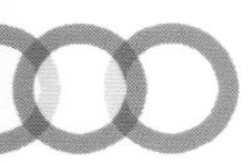

Answer

This is an avulsion fracture of the left anterior inferior iliac spine due to the sudden forceful contraction of the rectus femoris. Avulsion fractures occur in skeletally immature athletes with indirect trauma due to the force from sudden or unbalanced muscle contractions. Other commonly involved muscle and pelvic sites include the sartorius and anterior superior iliac spine and the hamstrings and ischial tuberosity. Initial management is conservative with rest and ice followed by limited protected weight-bearing with crutches and then light isometric stretching.

Keywords: orthopedics, trauma, extremity injury, blunt trauma, limp

Bibliography

Kocher MS, Tucker R. Pediatric athlete hip disorders. *Clin Sports Med* 2006;25(2):241–53.

Rossi F, Dragoni S. Acute avulsion fractures of the pelvis in adolescent competitive athletes: Prevalence, location and sports distribution of 203 cases collected. *Skeletal Radiol* 2001;30:127–31.

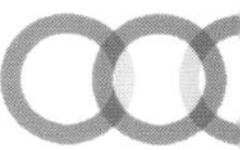

CASE 189

Barbara Pawel

Question

A 6-year-old male presents to the emergency department with a <1 cm laceration over his medial malleolus after falling onto broken glass. He refused to bear weight, or dorsiflex or plantarflex his ankle due to pain.

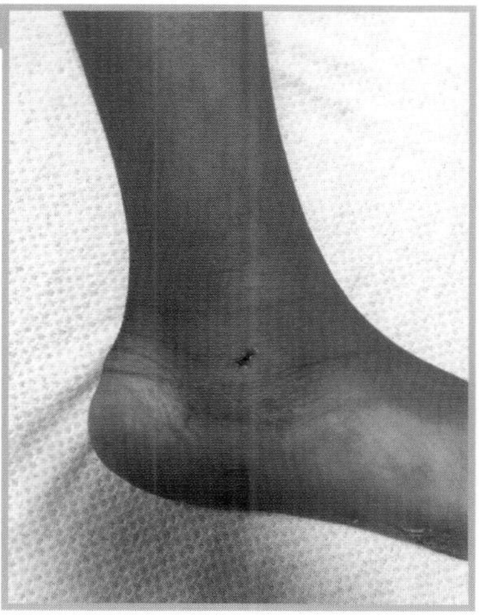

189.1

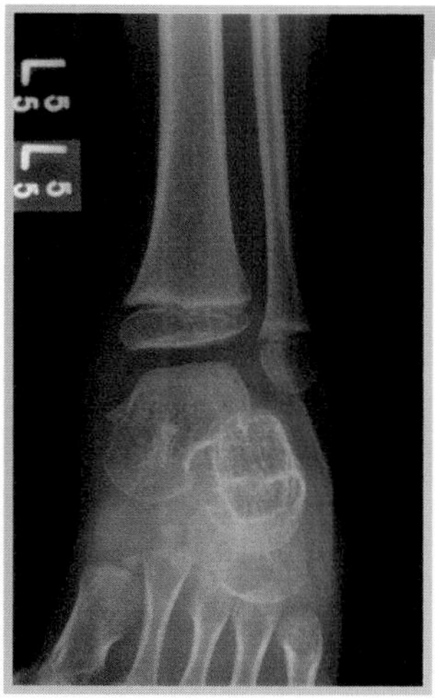

189.2

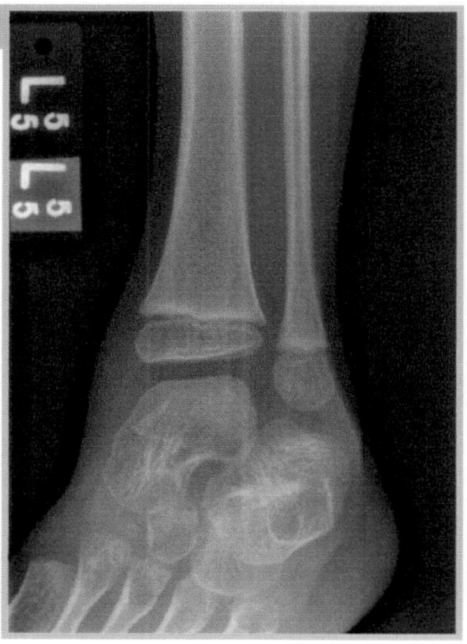

189.3

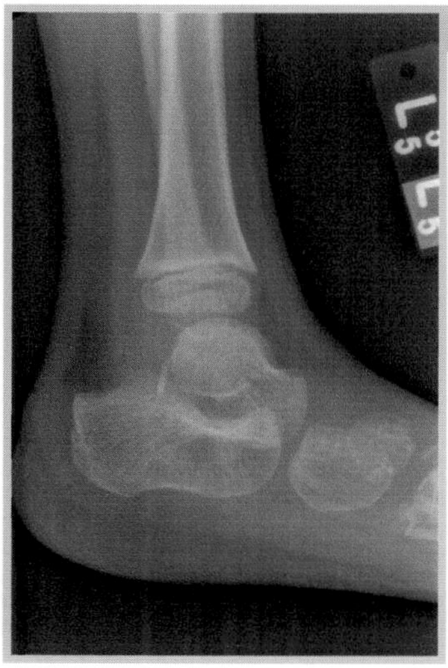

189.4

What are the indications for ordering an imaging study in this patient?

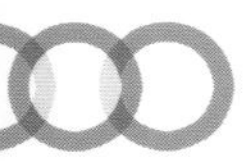

Answer

This patient presented with a history of sustaining a laceration on broken glass. Since the laceration is small it is not possible to visualize the base of the laceration to inspect for foreign bodies, penetration of the joint space, fractures, or tendon injuries. Plain radiographs can be helpful for visualization of radiopaque foreign bodies, including glass. An ultrasound can show both radiopaque and radiolucent foreign bodies.

Minor wounds can have a higher risk of infection if they are due to bites, associated with crush injuries/devitalized soft tissue, heavily contaminated, or have a retained foreign body. Comorbidities that affect wound healing such as diabetes, immunosuppression, or connective tissue disorders such as Ehlers-Danlos syndrome will also increase the risk of infection. Tendon function should be carefully checked since children may be unable to cooperate with the exam, and the ends of severed tendons may not be seen during inspection of the wound. Plain radiographs or ultrasound can locate superficial and deep foreign bodies that are missed during wound exploration. Subspecialty consultation is indicated if imaging reveals a large, deep foreign body or if there is concern for joint, nerve, flexor tendon, or major blood vessel involvement. Organic foreign bodies such as wood splinters require removal regardless of their size or depth due to the high likelihood of infection.

Keywords: ultrasound, penetrating trauma, extremity injury, limp

Bibliography

Mankowitz SL. Laceration Management. *J Emerg Med.* 2017;53(3):369–382.

Nwawka OK, Kabutey NK, Locke CM, Castro-Aragon I, Kim D. Ultrasound-guided needle localization to aid foreign body removal in pediatric patients. *J Foot Ankle Surg* 2014;53(1):67–70.

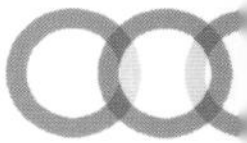

CASE 190

S. Margaret Paik

Question

An 11-year-old boy with a ventriculoperitoneal shunt is brought in by his mother with a complaint of vomiting and abdominal pain for the past 3 days. The vomitus is non-bilious and non-bloody. He has been unable to tolerate food or fluid well, and the mother notes some decreased urine output. He has been acting normally but does complain of a headache. The mother also notes mild scalp swelling at the site of the shunt insertion. His past medical history is significant for a history of prematurity born at 27 weeks gestational age and obstructive hydrocephalus, which required placement of a ventriculoperitoneal shunt at 4 weeks of age. He had one shunt revision 3 years ago for a shunt malfunction which presented with complaint of headache.

He is alert and cooperative. There is mild swelling at the base of his scalp without tenderness or overlying erythema. There is diffuse mild abdominal distension in the lower abdomen with voluntary guarding.

A head CT showed no acute change when compared to the previous head CT done one year ago. No disconnection of the shunt is seen in the shunt series radiographs. The opening pressure of the shunt reservoir is 30 cm of H_2O. An ultrasound of the abdomen is shown next.

190.1

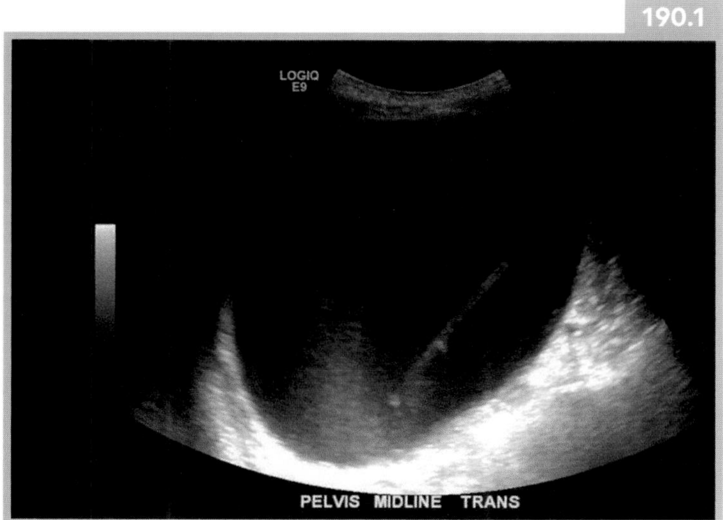

What is seen in the ultrasound?

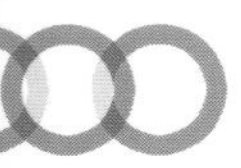

Answer

The ultrasound demonstrates a large pseudocyst in the mid and lower abdomen with visualization of the shunt catheter in the pseudocyst.

The reported incidence of abdominal pseudocyst from ventriculoperitoneal (VP) shunt is relatively rare (1%–4.5%) and requires a high index of suspicion. Patients will present with signs and symptoms of shunt malfunction (headache, vomiting, change in vision) in addition to complaints of abdominal pain and palpation of an abdominal mass. The true incidence of abdominal CSF (cerebrospinal fluid) pseudocyst is unknown as some patients are asymptomatic. Imaging to confirm the diagnosis is best done with either an abdominal ultrasound or CT scan.

Other complications associated with a VP shunt include infection, shunt obstruction, migration of the catheter (see Case 150), hemorrhage, subdural fluid collections, craniosynostosis, overdrainage of CSF, and stenosis and/or loculations of the ventricles.

Keywords: neurosurgery, abdominal pain, vomiting, ultrasound

Bibliography

Grosfeld JL, Cooney DR, Smith J, Campbell RL. Intra-abdominal complication following ventriculoperitoneal shunt procedures. *Pediatrics* 1974:54(6):791–6.

Roitberg BZ, Tomita T, McLone DG. Abdominal cerebrospinal fluid pseudocyst: A complication of ventriculoperitoneal shunt in children. *Pediatr Neurosurg* 1998;29:267–73.

Weprin BE, Swift DM. Complication of ventricular shunts. *Techn Neurosurg* 2002;7(3):224–42.

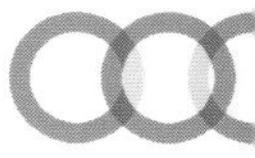

CASE 191

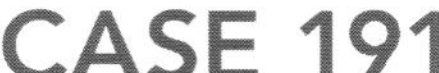

S. Margaret Paik

Question

A 3-year-old boy is brought in after his mother noticed redness to his left eye. The mother is concerned it is "pink eye." He has a 3-day history of runny nose and cough but no fever. He is in day care.

He is alert and well-appearing. There is mild erythema of the left upper eyelid without tenderness. There is chemosis with hyperemia of the bulbar and palpebral conjunctiva. The eye discharge is watery and thin.

191.1

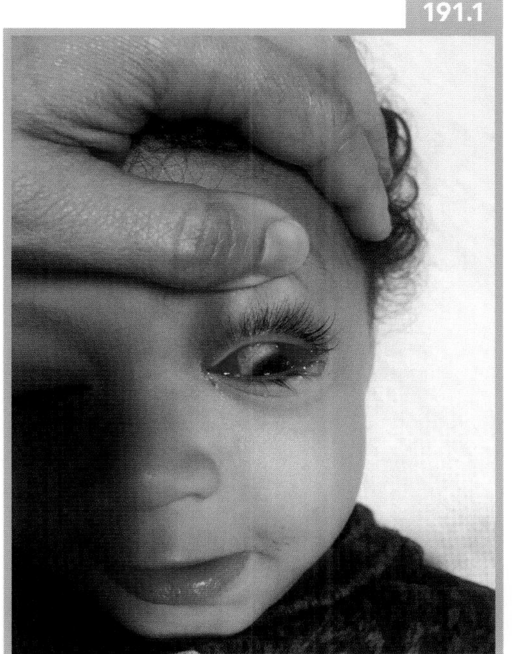

191.2

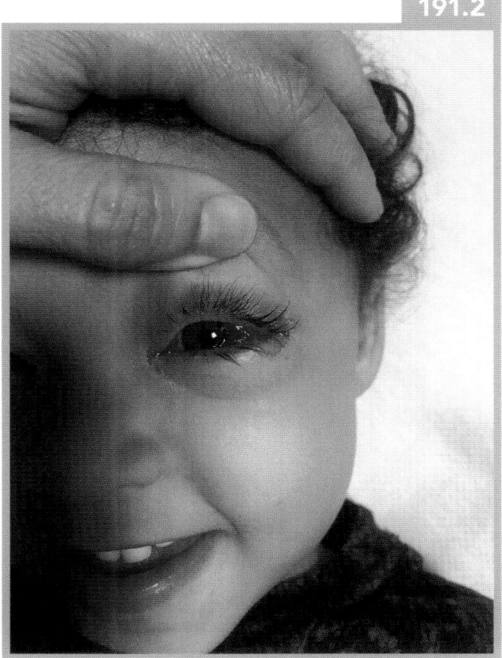

What is the most likely etiology? What is the treatment?

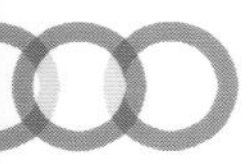

Answer

The patient has adenovirus conjunctivitis. Viruses cause up to 80% of acute conjunctivitis; the majority are due to adenovirus. Adenovirus is associated with pharyngoconjunctival fever (sudden onset high fever, pharyngitis, bilateral conjunctivitis, and periauricular lymphadenopathy) and epidemic keratoconjunctivitis (watery discharge, chemosis, hyperemia, and unilateral lymphadenopathy). Artificial tears and cold compresses can provide symptomatic relief. Topical antihistamines are used in some cases. Symptoms can last up to 2 weeks.

Patients with bacterial conjunctivitis present with persistent mucopurulent discharge. *Staphylococcus aureus*, *Streptococcus pneumoniae*, *Haemophilus influenzae*, and *Moraxella catarrhalis* are the common bacterial organisms. *Neisseria gonorrhoeae* causes a severe and sight-threatening conjunctivitis and presents with profuse purulent eye discharge in neonates and has a high risk of corneal perforation. Chlamydia can also cause conjunctivitis in infants. Herpes conjunctivitis is usually unilateral, with thin watery discharge and vesicular lesions on the eyelid and periorbital region. Allergic conjunctivitis is usually itchy with bilateral eye redness. The patient may also have a history of seasonal allergies or atopy.

Keywords: infectious diseases, infectious

Bibliography

Azari AA, Barney NP. Conjunctivitis: A systematic review of diagnosis and treatment. *JAMA* 2013;310(16):1721–30.

Leibowitz HM. The red eye. *N Engl J Med* 2000;343(5):345–51.

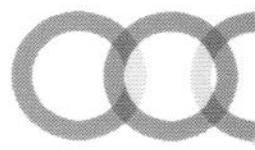

CASE 192

S. Margaret Paik

Question

A 4-year-old boy is brought in from the school playground after he fell off the swing onto his right shoulder. He is crying in pain and will not move his right upper extremity but is able to move his fingers normally. The right and left radial pulse are equal. The contour of his right shoulder is different when compared to his left.

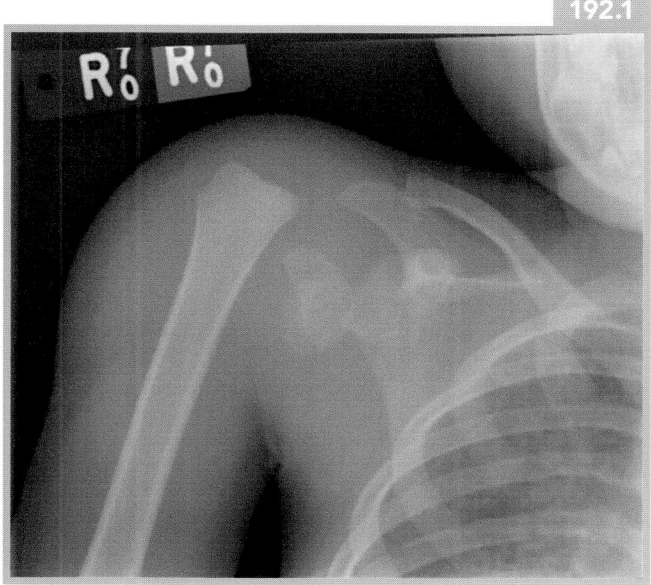

192.1

What does the radiograph of his shoulder show?

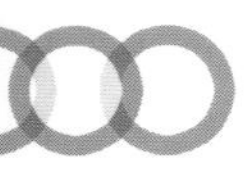

Answer

This is a Salter-Harris I fracture dislocation of the proximal humerus. Injuries to the pliable and porous pediatric bones can result in fractures unique to children. These include plastic deformities, buckle or torus fractures, greenstick fractures and physis fractures. The physis or growth plate in the long bones of children is a "weak link" with a potential for significant injuries. Physeal plate fractures are classified using the Salter-Harris classification (Table 192.1).

Table 192.1 Salter-Harris classification

Type I	Fracture through the growth of the physis Normal radiograph is seen with non-displaced fracture	Generally excellent prognosis
Type II	Fracture through the physis and metaphysis with a portion of metaphysis attached to the epiphysis The most common type of fracture	Generally excellent prognosis
Type III	Fracture begins intra-articular and travels through the epiphysis and into the physis	Prognosis is good with appropriate reduction
Type IV	Fracture through the epiphysis, physis, and metaphysis with intra-articular involvement	Associated with significant growth abnormalities
Type V	Physis is crushed Initial radiographs may be unremarkable History of an injury with significant axial load is vital	Poor prognosis with premature growth arrest

A Salter-Harris type I fracture of the humerus is usually seen in preschoolers or younger. Older children between 11 and 15 years of age are more likely to sustain a Salter-Harris type II fracture. Severe displacement of proximal humeral physeal as seen in this case requires reduction. Older patients may require internal fixation.

Keywords: orthopedics, extremity injury

Bibliography

Dobbs MB, Luhmann SL, Gordon JE, Strecker WB, Schoenecker PL. Severely displaced proximal humeral epiphyseal fractures. *J Pediatr Orthop* 2003;23(2):208–15.

Salter RB, Harris WR. Injuries involving the epiphyseal plate. *J Bone Joint Surg Am* 1963;45A:587–621.

Thorton MD, Della-Guistina K, Aronson PL. Emergency department evaluation and treatment of pediatric orthopedic injuries. *Emerg Med Clin North Am* 2015;33(2):423–49.

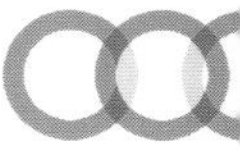

CASE 193

S. Margaret Paik

Question

A 10-year-old boy is brought with a complaint of a wart on the bottom of his right foot for the past 3 months. He has had pain with weight-bearing but the pain has increased in the last week. The mother tried soaking his foot in water as well as using an over-the-counter "wart" remover medication without improvement. She did notice a slight amount of drainage and thinks the bottom of his foot is a little red.

On examination the plantar surface of the right foot has a callus with surrounding erythema. No drainage is seen. The foot is slightly tender to palpation.

A radiograph is performed.

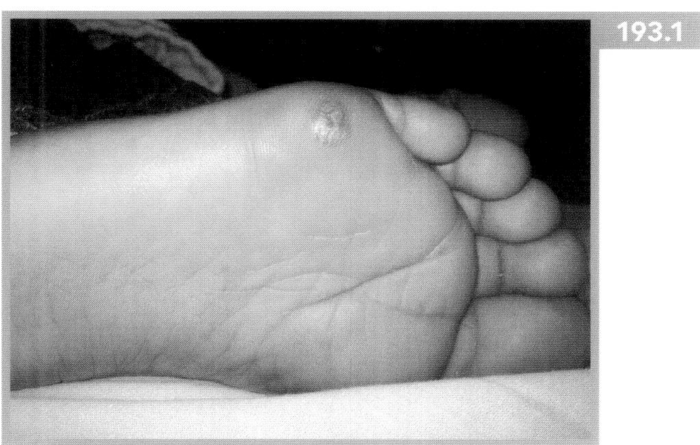

193.1

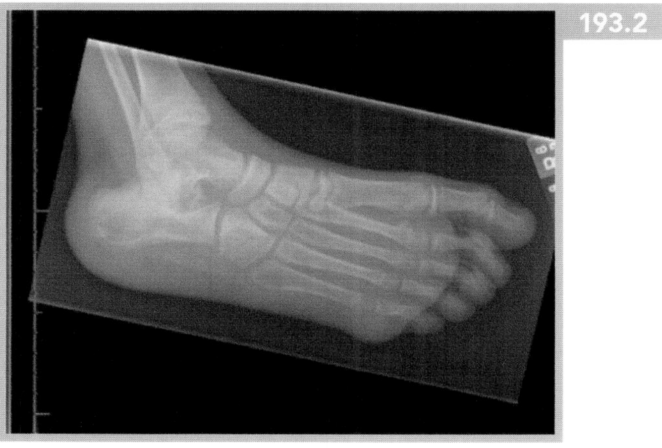

193.2

What is seen on the foot radiograph? What additional studies should be done? What are the treatment options?

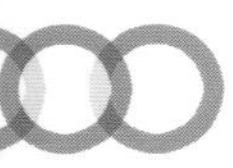

Answer

There is a radiopaque metallic foreign body. Evaluation for osteomyelitis and septic arthritis is necessary, even though there are no bony changes noted on the plain radiograph. Additional imaging with ultrasound, CT, or MRI can be done to evaluate for suspected deep infections. Tetanus immunization history will determine the need for tetanus prophylaxis.

Additional questions to the child reveal he had "stepped on something sharp" several months ago while running barefoot in the house. Empiric antibiotic coverage for gram-positive bacteria was started. Laboratory values showed a white blood cell count of 12.4 K/uL with an unremarkable differential. The erythrocyte sedimentation rate and C-reactive protein were not elevated. The child was taken to the operating room for wound exploration and removal of the foreign body. There was a small fluid collection which was cultured. A sewing needle was removed. Methicillin-sensitive *Staphylococcus aureus* was identified from the fluid collection 2 days later.

Keywords: orthopedics, penetrating trauma, extremity injury, skin and soft tissue infections, limp, foreign body

Bibliography

García-Gubern CF, Colon-Rolon L, Bond MC. Essential concepts of wound management. *Emerg Med Clin N Am* 2010;28(4):951–67.

Verdile VP, Freed HA, Gerard J. Puncture wounds to the foot. *J Emerg Med* 1989;7(2):193–9.

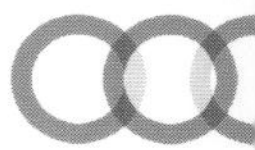

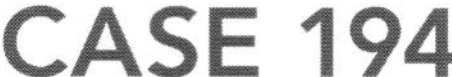

CASE 194

Barbara Pawel

Question

A 16-year-old boy presents to the emergency department with complaints of thigh and lower back pain, "sore muscles," and dark urine. His symptoms started 2 days after beginning post summer break football training camp. Workouts consisted of weight lifting and took place in a non-air-conditioned gym. He participated in a "dead lifting" contest with his friends during the workout.

What lab tests would be most diagnostic in this case?

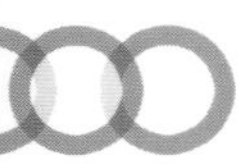

Answer

This patient's history is very concerning for exertional rhabdomyolysis. The creatine kinase (CK) is considered the defining biochemical marker with levels greater than four to five times the normal suggestive of this diagnosis. Myoglobinuria is also a diagnostic hallmark but results can be variable depending on sample timing due to its short serum half-life. The urine dipstick is positive for blood but there are <5 RBC/hpf microscopically. This makes the diagnosis of myoglobinuria more likely.

194.1

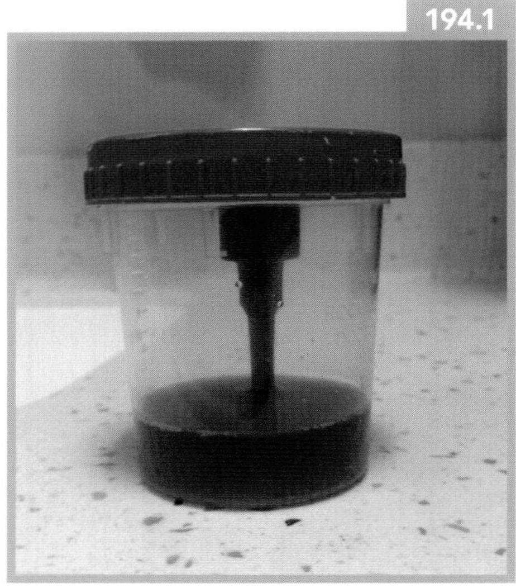

Rhabdomyolysis occurs when striated muscle breakdown releases cellular contents (myoglobin, creatine kinase, potassium, and phosphate) into the circulation. Calcium enters the cells causing continued myofiber contraction and further damage. Myoglobin is filtered through the kidneys and excreted into the urine (pigmenturia) resulting in the classic "tea-colored" urine. Myoglobin can also precipitate in the renal tubules causing acute kidney injury and can lead to renal failure.

Trauma (crush or high-voltage injuries, compartment syndrome) and medications (statins, amphetamines, cocaine, antipsychotics) are the causative etiologies for up to 80% of adult cases.

Infection is the leading cause in children. Influenza A and B (see Case 175), CMV (cytomegalovirus), and EBV (Epstein-Barr virus) are often associated along with other viral and bacterial infections. Congenital and genetic disorders of lipid or glycogen metabolism should also be considered. Rhabdomyolysis can be precipitated in these patients by fever, infections, exercise, or fasting.

Exertional rhabdomyolysis is common in teenagers due to the growing popularity of highly strenuous exercise regimens and increasing intensity in youth sports programs. Heavy weight lifting is particularly damaging especially in the unconditioned person exercising in high temperatures with some element of dehydration.

Treatment is aimed at early and aggressive IV rehydration while monitoring urine output serum pH and electrolytes.

Keywords: renal/nephrology, hematuria, mimickers

Bibliography

Elsayed EF, Reilly RF. Rhabdomyolysis: A review, with emphasis on the pediatric population. *Pediatr Nephrol* 2010;25:7–18.

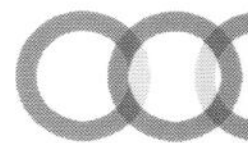

CASE 195

S. Margaret Paik

Question

A 10-day-old baby girl is brought into the emergency department by the parents after they noted redness and swelling around the umbilical stump. The baby is a term infant, born via vaginal delivery at 38 weeks gestational age. The mother had prenatal care and denies any perinatal infections or complications. The mother has had a history of "boils" in the past but did not have any during her pregnancy. The baby has been feeding well and there is no history of fever.

On physical examination, there is swelling to the umbilicus with surrounding erythema, approximately 1 cm circumferentially without streaking. There is no purulent discharge. The abdomen and umbilicus are not tender to touch. There is a residual umbilical cord.

195.1

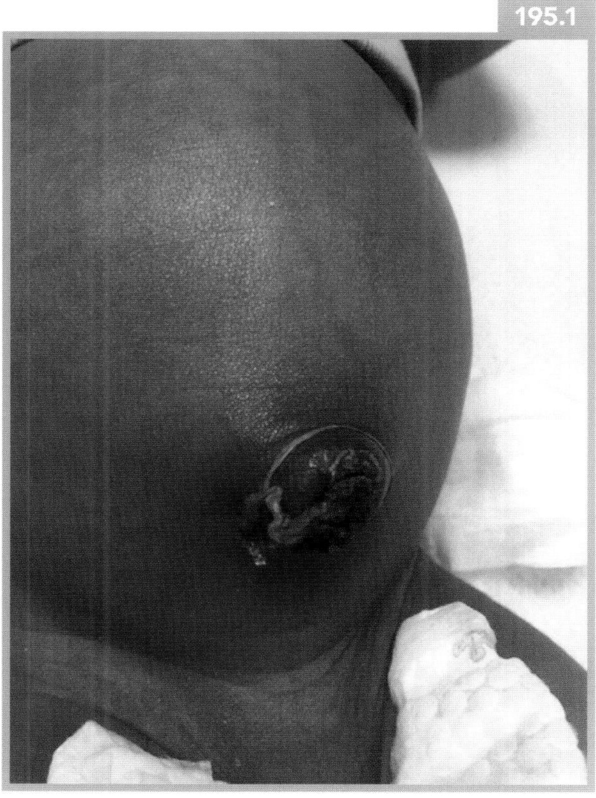

What is this condition? What are some complications associated with this condition?

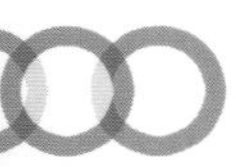

Answer

This is omphalitis, an infection of the umbilicus and the surrounding soft tissue. Findings include surrounding induration, erythema, purulent discharge, and tenderness. Although rare in developed countries, risk factors include prolonged rupture of membranes, chorioamnionitis, low birth weight, home birth, and catheterization of the umbilicus. Infants can present with fever, irritability, and poor feeding, especially in cases of complicated omphalitis.

Causative organisms include *Staphylococcus aureus, Staphylococcus epidermidis*, groups A and B *streptococcus, Escherichia coli, Klebsiella, Pseudomonas*, and *Clostridium difficile*. Major complications associated with omphalitis include septicemia, necrotizing fasciitis, peritonitis, adhesive small bowel obstruction, retroperitoneal and pelvic abscesses, and hepatic venous thrombosis.

Initial management consists of evaluation for sepsis and parenteral antibiotics. Evaluation for infectious focus (e.g. patent urachus) is warranted for infants unresponsive to appropriate parenteral antibiotic therapy.

Keywords: neonate, infectious diseases, dermatology, do not miss

Bibliography

Fraser N, Davies BW, Cusack J. Neonatal omphalitis: A review of its serious complications. *Acta Pædiatr,* 2006;95:519–22.

Imdad A, Bautista RMM, Senen KAA, Uy MEV, Mantaring III JB, Bhutta ZA. Umbilical cord antiseptics for preventing sepsis and death among newborns. *Cochrane Database System Rev* 2013;(5). Art. No.: CD008635. doi:10.1002/14651858.CD008635.pub2.

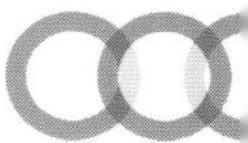

CASE 196

S. Margaret Paik

Questions

A 14-year-old boy is brought to the emergency department (ED) with complaints of coughing up blood and left-sided chest pain for several weeks. He had been seen in an ED 12 days earlier with the complaint of left-sided chest pain, a nonproductive cough, and feeling warm. The pain was made worse with movement and leaning forward. He had a temperature of 38.5°C and a respiratory rate of 20. A chest radiograph was done during the previous ED encounter showing left lower lobe subsegmental atelectasis (see Images 196.1 and 196.2). He was discharged home with instructions to follow-up with his primary care physician and to return to the ED if his symptoms worsened.

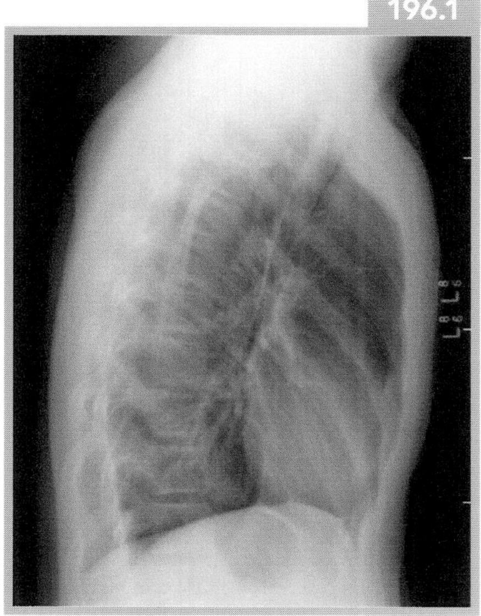

196.1

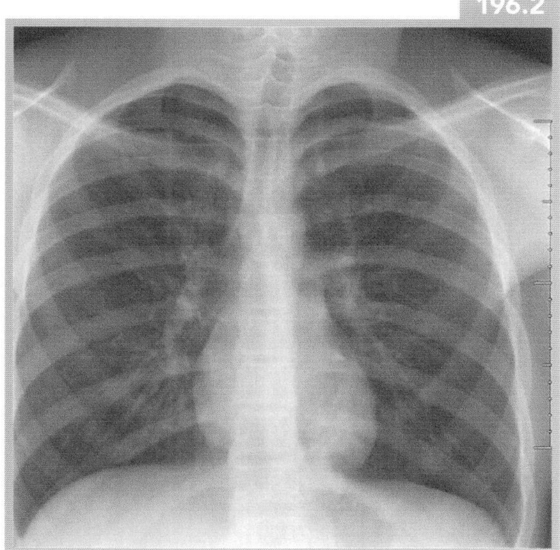

196.2

The patient states the cough became productive 10 days ago and today there was bright red blood in the sputum. The left-sided chest pain is worse and he has had back pain for the past week. There is a 5 lb/2.5 kg weight loss. His temperature is 37.3°C with a pulse rate of 112. His respiratory rate is 18 and the room air saturation is 97%. A second chest radiograph is ordered (see Images 196.3 and 196.4).

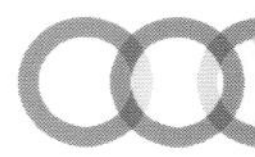

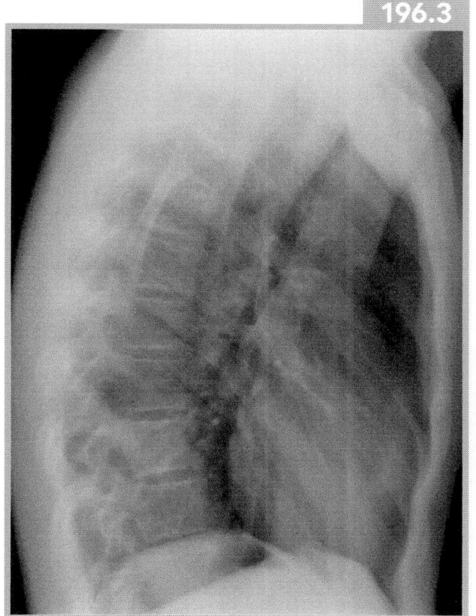
196.3

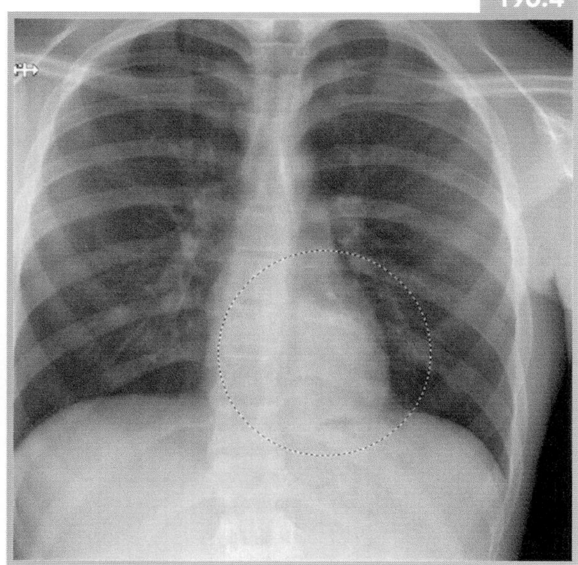
196.4

1. What do the chest radiographs show?
2. What are some types of complicated pneumonia? What are the bacterial causes?

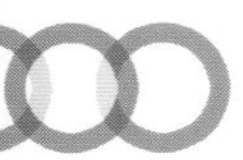

Answers

1. There is airspace opacity in the left lower lobe without pleural effusion or pneumothorax. A CT with IV contrast is performed and shows the opacity of the left lower lobe with multifocal areas of hypoattenuation, concerning for necrotizing pneumonia.

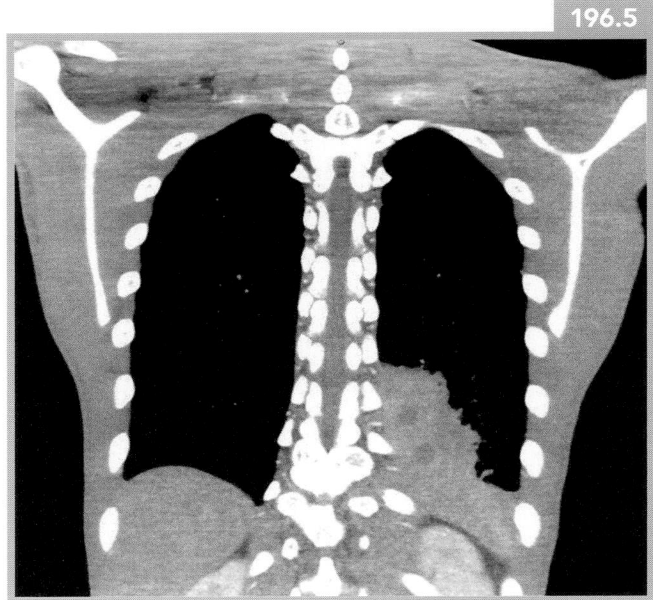

2. A simple parapneumonic effusion is fluid within the pleural cavity without loculations. Fibrin deposition in the pleural space can lead to a loculated parapneumonic effusion and is best visualized on ultrasound or CT. Empyema is a purulent parapneumonic fluid collection. Lung entrapment with pleural rind formation is seen with an organized multiloculated empyema. Necrotizing pneumonia is usually a result of localized infection and is associated with aspiration. Lung abscess can be the result of aspiration of foreign body or heavily infected oral secretions. Bacterial causes included *Streptococcus pneumoniae*, methicillin-resistant *Staphylococcus aureus*, *Streptococcus pyogenes*, and *Mycoplasma pneumoniae*.

Keywords: pulmonary, infectious diseases, chest pain, CT

Bibliography

Eastham KM, Freeman R, Kearns AM, Eltringham G, Clark J, Leeming J, Spencer DA. Clinical features, aetiology and outcome of empyema in children on the north east of England. *Thorax* 2004;59:522–5.

Mani CS, Murray DL. Acute pneumonia and its complications. In *Principles and Practice of Pediatric Infectious Diseases*, 4th ed., Long SS, Pickering LK, Prober CG, eds. Edinburgh: Elsevier Saunders, 2012:235–45.

Wexler ID, Knoll S, Picard E, Villa Y, Shoseyov D, Engelhard D, Kerem E. Clinical characteristics and outcome of complicated pneumococcal pneumonia in a pediatric population. *Pediatr Pulmonol* 2006;41(8):726–34.

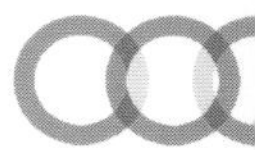

CASE 197

S. Margaret Paik

Questions

A 2-year-old girl is brought in for evaluation for a cough for the past week. She has had fever to 38–39°C and only fair oral intake for the past 3 days. Her immunizations are up to date and she does not have a significant past medical history and has no known drug allergies. On physical examination she has a respiratory rate of 30 with an oxygen saturation of 97% on room air. Crackles are heard in the left side. The chest radiograph shows focal opacities in left lower lobe.

197.1

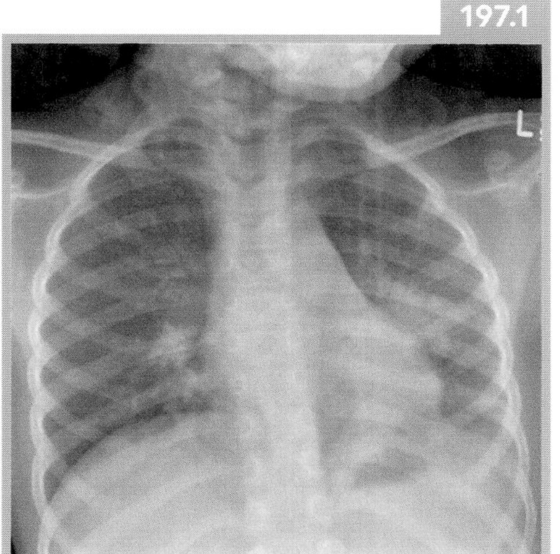

197.2

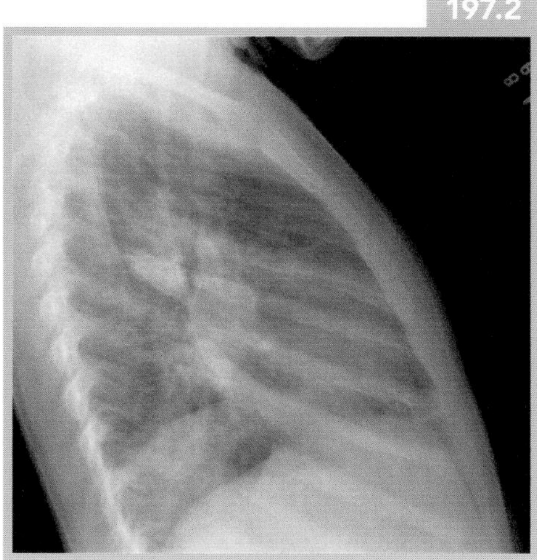

1. What are the presenting signs and symptoms of pneumonia in young children?
2. Can this child be treated as an outpatient with empiric antibiotics? Are additional laboratory studies or blood cultures indicated?

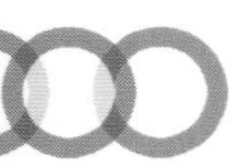

Answers

1. Children with pneumonia may present with fever, tachypnea, cough, and may be ill-appearing. They may also have poor oral intake and be fussy. Physical examination findings include presence of rales or decreased breath sounds with signs of respiratory distress (grunting, retractions, nasal flaring) and hypoxemia.
2. This child has community-acquired pneumonia. Because she has no hypoxia, is not dehydrated, and has no signs of respiratory insufficiency, she can be treated as an outpatient with oral amoxicillin, preferably high dose (80–90 mg/kg/day) to cover for resistant *Streptococcus pneumoniae*. Laboratory studies are usually not indicated in uncomplicated pneumonia. Blood cultures are strongly indicated in current guidelines but identify a bacterial organism in only a small number of patients.

Keywords: pulmonary, infectious diseases, cough, fever

Bibliography

Bradley JS, Byington CL, Shah SS, Alverson B et al. The management of community-acquired pneumonia in infants and children older than 3 months of age: Clinical practice guidelines by the Pediatric Infectious Diseases Society and the Infectious Diseases Society of America. *Clin Infect Dis* October 2011;53(7):e25–76.

Iroh Tam PY, Bernstein E, Ma X, Ferrieri P. Blood culture in evaluation of pediatric community-acquired pneumonia: A systematic review and meta-analysis. *Hosp Pediatr* 2015;5(6):324–36.

Murphy CG, Van De Pol AC, Harper MB, Bachur RG. Clinical predictors of occult pneumonia in the febrile child. *Acad Emerg Med* 2007;14(3):243–9.

Shah SN, Bachur RG, Simel DL, Neuman ML. Does this child have pneumonia? The Rational Clinical Examination Systematic Review. *JAMA* 2017;318(5):462–71.

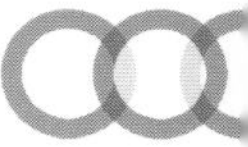

CASE 198

Barbara Pawel

Questions

A 3-year-old female presents to the emergency department with 1 week of fever, cough, and progressive increased work of breathing. She was started on antibiotics by her physician 4 days ago without improvement. Her vital signs were T39°, RR 50, Sat 88% on RA. On examination she was ill-appearing with dry mucous membranes. Her respiratory exam revealed grunting, nasal flaring, and suprasternal/intercostal/subcostal retractions. On auscultation she had crackles in the left lung field and distant breath sounds with dullness to percussion on the right. Her chest radiographs are shown. A chest CT was done after visualization of the chest radiographs.

198.1

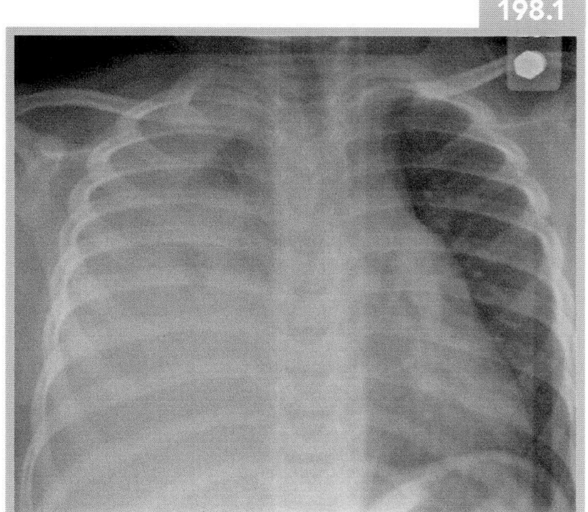

198.2

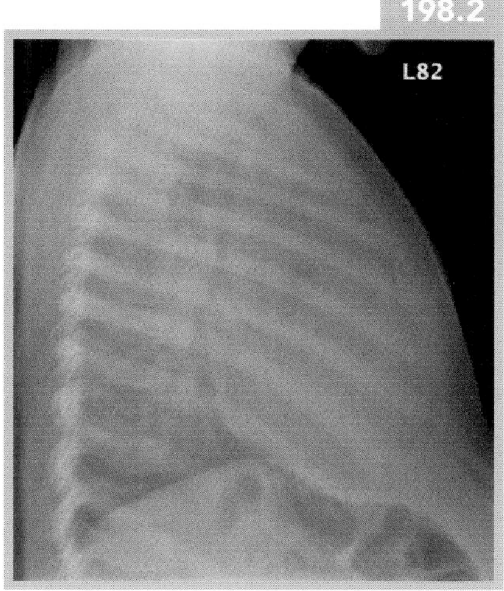

198.3

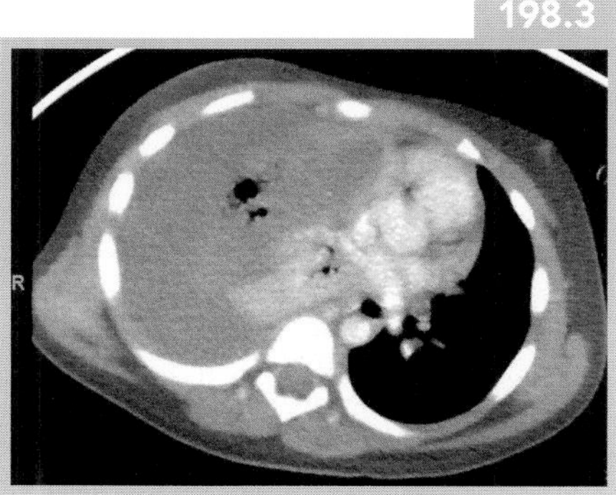

1. Which subset of patients with community-acquired pneumonia (CAP) requires hospitalization?
2. Which subset of patients with CAP requires admission to the intensive care unit?

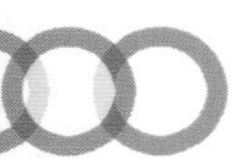

Answers

1. Children with any of these features should be hospitalized:
   - Moderate to severe CAP
     - Tachypnea
     - Retractions and grunting
     - Hypoxemia (<90% on initial visit)
   - Young age: <3–6 months
   - Pathogen with increased virulence (e.g. community-acquired methicillin-resistant *Staphylococcus aureus*)
   - Dehydration, vomiting, or unable to take oral meds
   - Significant comorbidity
   - Psychosocial concerns (noncompliance, lack of follow-up)
2. Children with any of these features should be admitted to an intensive care unit:
   - Impending respiratory failure
   - Requires non-invasive ventilation or intubation
   - Altered mental status due to hypoxia or hypercarbia
   - Requires blood pressure/perfusion support
   - Pulse oximetry ≤92% with inspired oxygen ≥50%

Community-acquired pneumonia is caused by multiple pathogens. Viruses are responsible for CAP in 50% of children <5 years of age. *Streptococcus pneumoniae* is the most common bacterial pathogen. Mycoplasma/chlamydia pneumonia is more common over the age of 5 years. Community-acquired methicillin-resistant *Staphylococcus aureus* is associated with more complications. Mild pneumonia does not require imaging or labs and can be treated as an outpatient. Preschool-age children only need antibiotics if a bacterial infection is suspected. CBC and blood culture is recommended for moderate to severe CAP requiring admission. Chest radiograph should be done on patients who are admitted or fail outpatient therapy, and to document CAP complications such as parapneumonic effusions, necrotizing pneumonia, and pneumothorax. Effusions occur more frequently with bacterial pneumonia. Effusions should be assessed for loculations using US or CT. Small uncomplicated effusions usually resolve with antibiotics. Larger or purulent effusions require a drainage procedure such as a chest tube with fibrinolytic agents or video-assisted thoracoscopic surgery.

Keywords: pulmonary, infectious diseases, CT, respiratory distress, fever

Bibliography

Bradley JS, Byington CL, Shah SS, Alverson B et al. The management of community-acquired pneumonia in infants and children older than 3 months of age: Clinical Practice Guidelines by the Pediatric Infectious Diseases Society and the Infectious Diseases Society of America. *Clin Infect Dis* 2011:e1–e52.

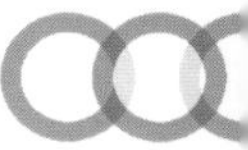

CASE 199

S. Margaret Paik

Question

A 4-year-old boy is brought in by paramedics after a fall from the third story of an apartment building. The child is put into a cervical collar, immobilized on a backboard, and transported to a pediatric trauma center. Upon arrival the child has grunting respirations. The Glasgow Coma Scale score is 6 (see Case 40). The child is intubated with inline cervical spine immobilization. The cervical spine posteroanterior and lateral radiograph show the alignment of the cervical spine to be within normal limits but with significant prevertebral soft tissue swelling.

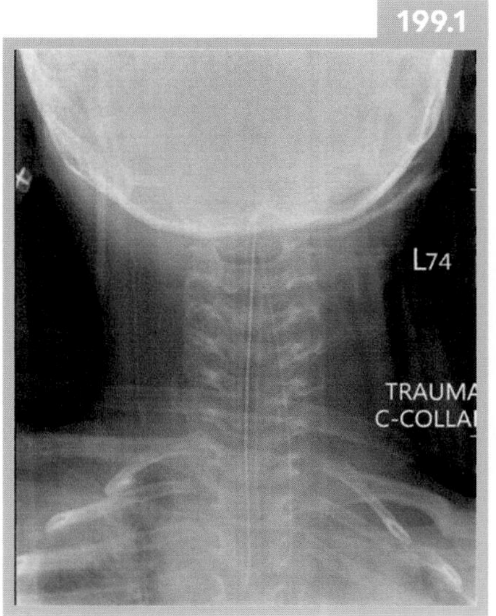

199.1

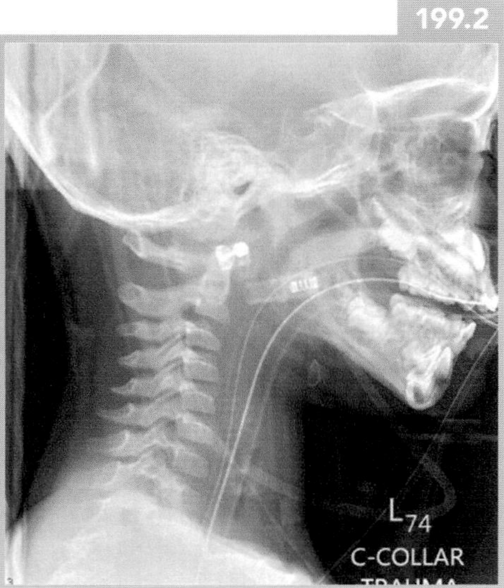

199.2

1. What are the four contour lines seen on a lateral neck radiograph that are used to evaluate the cervical spine?
2. How does the cervical spine for a child differ from an adult and what are the different types of injuries seen because of these differences?

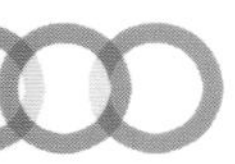

Answer

1.
   i. Anterior vertebral bodies
   ii. Posterior vertebral bodies
   iii. Spinolaminal line/posterior spinal canal
   iv. Spinous process tips

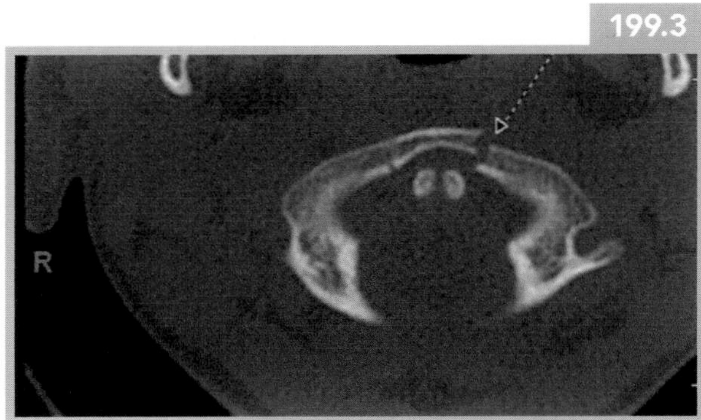

The cervical spine CT is done and shows diastasis between the ossification centers on the left aspect of C1 anterior arch with anterior displacement of the medial fragment.

2. The fulcrum of motion for younger children (<8 years old) is higher at the level of C2-C3 compared to adults. Ligamentous laxity, angled and shallow facet joints, anterior wedging of the vertebral bodies, and underdeveloped spinous processes contribute to the hypermobility of the pediatric spine. Additionally, the young child has a relatively large head and weaker neck muscles. The fulcrum is lower at C5-C6 in adults.

Keywords: neck injury, blunt trauma, CT, do not miss

Bibliography

Bonadio WA. Cervical spine trauma in children: Part I. General concepts, normal anatomy, radiographic evaluation. *Am J Emerg Med* 1993;11(2):58–65.

Lustrin ES, Karakas SP, Ortis AO, Cinnamon J, Castillo M, Vheesan K, Brown JH, Diamond AS, Black K, Singh S. Pediatric cervical spine: Normal anatomy, variants and trauma. *RadioGraphics* 2003;23(3):539–60.

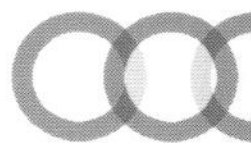

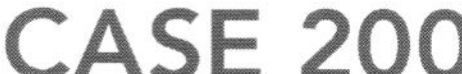

CASE 200

Barbara Pawel

Question

A 14-year-old male landed on his neck while doing backflips on a trampoline. He complained of neck, left shoulder, and arm pain with paresthesia. The lateral cervical spine radiograph demonstrated step-offs at C3-4 of both the anterior and posterior vertebral lines suggestive of ligamentous injury. A CT revealed a C4 compression deformity, grade 2 anterolisthesis, and a jumped C3/C4 facet. The patient underwent an open anterior cervical discectomy and fusion.

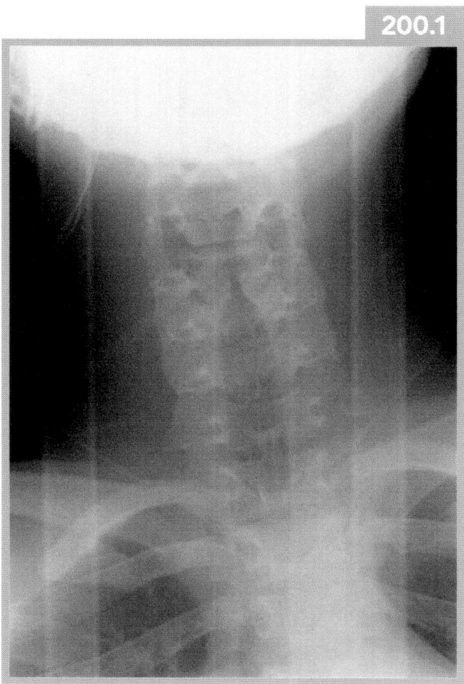

200.1

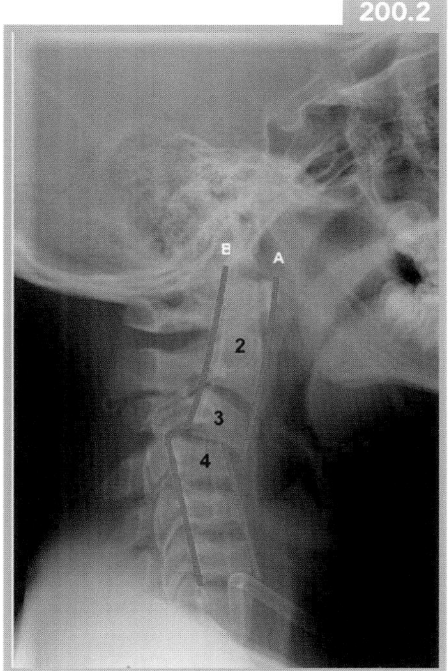

200.2

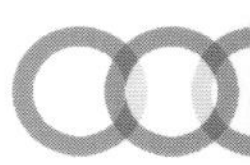

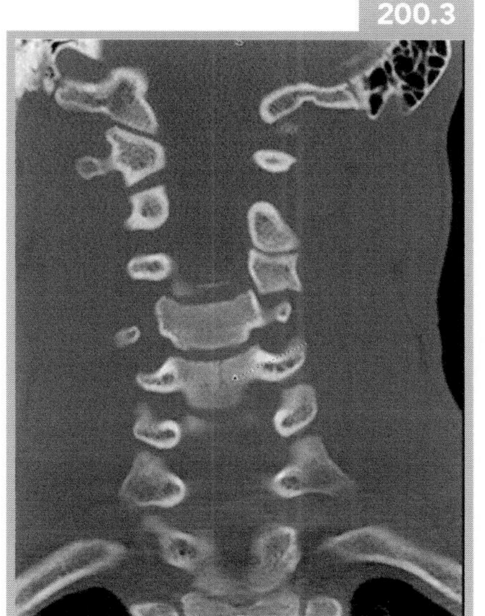
200.3

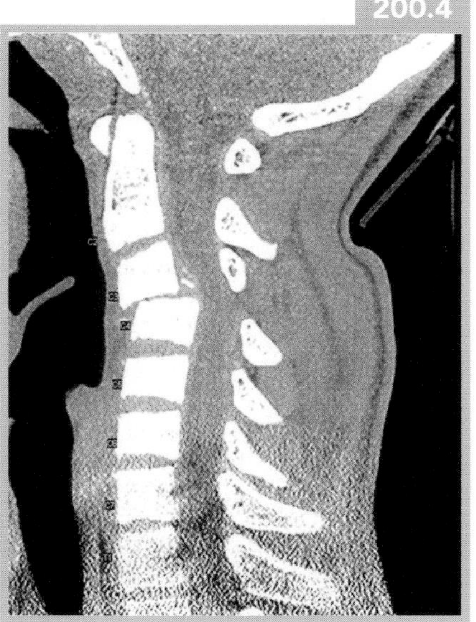
200.4

Which activities are associated with the most neck injuries in pediatric patients?

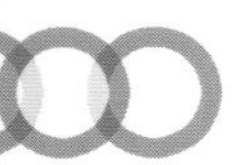

Answer

- All ages: Motor vehicle crashes (MVCs) cause 35% of spinal cord injuries
- Gunshot wound (GSW)
- Falls
- Sports related: 25% of c-spine (cervical spine) fractures in children and adolescents
  - High risk: football, gymnastics, cheerleading, and ice hockey

The incidence of pediatric neck injuries increases with age. Adolescents are more likely to sustain fractures/injuries to the lower cervical spine, whereas younger children sustain more ligamentous injuries to the upper cervical spine. Organized sports–related injuries are well publicized, but many spine injuries occur during unsupervised activities such as diving, skiing, surfing, and trampoline use.

All trauma patient evaluations begin with the primary survey focusing on life-threatening conditions. Airway patency interventions are routinely instituted while protecting the cervical spine.

A careful history can help differentiate between neurologic pain (burning, paresthesia, upper arm pain) and musculoskeletal injuries including unstable fractures (neck tightness/spasm). Flexion injuries cause fractures and dislocations anteriorly through compression and disrupt the ligaments posteriorly. Extension injuries do the reverse with bony injuries posteriorly (spinous process, facets) and ligamentous disruption anteriorly. Both mechanisms can cause disc rupture and cord compromise. A careful neurologic assessment (motor, sensory, DTRs [deep tendon reflexes), and perineal evaluation to assess for sacral sparing) is critical to evaluating a spinal cord injury. All patients with suspected spine injury should remain immobilized until imaged. Plain radiographs include three views. An MRI to evaluate the spinal cord or a CT to evaluate fractures may be necessary.

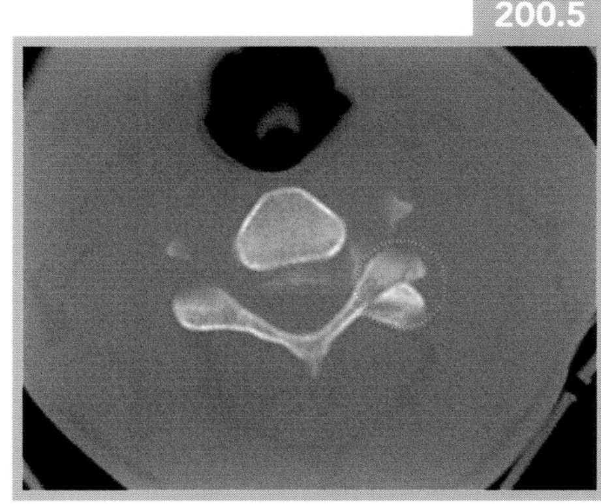

Lateral c-spine. (A) Anterior vertebral line, (B) posterior vertebral line.

Keywords: neck injury, blunt trauma, CT, do not miss

Bibliography

American College of Surgeons Committee on Trauma. *Advanced Trauma Life Support (ATLS) Student Course Manual.* 9th ed. Chicago: American College of Surgeons, 2012.

Nigrovic LE, Rogers AJ, Adelgais KM, Olsen CS, Leonard JR, Jaffe DM, Leonard JC, Pediatric Emergency Care Applied Research Network (PECARN) Cervical Spine Study Group. Utility of plain radiographs in detecting traumatic injuries of the cervical spine in children. *Pediatric Emer Care* 2012;28:26–32.

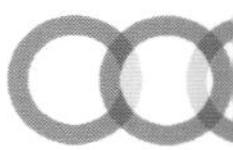

INDEX

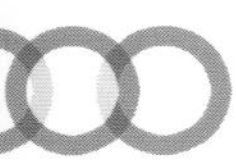

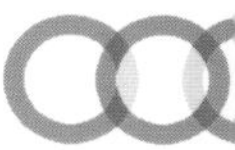

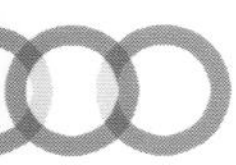

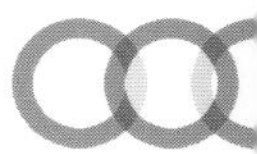

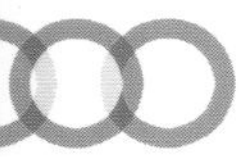

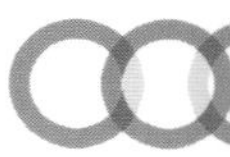

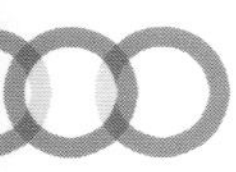

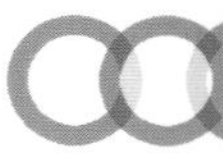

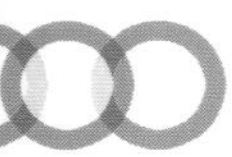

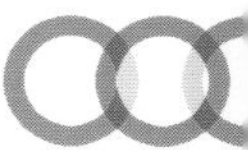

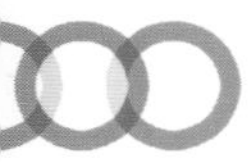

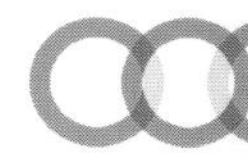